# Surgery for Cancers of the Gastrointestinal Tract

Joseph Kim • Julio Garcia-Aguilar
Editors

# Surgery for Cancers of the Gastrointestinal Tract

## A Step-by-Step Approach

Springer

*Editors*
Joseph Kim
Division of Surgical Oncology
City of Hope
Los Angeles, CA, USA

Julio Garcia-Aguilar
Department of Surgery
Memorial Sloan-Kettering Cancer Center
New York, NY, USA

Videos to this book can be accessed at
http://www.springerimages.com/videos/978-1-4939-1892-8

ISBN 978-1-4939-4840-6 ISBN 978-1-4939-1893-5 (eBook)
DOI 10.1007/978-1-4939-1893-5
Springer New York Heidelberg Dordrecht London



Printed on acid-free paper

Springer is part of Springer Science+Business Media (www.springer.com)

# Preface

Cancers of the gastrointestinal tract are among the leading causes of cancer-related deaths in the USA and worldwide. Surgical intervention remains the only means for cure in these cancers. Tremendous advances in surgical technology have changed the way that we perform the operations to remove these cancers. Minimally invasive and robotic technologies are now routinely used, yet open operations remain the gold standard. This surgery textbook will provide an educational resource of modern and advanced operative techniques for patients with cancers of the gastrointestinal tract. The textbook will provide a step-by-step surgical approach, highlighting key learning points and potential operative pitfalls. When appropriate, two or more approaches to an operative procedure will be presented to provide perspective on different surgical techniques. In select circumstances the written descriptions will be paired with video presentations of the cancer operation. This textbook will serve as a reference manual for surgeons at all levels of training and also for surgeons in practice who seek to reinforce or learn new surgical techniques. The chapters have been written by experts in their fields and include up-to-date scientific and clinical information.

For the time necessary to complete this book, we are indebted to Nicole Herrera for her organizational support. We are also grateful to J. Blair Hamner, Steve Sentovich, and Audrey Choi for their assistance; and the book could not have been completed without the unending dedication from Lily Li.

We would like to thank Springer-Verlag for giving us the opportunity of completing this book, including Richard Hruska (Senior Editor, Clinical Medicine), Maria Smilios (Development Editor), Joanna Perey (Associate Editor), Alice Essenpreis (Rights and Permissions), and Wendy Vetter (illustrator).

Finally, we could not have completed this work without the love and understanding of our families (Sarah, Anderson, Lauren, and Elsa).

Los Angeles, CA, USA — Joseph Kim, MD, FACS

New York, NY, USA — Julio Garcia-Aguilar, MD, PhD, FACS

# Contents

# Contributors

**Syed A. Ahmad, M.D.** Division of Surgical Oncology, Department of Surgery, University of Cincinnati College of Medicine, Cincinnati, OH, USA

**Bestoun Ahmed, M.D., F.A.C.S.** Division of General Surgery, Department of Surgery, University of Florida College of Medicine—Jacksonville, Jacksonville, FL, USA

**Nasser K. Altorki, M.D.** Department of Cardiothoracic Surgery, New York Presbyterian Hospital, Weill Cornell Medical Center, New York, NY, USA

**Avo Artinyan, M.D., M.S.** Division of Surgical Oncology, Department of Surgery, Baylor College of Medicine, Houston, TX, USA

**Brian Badgwell, M.D., M.S.** Department of Surgical Oncology, The University of Texas MD Anderson Cancer Center, Houston, TX, USA

**Brian K. Bednarski, M.D.** Department of Surgical Oncology, The University of Texas MD Anderson Cancer Center, Houston, TX, USA

**Ronald Bleday, M.D.** Division of Colorectal Surgery, Department of Surgery, Brigham and Women's Hospital, Harvard Medical School, Boston, MA, USA

**Raul M. Bosio, M.D., M.S.B.S.** Department of Surgery, University of California, Irvine School of Medicine, Orange, CA, USA

**George J. Chang, M.D., M.S., F.A.C.S., F.A.S.C.R.S.** Department of Surgical Oncology, The University of Texas MD Anderson Cancer Center, Houston, TX, USA

**Callisia Clarke, M.D.** Department of Surgical Oncology, The University of Texas MD Anderson Cancer Center, Houston, TX, USA

**Conor P. Delaney, M.D., M.Ch., Ph.D., F.R.C.S.I., F.A.C.S., F.A.S.C.R.S.** Digestive Health Institute, University Hospitals Case Medical Center, Cleveland, OH, USA

**Leandro Feo, M.D.** Department of Surgery, Memorial Sloan Kettering Cancer Center, New York, NY, USA

**Julio Garcia-Aguilar, M.D., Ph.D.** Department of Surgery, Benno C. Schmidt Chair in Surgical Oncology, Memorial Sloan Kettering Cancer Center, New York, NY, USA

**Gemma Gossedge, M.B.Ch.B., M.R.C.S.** Leeds Institute for Biological and Clinical Sciences, University of Leeds, Leeds, UK

**Jin Gu, M.D., F.A.C.S.** Department of Colorectal Surgery, Peking University Cancer Hospital, Beijing, People's Republic of China

**John B. Hamner, M.D., F.A.C.S.** Division of Surgical Oncology, City of Hope, Duarte, CA, USA

**Wayne L. Hofstetter, M.D.** Department of Thoracic and Cardiovascular Surgery, The University of Texas MD Anderson Cancer Center, Houston, TX, USA

**Melissa E. Hogg, M.D.** Division of Surgical Oncology, University of Pittsburgh Medical Center, Pittsburgh, PA, USA

**Mark D. Iannettoni, M.D., M.B.A.** Department of Cardiovascular Sciences, East Carolina Heart Institute, Brody School of Medicine at East Carolina University, Greenville, NC, USA

**David Jayne, B.Sc., M.B.B.Ch., M.D., F.R.C.S.** St. James's University Hospital, Leeds LS9 7TF, UK

**John C. Keech, M.D.** Department of Cardiothoracic Surgery, University of Iowa Hospitals and Clinics, Iowa City, IA, USA

**Kaitlyn J. Kelly, M.D.** Division of Surgical Oncology, Moores Cancer Center, University of California, San Diego, La Jolla, CA, USA

**Jae Y. Kim, M.D.** Division of Thoracic Surgery, Department of Surgery, City of Hope, Duarte, CA, USA

**Joseph Kim, M.D., F.A.C.S.** Division of Surgical Oncology, City of Hope, Duarte, CA, USA

**Young Tae Kim, M.D., Ph.D.** Department of Thoracic and Cardiovascular Surgery, Seoul National University Hospital, Seoul National University College of Medicine, Seoul, South Korea

**Antonio M. Lacy, M.D., Ph.D.** Department of Gastrointestinal Surgery, University of Barcelona School of Medicine, Clinic Hospital, Quiron Hospital, Barcelona, Spain

Centro Esther Koplowitz, University of Barcelona, Villarroel, Barcelona, Spain

**Paul C. Lee, M.D.** Department of Cardiothoracic Surgery, New York Presbyterian Hospital, Weill Cornell Medical Center, New York, NY, USA

**Andrew M. Lowy, M.D.** Division of Surgical Oncology, Moores Cancer Center, University of California, San Diego, La Jolla, CA, USA

**Robert D. Madoff, M.D., F.A.C.S., F.A.S.C.R.S.** Division of Colon and Rectal Surgery, Department of Surgery, University of Minnesota, Minneapolis, MN, USA

**Laura Mora-Lopez, M.D.** Coloproctology Unit, Department of General and Digestive Surgery, Parc Tauli University Hospital, Barcelona, Spain

**Michael S. Nussbaum, M.D., F.A.C.S.** Division of General Surgery, Department of Surgery, University of Florida College of Medicine—Jacksonville, Jacksonville, FL, USA

**Seung-Young Oh, M.D.** Department of Surgery, Seoul National University College of Medicine, Seoul, South Korea

**Chinnusamy Palanivelu, M.S., MCh GI Surgery, F.A.C.S., F.R.C.S.** Division of Minimally Invasive & HPB Surgery, GEM Centre for Liver and Pancreas, GEM Hospital & Research Centre, Coimbatore, Tamilnadu, India

**Philip Paty, M.D.** Division of Colon & Rectal Surgery, Department of Surgery, Memorial Sloan Kettering Cancer Center, New York, NY, USA

**Alessio Pigazzi, M.D., Ph.D.** Department of Surgery, University of California, Irvine School of Medicine, Orange, CA, USA

**Jeffrey L. Ponsky, M.D.** Surgical Education, Case Western Reserve University, Cleveland, OH, USA

**Vitaliy Poylin, M.D.** Division of Colon and Rectal Surgery, Beth Israel Deaconess Medical Center, Boston, MA, USA

Beth Israel Deaconess Medical Center, Harvard Medical School, Boston, MA, USA

**Dan J. Raz, M.D., M.A.S.** Division of Thoracic Surgery, Department of Surgery, City of Hope, Duarte, CA, USA

**Andrew Russ, M.D.** Department of Surgery, University of Tennessee Medical Center, Knoxville, TN, USA

**Tushar Samdani, M.D.** Department of Surgery, Memorial Sloan Kettering Cancer Center, New York, NY, USA

**Palanisamy Senthilnathan, M.S., DNB GI Surgery, F.A.C.S.** Division of Minimally Invasive & HPB Surgery, GEM Centre for Liver and Pancreas, GEM Hospital & Research Centre, Coimbatore, Tamilnadu, India

**Stephen M. Sentovich, M.D., M.B.A.** Division of Surgical Oncology, City of Hope, Duarte, CA, USA

**Boris Sepesi, M.D.** Department of Thoracic and Cardiovascular Surgery, The University of Texas MD Anderson Cancer Center, Houston, TX, USA

**Xavier Serra-Aracil, M.D.** Coloproctology Unit, Department of General and Digestive Surgery, Parc Tauli University Hospital, Universitat Autònoma de Barcelona, Barcelona, Spain

**Bhavin C. Shah, M.D.** Division of Surgical Oncology, University of Pittsburgh Medical Center, Pittsburgh, PA, USA

**J. Joshua Smith, M.D., Ph.D.** Department of Surgery, Memorial Sloan Kettering Cancer Center, New York, NY, USA

**Vivian E. Strong, M.D., F.A.C.S.** Memorial Sloan-Kettering Cancer Center, New York, NY, USA

Weill Medical College of Cornell University, New York, NY, USA

**Mark Y. Sun, M.D.** Division of Colon and Rectal Surgery, Department of Surgery, University of Minnesota, Saint Paul, MN, USA

**Erin Teeple, M.D.** Department of Surgery, Thomas Jefferson University/AI DuPont Hospital for Children, Wilmington, DE, USA

**Marta Jiménez Toscano, M.D.** Department of Gastrointestinal Surgery, University of Barcelona School of Medicine, Clinic Hospital, Barcelona, Spain

**Lin Wang, M.D.** Department of Colorectal Surgery, Peking University Cancer Hospital, Beijing, People's Republic of China

**Dilendra H. Weerasinghe, M.D., M.R.C.S.Ed., M.R.C.S.** Division of General Surgery, Department of Surgery, University of Florida College of Medicine—Jacksonville, Jacksonville, FL, USA

**Gregory C. Wilson, M.D.** Division of Surgical Oncology, Department of Surgery, University of Cincinnati Medical Center, Cincinnati, OH, USA

**Han-Kwang Yang, M.D., Ph.D., F.A.C.S.** Department of Surgery, Seoul National University College of Medicine, Seoul, South Korea

**James Yoo, M.D.** Division of Colon and Rectal Surgery, Department of Surgery, Tufts Medical Center, Tufts University School of Medicine, Boston, MA, USA

**Herbert J. Zeh III, M.D.** Division of Surgical Oncology, University of Pittsburgh School of Medicine, University of Pittsburgh Medical Center, Pittsburgh, PA, USA

**Amer H. Zureikat, M.D.** Division of Surgical Oncology, University of Pittsburgh School of Medicine, University of Pittsburgh Medical Center, Pittsburgh, PA, USA

# Part I

# Esophagus

# 1 Open Technique for Ivor Lewis Esophagectomy

Boris Sepesi and Wayne L. Hofstetter

## Historical Perspective

The first successful resection of the thoracic esophagus was performed by Franz Torek in Germany on March 14, 1913, under chloroform and ether anesthesia [1]. The patient, who suffered from squamous cell carcinoma of the esophagus, was effectively cured by this resection and survived for an additional 12 years. He died of pneumonia without cancer recurrence. Unfortunately, many esophageal cancer patients who underwent esophagectomy at the beginning of the twentieth century succumbed in the early postoperative period. However, Torek's success gave first hope that resection of the esophagus for carcinoma may become a feasible treatment modality as anesthesia and perioperative care evolved.

The main complexity of esophageal surgery at the beginning of the twentieth century was related to the intrathoracic location of the esophagus and patient tolerance of intraoperative pneumothorax, since positive pressure ventilation or selective lung ventilation did not exist. Another complex issue was associated with a reliable reconstruction of the alimentary tract following esophagectomy. Since then many operative techniques have been developed for the resection and reconstruction of the esophagus. The one technique that is commonly used and has withstood the test of time was presented by British surgeon Ivor Lewis in 1946 at the Royal College of Surgeons Hunterean Lecture [2]. Lewis proposed the combination of laparotomy and right thoracotomy for the resection of cancer of the esophagus. The operation was performed in two stages. First, laparotomy was performed with gastric mobilization followed by right thoracotomy 10–15 days later. During right thoracotomy the esophagus and tumor were resected, and alimentary continuity was reestablished with esophagogastric anastomosis. Lewis' series described successful postoperative outcome in five of seven patients, a rare surgical triumph at the time. Nearly 70 years later, although performed as a single-stage procedure and with additional modifications, Ivor Lewis esophagectomy continues to be an applicable and widely used technique for the resection of middle or distal esophageal carcinoma.

## Anatomical Highlights

Ivor Lewis esophagectomy consists of abdominal dissection followed by right thoracotomy (Fig. 1.1). Understanding the abdominal and thoracic anatomy is therefore paramount to the performance of the operation.

B. Sepesi, M.D. • W.L. Hofstetter, M.D. (✉)
Department of Thoracic and Cardiovascular Surgery, The University of Texas, MD Anderson Cancer Center, 1515 Holcombe Boulevard, Houston, TX 77030, USA
e-mail: whofstetter@mdanderson.org

J. Kim and J. Garcia-Aguilar (eds.), *Surgery for Cancers of the Gastrointestinal Tract: A Step-by-Step Approach*, DOI 10.1007/978-1-4939-1893-5_1, © Springer Science+Business Media New York 2015

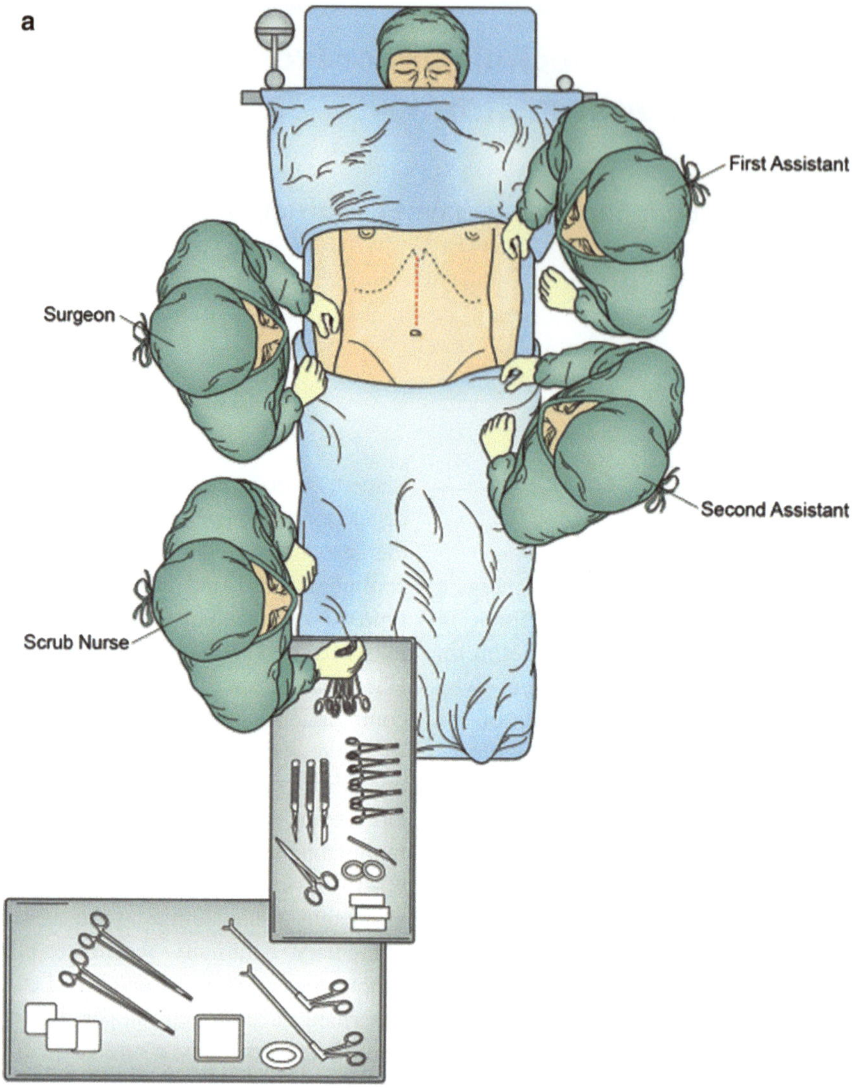


**Fig. 1.1** Operative positioning for (**a**) upper midine laparotomy and (**b**) right fifth interspace thoracotomy

## Abdominal Anatomy

Knowledge of the upper abdominal anatomy is crucial to safe and effective esophageal and gastric mobilization, performance of adequate lymphadenectomy, and creation of the gastric conduit. Relationship of the esophagus and stomach to solid organs, vascular structures, and ligamentous attachments must be considered. The esophagus enters the abdomen via the esophageal hiatus located at the level of the T8 vertebra. It is attached to the diaphragmatic crus via the phrenoesophageal ligament, which extends onto the proximal portion of the stomach. The structures considered during the dissection on the right side of the crus include the inferior vena cava, left lobe of the liver, caudate lobe of the liver, pars flaccida, duodenum, porta hepatis, and right gastric artery.

Posteriorly, the abdominal esophagus and stomach are closely related to the abdominal aorta, celiac axis, left gastric artery and vein, common hepatic and splenic arteries, pancreas,

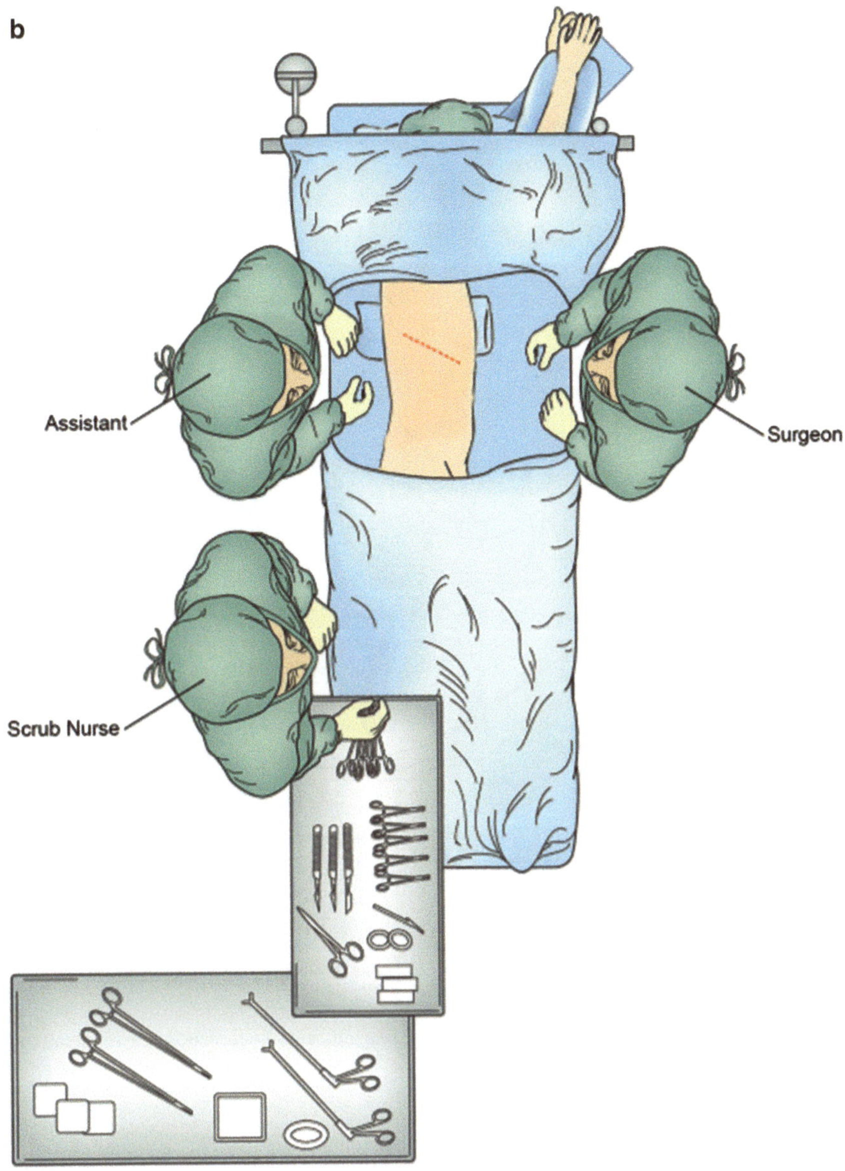


**Fig. 1.1** (continued)

and branches of the cisterna chyle (Fig. 1.2). Inferiorly, the important structures include the right gastro-epiploic artery, greater omentum, and transverse colon and mesocolon. On the left side, the greater curvature of the stomach has attachments to the colon and spleen. After mobilization of the short gastric arteries, the tail of the pancreas and left crus come into view.

## Thoracic Anatomy

Important structures within the right thorax related to the esophagus include the thoracic aorta, azygos vein and azygos arch, thoracic duct, inferior pulmonary vein, posterior pericardium, left and right mainstem bronchi, vagus nerves along with their bronchial branches, trachea, and

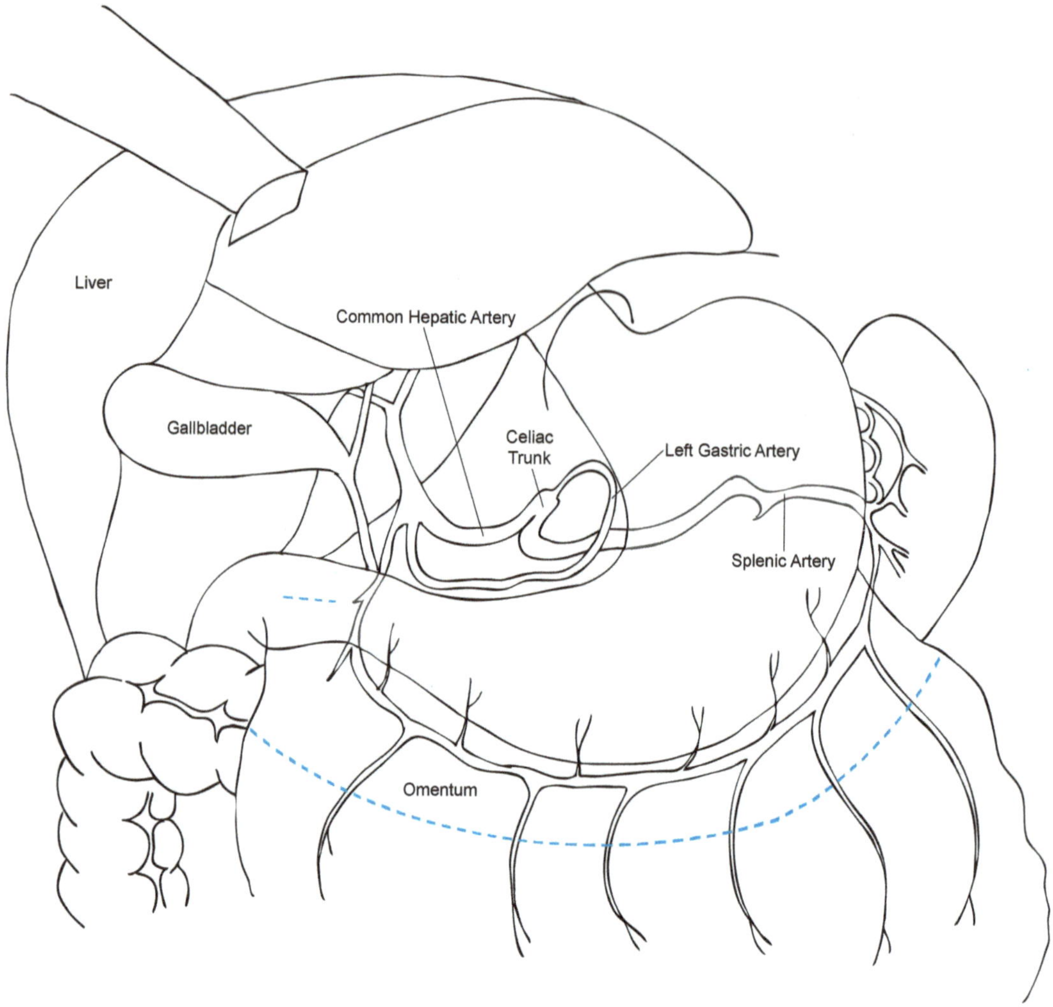


**Fig. 1.2** The arterial cascade of the stomach. The *blue dashed line* indicates the resection line for creation of the gastric conduit and omental flap

left recurrent laryngeal nerve. Important lymphatic basins include mediastinal level 8 and 9 lymph nodes, subcarinal level 7 lymph nodes, and paratracheal level 4 lymph nodes.

## Indications for the Operation

Currently, there are several surgical techniques utilized for the resection and reconstruction of the esophagus. Ivor Lewis esophagectomy is one of those techniques; however, it does not fit all clinical scenarios in which esophageal resection may be indicated. The main decision points about the utility of the Ivor Lewis approach are the location of tumor within the esophagus and subsequently the level of anticipated esophagogastric anastomosis. Generally, the most common indication for Ivor Lewis esophagectomy is carcinoma of the esophagus located in the middle or distal esophagus and as low as the gastroesophageal junction (GEJ) and upper cardia. Other potential indications include severe esophageal stricture from gastroesophageal reflux disease or end-stage achalasia. Tumors located proximal to the level of the carina or azygos arch, or less than 25 cm from the incisors on esophagoscopy require an anastomosis in the neck and are not suitable for the Ivor Lewis approach.

## Preoperative Evaluation and Imaging

Considering that esophageal carcinoma is the most frequent indication for Ivor Lewis esophagectomy, the preoperative evaluation includes adequate clinical staging along with the assessment of physiologic fitness and nutritional status of the patient. Staging of esophageal carcinoma includes esophago-gastro-duodenoscopy (EGD) with endoscopic ultrasound (EUS) to define the location of the tumor within the esophagus and the depth of esophageal wall penetration. EUS is also useful for the assessment of regional and some non-regional lymph nodes. Positron emission tomography combined with computed tomography (PET/CT) supplements staging by searching for distant metastatic disease. Ivor Lewis esophagectomy may be utilized in patients with Tis-4a, N0-3 stages.

Evaluation of the physiologic fitness and suitability for the operation is based on the surgeon's judgment which is guided by a thorough medical history and physical examination. Adjunctive studies such as pulmonary function tests and stress echocardiogram may further help with the decision-making process. The preoperative nutritional status is very important to the overall success of the operation. Patients with esophageal adenocarcinoma usually demonstrate more robust physiognomy than patients with squamous cell carcinoma who often present in an emaciated condition. However, prolonged dysphagia due to tumor obstruction or esophagitis related to neoadjuvant radiation therapy are frequent reasons for weight loss, and must be addressed prior to definitive surgical procedure.

## Perioperative Preparation

Bowel preparation or chlorhexidine shower the day before the operation are left to the discretion of the operating surgeon; they are likely more dogmatic than necessary. Clinical judgment is the best guide. While formal bowel prep is likely not necessary, preoperative constipation may manifest as significant postoperative ileus that may hinder nutrition and progress toward discharge. Our practice is to place patients on a liquid diet for 2 days prior to surgery and to use a cathartic if there is history of constipation. From an anesthesia standpoint, patients should be prepared to tolerate single lung ventilation. Epidural analgesia has become an extremely useful tool for postoperative pain control but its use must be tempered to the downside of perioperative hypotension from a sympatholytic effect. Long acting local blocks as part of a pain control cocktail are also acceptable.

## Description of the Operation

Ivor Lewis esophagectomy consists of a series of operative steps and maneuvers, some which have been the source of fervent discussion and even randomized trials. Herein, we describe our modifications and approach to open Ivor Lewis esophagectomy, which can be divided into following steps: abdominal incision, mobilization of the abdominal esophagus and stomach, mobilization of the greater omental pedicle flap, dissection of the left gastric artery and D2 lymphadenectomy, pylorus draining procedure, gastric conduit creation, and feeding jejunostomy. The thoracic part of the operation can be divided into: muscle-sparing right thoracotomy incision, esophageal mobilization, thoracic duct ligation, lymphadenectomy, esophagogastric anastomosis, and omental pedicle transposition and envelope.

### Abdominal Incision and Exposure

An upper midline laparotomy incision extending from just above the xiphoid process to the level of the umbilicus provides adequate exposure of the upper abdominal viscera and the omentum. In patients with central obesity, a bilateral subcostal incision with the division of the bilateral rectus abdominis muscles is an excellent alternative of exposing the upper abdomen to avoid subsequent risk of ventral incisional hernia. The blades of the Thompson retractor are placed in bilateral subcostal regions to aid the exposure of the diaphragm and the GEJ. To avoid tearing the liver capsule from excessive retractor traction, the falciform ligament may be divided to the level of the diaphragmatic attachments.

## Gastric and Esophageal Mobilization

The left lobe of the liver overlying the GEJ is retracted anteriorly. Mobilization of the triangular ligament is also an option but is rarely necessary. The pars flaccida is opened, exposing the caudate lobe of the liver and the right diaphragmatic crus within the lesser sac. Then, the phreno-esophageal ligament overlying the diaphragmatic crus is incised and the crus is dissected free from the GEJ. If involved with carcinoma, a part of the crus is resected en bloc with the operative specimen to ensure negative radial margins. A penrose drain is passed around the GEJ to aid with manipulation of the esophagus and further dissection proceeds in the superior and lateral periaortic planes and along the pleural surfaces laterally reaching up into the mediastinum. This maneuver facilitates intrathoracic esophageal mobilization; however, care must be taken not to inadvertently injure or partially divide the inferior pulmonary veins on either side.

## Mobilization of the Omental Pedicle

The transverse colon is lifted out of the body cavity and retracted inferiorly as the omentum is retracted superiorly. The avascular plane between the omentum and colon is opened while carefully avoiding injury to the colon, mesocolon, omentum, and greater curvature blood supply (i.e., the right gastro-epiploic vessels). The omentum is fully mobilized off the transverse colon and mesocolon after entering the lesser sac to the level of the gastroduodenal artery. Care is taken to preserve the entire course of the right gastro-epiploic artery during omental mobilization by careful palpation and/or visualization of this artery. The omental pedicle flap, based on 2–3 perforating omental arterial branches off the right gastro-epiploic artery, is created along the left side of the greater curvature (Fig. 1.2). Gastric mobilization along the greater curvature is completed with the division of the short gastric arteries staying relatively close to the stomach to avoid inadvertent splenic injury.

## Abdominal D2 Lymphadenectomy and Left Gastric Artery Division

With the aid of a nasogastric tube in the stomach stretching along the greater curvature, the stomach is elevated to approach the celiac axis and left gastric artery from the lesser sac in the dissection plane created above the mesocolon. The peritoneum overlying the superior edge of the pancreas is incised to reveal the common hepatic and splenic arteries. The tissues anterior and cranial to the common hepatic and splenic arteries is included in the lymph node dissection and lymph node tissues along the left gastric artery is dissected and swept anteriorly with the specimen. The left gastric vein and artery are then divided at their origin (doubly ligated or stapled) after ensuring a good palpable pulse in both splenic and common hepatic arteries. The boundaries of dissection from right to left are the porta hepatis/vena cava to the splenic hilum, respectively; and periaortic tissues from the celiac artery inferiorly up to the extent of the mediastinal resection (Fig. 1.3). Clips should be placed on the larger lymphatics in the area of the porta hepatis to avoid chylous ascites.

## Pylorus Draining Procedure

Controversy surrounds this portion of the procedure [3]. Some experts leave the pylorus completely intact, whereas others favor pyloromyotomy, botox injection, selective balloon dilation postoperatively, or formal pyloroplasty. Emptying of the gastric conduit through the pylorus may be related to the width of the conduit, however conclusive evidence is lacking.

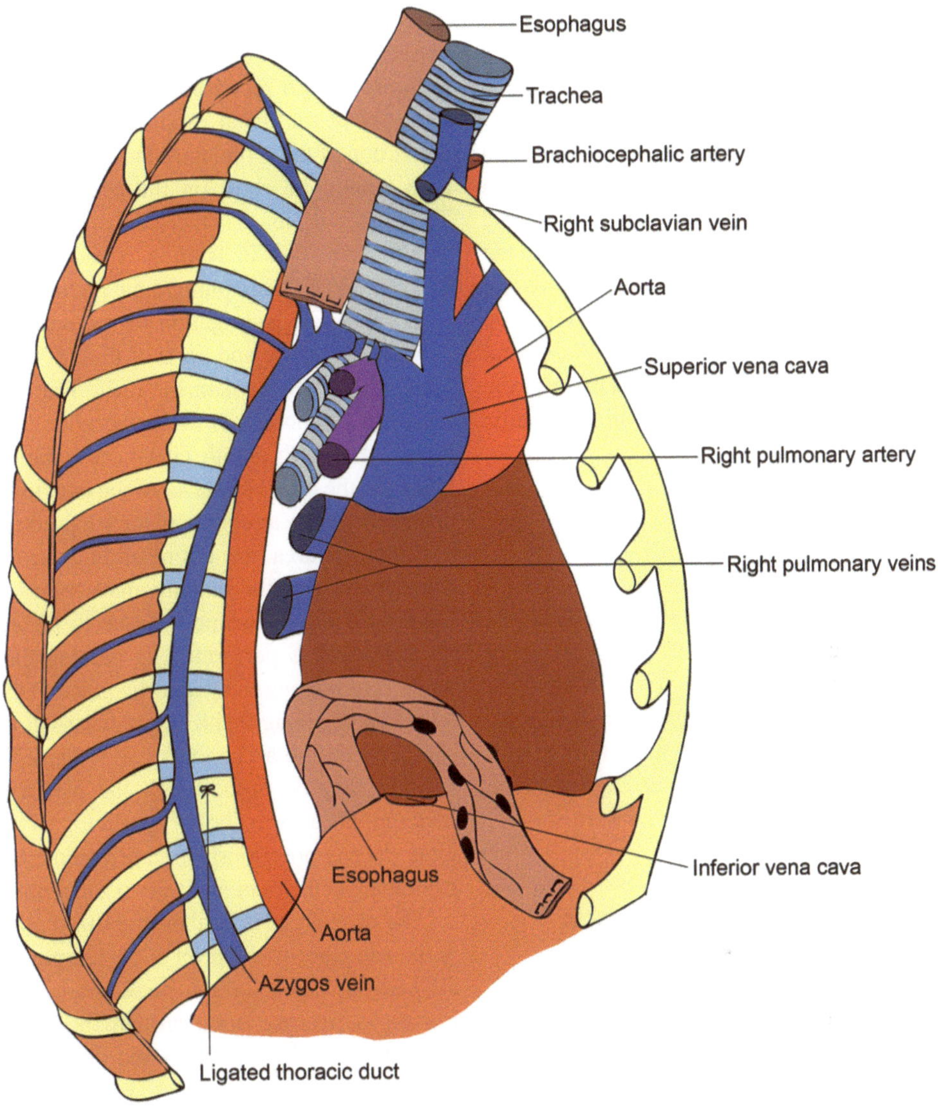


**Fig. 1.3** Thoracic dissection showing ligation of the azygos arch, ligation of the thoracic duct, and resection of the esophagus with surrounding lymphatic tissues

Our preference has been to perform either pyloromytomy or pyloroplasty.

The pylorus is identified and a 00 silk suture is placed at the superior and inferior border of the pylorus. With the cutting cautery current at 15 V the muscle tissue of the pyloric sphincter is divided and pyloromyotomy is performed; or alternatively, a Heineke-Mikulicz pyloroplasty is performed. The pyloromyotomy or pyloroplasty may be covered with a piece of omentum or previously mobilized falciform ligament and secured in place with previously placed 00 silk sutures.

## Gastric Pedicle Creation

The incisura is identified at the lesser curvature of the stomach and the right gastric artery is divided above the incisura. Multiple fires of green 4.5 mm linear stapler loads aiming towards the angle of His are used to create a gastric conduit approximately 4 cm in width. In cases where the tumor extends into the stomach, care must be taken to ensure an adequate distal margin. A second staple line can be fired parallel to the first to supply the pathologist with specimen to determine the distal margin status on frozen section examination. The conduit can be completely formed in the abdomen and transferred to the chest with traction sutures, or alternatively partially formed in the abdomen with completion of the tubularization in the chest after formation of the anastomosis. Using 000 silk sutures, the omental pedicle that is to be transferred into the chest is tacked to the staple line on the proximal stomach to facilitate transposition of the gastric conduit and omentum to the chest. A feeding jejunostomy catheter is placed 30 cm from the ligament of Treitz in Witzeled fashion. Finally, the abdomen is closed.

## Right Thoracotomy

The patient is positioned in the left lateral decubitus position and right, muscle-sparing thoracotomy is performed (Fig. 1.1b). Neither the latissimus dorsi nor the serratus anterior muscles is divided. The chest cavity is entered in the fifth interspace and the sixth rib may be cut behind the paraspinous muscle to aid with exposure.

## Esophageal Mobilization, Thoracic Duct Ligation, and Lymphadenectomy

Esophageal mobilization begins with incision of the inferior pulmonary ligament. The right lung is retracted anteriorly and the mediastinal pleura is incised along the anterior surface of the esophagus at the edge of the lung parenchyma. Continuing superiorly and staying close to the posterior pericardium, the subcarinal level 7 lymph node compartment is mobilized en bloc with the esophagus. Care must be used with any cautery device in the subcarinal region to avoid thermal airway injury. Scissor dissection is another option with vascular clip control of bronchial vessels supplying the level 7 LNs.

The azygos arch is then mobilized and divided with a vascular 2.5 mm linear stapler load. The mediastinal pleura above the azygos arch is then incised and the esophagus is further mobilized away from the trachea using both sharp and blunt dissection. Care must be taken in this region not to injure the left recurrent laryngeal nerve. If the tumor is in the distal esophagus or below, any dissection of the esophagus above the level of the arch should be right on the esophageal wall. The posterior pleura is incised just anterior to the azygos vein. This incision is extended inferiorly to the level of the diaphragmatic hiatus.

For thoracic duct ligation we focus on the area between the spine and aorta at the T10 vertebral level which will contain the duct. The duct traverses the diaphragm with the aorta in the aortic hiatus. Above the ninth interspace there is variability in the crossover level of the duct to the left chest, therefore attempts at duct ligation in the mid-thoracic area may not result in control of the duct. Just above the diaphragmatic hiatus, mass ligation of the paraspinous tissue to include the thoracic duct is performed by passing the right angle clamp along the periaortic plane to the vertebral body. Using 0 silk suture material, the tissue between the aorta and spine is ligated. Duct ligation may be optimized if the pleura is left intact in this area to "hold" the suture, as the thoracic duct is notoriously friable and the ligature itself can cut the duct and lead to a chylothorax.

The esophagus is further mobilized along the periaortic plane to the level of the left pleura with all periesophageal lymph node bearing tissues. Passing a penrose drain around the esophagus may facilitate the retraction and dissection. The boundaries of the modified en bloc thoracic esophageal dissection are from right to left, the pleura to pleura, diaphragm to azygos arch, and azygos vein/spine to pericardium, respectively (Figs. 1.4 and 1.5).

## Anastomosis

The esophagus is divided for approximately 75 % of its circumference at or above the level of the azygos arch. We typically employ an intraluminal stapling device for an end-to-side esophagogastrostomy. Depending on the size of the esophagus, either a 25 or 29 mm anvil of a circular stapler is placed within the esophagus. 00 or 000 prolene

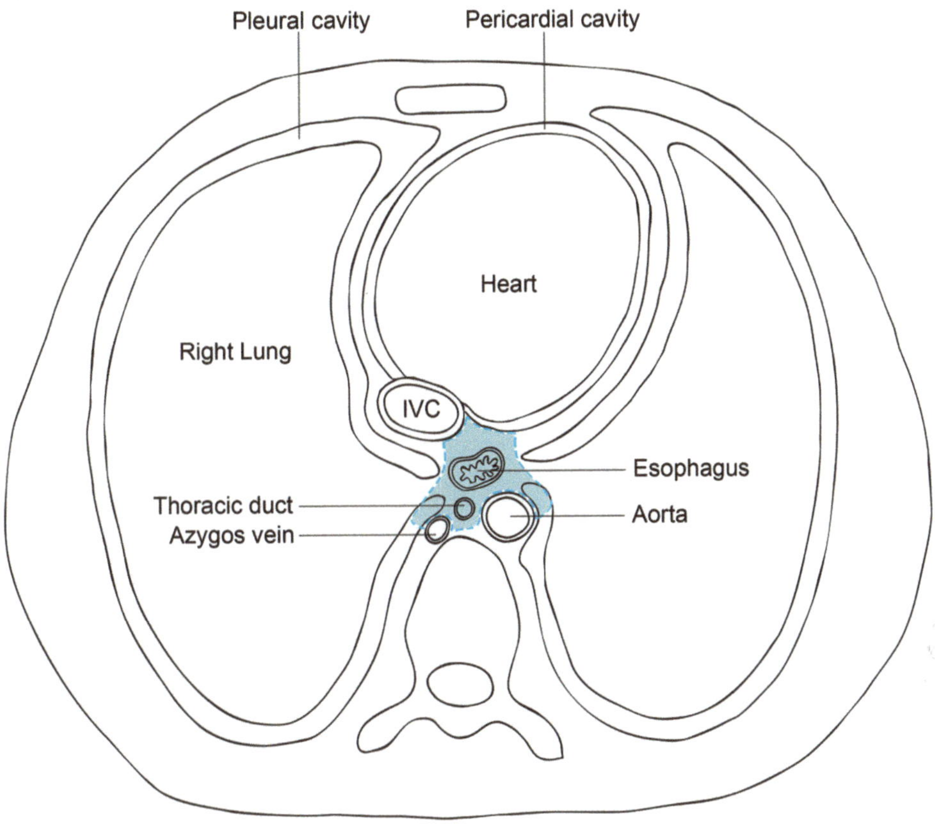


**Fig. 1.4** Axial image depicting the boundaries of the thoracic dissection from pleura to pleura, diaphragm to azygos arch, and azygos vein/spine to pericardium

suture is sewn in a continuous horizontal mattress fashion approximately 2 mm from the cut esophageal wall incorporating full thickness esophageal wall to purse-string the esophagus around the staple anvil. The esophagus is then fully divided and at this point a proximal esophageal margin can be sent for frozen section analysis as necessary. The same prolene suture is then continued as a second over-and-over layer (i.e., baseball stitch) to further align the esophageal wall around the anvil.

The resected portion of the esophagus, stomach, and the omentum are delivered to the chest cavity in the anatomic position. It is important to ensure that the conduit is not twisted. The staple line of the lesser curvature of the stomach should be pointing laterally, directly towards the surgeon's view. The stitches between the surgical specimen and gastric conduit and omentum are cut and the specimen is removed. Alternatively, the gastric conduit may be partially created within the abdomen and delivered to the chest cavity, where the gastric conduit is completed in the chest after esophagogastric anastomosis.

The gastric conduit is inspected and stretched superiorly inside the thoracic cavity to avoid redundancy of the conduit. A suitable well perfused area for the anastomosis is selected on the greater curvature of the stomach. Gastrotomy is performed at the tip of the gastric conduit, a circular stapler is placed inside the conduit, and the stapler is opened with the spike penetrating the conduit in the preselected anastomotic area opposite the staple line on the lesser curvature. The anvil and spike of the stapler are aligned while ensuring that no other tissues such as lung parenchyma are trapped inside the anastomosis. The stapler is closed, fired, and removed through

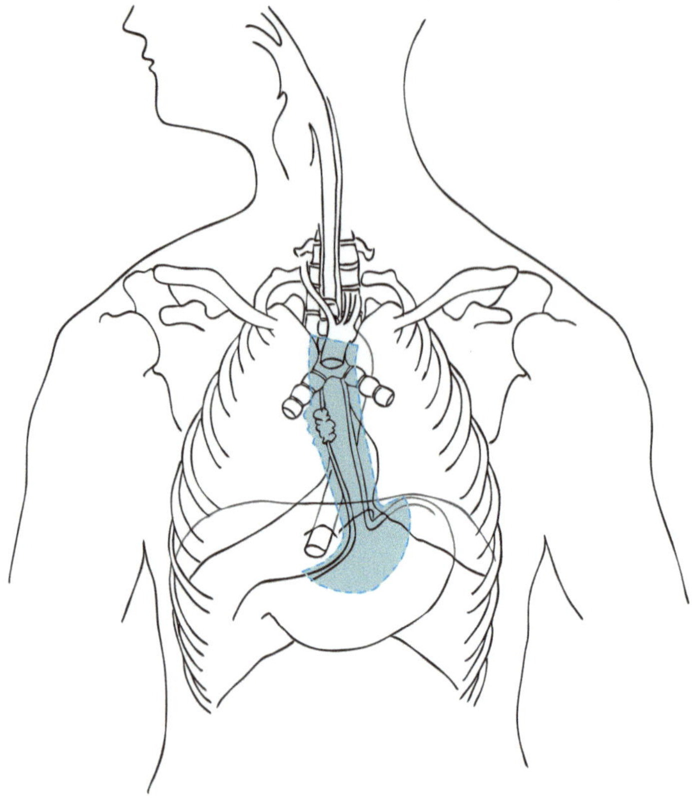

**Fig. 1.5** Coronal image depicting the extent of resection from the intra-abdominal stomach to the thoracic esophagus

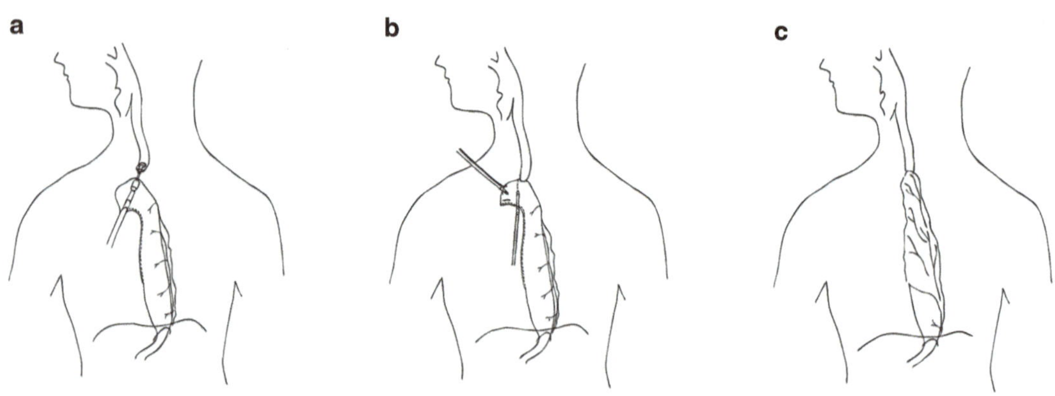


**Fig. 1.6** The creation of the esophagogastrostomy. (**a**) The circular stapler is used to create the anastomosis. (**b**) The tip of the gastric conduit where the circular stapler was introduced is resected. (**c**) The omental flap covers the anastomosis and staple line of the gastric conduit

the gastrotomy. The anastomosis is visually inspected through the gastrotomy site and a nasogastric tube is advanced under direct vision across the anastomosis into the gastric conduit. An additional green linear stapler load is used to amputate the tip of the conduit thus removing the gastrotomy site. This staple line should be sufficiently away from the circular staple line of the esophagogastric anastomosis to avoid tissue ischemia between the staple lines (Fig. 1.6).

## Omental Envelope

An omental pedicle flap is placed underneath, between the anastomosis and the airway to circumferentially envelop the anastomosis and gastric staple line. A few 000 silk sutures are used to secure the omentum around the anastomosis. The chest cavity is then irrigated and chest tubes are placed in the pleural spaces. Prior to approximating costal sutures, the lung is insufflated and it is ensured that all three lobes of the right lung are anatomically aligned and expanded without evidence of trapping or atelectasis. The thoracotomy incision is closed in routine fashion.

## Postoperative Management

The patient is extubated in the operating room and transferred to the postanesthesia care unit (PACU) and then to a monitored step-downward. Portable chest x-ray is obtained in PACU and formal upright postero-anterior and lateral chest x-rays are obtained on postoperative day (POD) #1. Intravenous fluids are usually infused at a rate of 125 mL/h for the first 2 days. However, the fluid management is guided by the clinical status and urine output. It is important to maintain adequate blood pressure/perfusion to the newly created gastric conduit. The nasogastric tube is kept to continuous low wall suction for a few days, then placed to gravity and then removed on POD 4–5 as long as there are no signs of early anastomotic leak or ileus. Chest tubes are removed after nasogastric tube removal, as long as there is no evidence of chyle leak, bile leak, or air leak; and the volume of the output is less than 400 mL for 24 h.

Feeding via the jejunostomy catheter is initiated on POD #3, initially at a rate of 15 mL/h and advanced to goal by 15 mL daily. When bowel function returns, feeds can be advanced fairly rapidly to goal. Pain is transitioned to liquid pain medicines via the jejunostomy tube when the patient is tolerating feeds well. Generally, patients are discharged from the hospital on POD #7 after receiving instructions on tube feedings and jejunostomy tube care.

A barium swallow is performed between POD #10 to 14 prior to the first outpatient visit. If there is no sign of anastomotic leak, a diet is initiated and the patient has a formal consultation with a nutritionist to discuss oral transitioning, weaning tube feeds, and postesophagectomy dietary habits.

## Complications

Esophagectomy is associated with a relatively high potential risk (approximately 50 %) for postoperative morbidity and a relatively small but significant (approximately 4 % 90-day) risk of mortality [4]. Postoperative morbidity may be related to virtually any organ system. Pneumonia, atelectasis, acute respiratory failure, atrial fibrillation, ileus, wound complications, recurrent laryngeal nerve injury, myocardial infarction, stroke, pulmonary embolism, bowel ischemia, and conduit necrosis are all possible postoperatively. However, the most common complication, which most often determines the postoperative course, is anastomotic leak. Successful healing of the esophagogastric anastomosis depends on many factors, of which relative ischemia is likely the most important. To maximize the chance for healing and minimize potential anastomosis related complications, surgeons have experimented with constructing the anastomosis in the neck or chest, stapling the anastomosis linearly or circularly, or sewing the anastomosis in one or two layers. The Ivor Lewis esophagectomy anastomosis is constructed within the right chest, and our preference has been a circular anastomosis at or above the level of the azygos vein to minimize postoperative reflux. If neoadjuvant therapy was employed, placing the anastomosis in an area of nonirradiated esophagus may help to avoid a leak. We also favor enveloping the anastomosis with an omental pedicle [5]. Using this technique, our leak rate has decreased from 8 to 4 %. Importantly, severe leaks requiring reoperative intervention are now extremely rare with the use of the omental buttress.

The management of an anastomotic leak varies depending on the severity of the leak and the clinical and hemodynamic characteristics. Experience and clinical judgment is required in this setting. The management strategy may range from nonoperative to endoscopic to operative treatments. Contained anastomotic leaks without signs of systemic inflammation or sepsis are usually treated with *nil per os* and occasional antibiotics. Anastomotic leaks draining into the pleural cavity or stimulating systemic inflammatory response or sepsis require more aggressive management. The main principle is sepsis control, which may be accomplished with endoscopic, image-guided, or operative techniques. Over the last decade, endoscopic stenting of an anastomotic leak has become popular, and few studies suggest success with this approach [6]. Operative approach is occasionally necessary and usually necessitates decortication of the lung, along with anastomotic reinforcement with a vascularized muscle flap. Intercostal, serratus anterior, or latissimus dorsi muscles provide excellent choices for coverage of the defect [7]. Necrosis of the gastric conduit is a rare but life threatening complication [8]. Early recognition is important, and treatment involves resection of the conduit and esophagostomy. Enteral reconstruction can be subsequently achieved either with colon or jejunal interposition depending on the institutional experience and expertise [9].

## Conclusion

Open Ivor Lewis esophagectomy remains an excellent and reproducible procedure for the treatment of middle and distal esophageal carcinoma. With the addition of omental transposition, the perioperative anastomosis leak rate and leak-associated complications have further declined. However, principles of careful gastric mobilization based on the right gastro-epiploic artery, conduit creation, and meticulous anastomosis construction within the chest remain the core maneuvers of this time-honored surgical procedure.

## References

1. Dubecz A, Schwartz SI. Franz John A. Torek. Ann Thorac Surg. 2008;85(4):1497–9. doi:10.1016/j.athoracsur.2007.10.106.
2. Lewis I. The surgical treatment of carcinoma of the oesophagus; with special reference to a new operation for growths of the middle third. Br J Surg. 1946;34:18–31.
3. Gaur P, Swanson SJ. Should we continue to drain the pylorus in patients undergoing an esophagectomy? Dis Esophagus. 2013. doi:10.1111/dote.12035.
4. Low DE, Bodnar A. Update on clinical impact, documentation, and management of complications associated with esophagectomy. Thorac Surg Clin. 2013;23(4):535–50. doi:10.1016/j.thorsurg.2013.07.003.
5. Sepesi B, Swisher SG, Walsh GL, Correa A, Mehran RJ, Rice D, et al. Omental reinforcement of the thoracic esophagogastric anastomosis: an analysis of leak and reintervention rates in patients undergoing planned and salvage esophagectomy. J Thorac Cardiovasc Surg. 2012;144(5):1146–50. doi:10.1016/j.jtcvs.2012.07.085.
6. Dasari BV, Neely D, Kennedy A, Spence G, Rice P, Mackle E, et al. The role of esophageal stents in the management of esophageal anastomotic leaks and benign esophageal perforations. Ann Surg. 2014;259(5):852–60. doi:10.1097/sla.0000000000000564.
7. Martin LW, Hofstetter W, Swisher SG, Roth JA. Management of intrathoracic leaks following esophagectomy. Adv Surg. 2006;40:173–90.
8. Wormuth JK, Heitmiller RF. Esophageal conduit necrosis. Thorac Surg Clin. 2006;16(1):11–22. doi:10.1016/j.thorsurg.2006.01.003.
9. Marks JL, Hofstetter WL. Esophageal reconstruction with alternative conduits. Surg Clin North Am. 2012;92(5):1287–97. doi:10.1016/j.suc.2012.07.006.

## Key Operative Steps

1. Create upper midline incision from the xiphoid to the umbilicus.
2. Retract the left lobe of the liver anteriorly and superiorly over the gastroesophageal junction.
3. Open the pars flaccida exposing the caudate lobe and right diaphragmatic crus.
4. Incise the phreno-esophageal ligament over the diaphragmatic crus and dissect the crus free from the gastroesophageal junction.
5. Pass a penrose drain around the gastroesophageal junction to aid with dissection.
6. Divide the avascular plane between the omentum and colon. Preserve the entire course of the right gastro-epiploic artery.

7. Create an omental pedicle flap, based on 2–3 perforating omental arterial branches off the right gastroepiploic artery.
8. Complete gastric mobilization along the greater curvature by dividing short gastric arteries.
9. Perform D2 lymphadenectomy and divide the left gastric vessels.
10. Perform either pyloromyotomy or pyloroplasty.
11. Create the gastric conduit with multiple fires of linear stapler from incisura towards the angle of His.
12. Create feeding jejunostomy 30 cm from the ligament of Treitz.
13. Close the abdomen.
14. Perform right thoracotomy.
15. Mobilize the esophagus by incising the inferior pulmonary ligament, retracting the lung anteriorly and medially, and incising the mediastinal pleura along the anterior surface of the esophagus.
16. Mobilize the subcarinal/level 7 lymph node compartment en bloc with the esophagus.
17. Mobilize the azygos arch and divide it with vascular stapler.
18. Mobilize the esophagus away from the trachea.
19. Incise the posterior pleura anterior to the azygos vein and extend inferiorly to the diaphragmatic hiatus.
20. Ligate the thoracic duct between the spine and aorta at T10.
21. Mobilize the esophagus along the periaortic plane to the left pleura with all periesophageal lymphatic tissues.
22. Divide the esophagus at or above the level of the azygos arch.
23. Purse-string the esophagus around the anvil of the stapler.
24. Create gastrotomy at the tip of the gastric conduit and place the circular stapler into the conduit.
25. Open the stapler extending the spike along the greater curvature of the stomach. Align the anvil with the spike and staple the anastomosis.
26. Amputate the tip of the conduit removing the gastrotomy site.
27. Place the omental pedicle flap between the anastomosis and the airway and circumferentially envelop the anastomosis and gastric staple line.
28. Irrigate the chest cavity and place chest tubes in the pleural spaces.
29. Close thoracotomy incision in routine fashion.

# 2 Minimally Invasive Ivor Lewis Esophagectomy

Dan J. Raz and Jae Y. Kim

## Technical Considerations

We perform minimally invasive Ivor Lewis esophagectomy through a hybrid approach. The abdominal portion is performed laparoscopically without the robot and the thoracic portion is performed robotically. We have found little advantage in using the robot for gastric mobilization and additional ports would be required. In the abdomen there is also the disadvantage of the having to undock the robot when adjustments are made in the position of the patient table. In the chest, there is less need to adjust patient positioning during the course of the procedure. The wristed instrumentation makes the circumferential esophageal mobilization easier. Likewise, placing an esophageal purse-string suture for the esophagogastric anastomosis is also facilitated by the robot.

## Positioning and Preoperative Esophagoscopy

The patient is positioned on the operating room table with both arms tucked and a foot board well secured below the feet. Before prepping the patient, the table should be put in steep reverse Trendelenburg to test positioning. Esophagogastroduodenoscopy (EGD) should be performed intraoperatively prior to surgical resection. It is important to assess the length of tumor and Barrett's disease and to inspect the stomach for ulcerations or other lesions. Excessive insufflation should be avoided. Some surgeons may choose to inject botulinum toxin (200 units) into the pylorus endoscopically and to dilate the pylorus during the endoscopy. We do not perform pyloroplasty or pyloromyotomy. We favor preoperative botulinum toxin injection and pyloric dilatation. Alternatively, botulinum toxin can be injected into the pylorus during the laparoscopic procedure using an aspiration needle. A nasogastric tube (NGT) is then placed.

## Laparoscopic Mobilization of Gastric Conduit

### Port Placement

The surgeon stands on the patient's right side with the assistant on the patient's left (Fig. 2.1). A 12-mm camera port is placed two-thirds of the

Electronic supplementary material: Supplementary material is available in the online version of this chapter at 10.1007/978-1-4939-1893-5_2. Videos can also be accessed at http://www.springerimages.com/videos/978-1-4939-1892-8.

D.J. Raz, M.D., M.A.S. • J.Y. Kim, M.D. (✉)
Division of Thoracic Surgery, Department of Surgery, City of Hope, 1500 East Duarte Road, Duarte, CA 91010, USA
e-mail: jaekim@coh.org

J. Kim and J. Garcia-Aguilar (eds.), *Surgery for Cancers of the Gastrointestinal Tract: A Step-by-Step Approach*, DOI 10.1007/978-1-4939-1893-5_2, © Springer Science+Business Media New York 2015

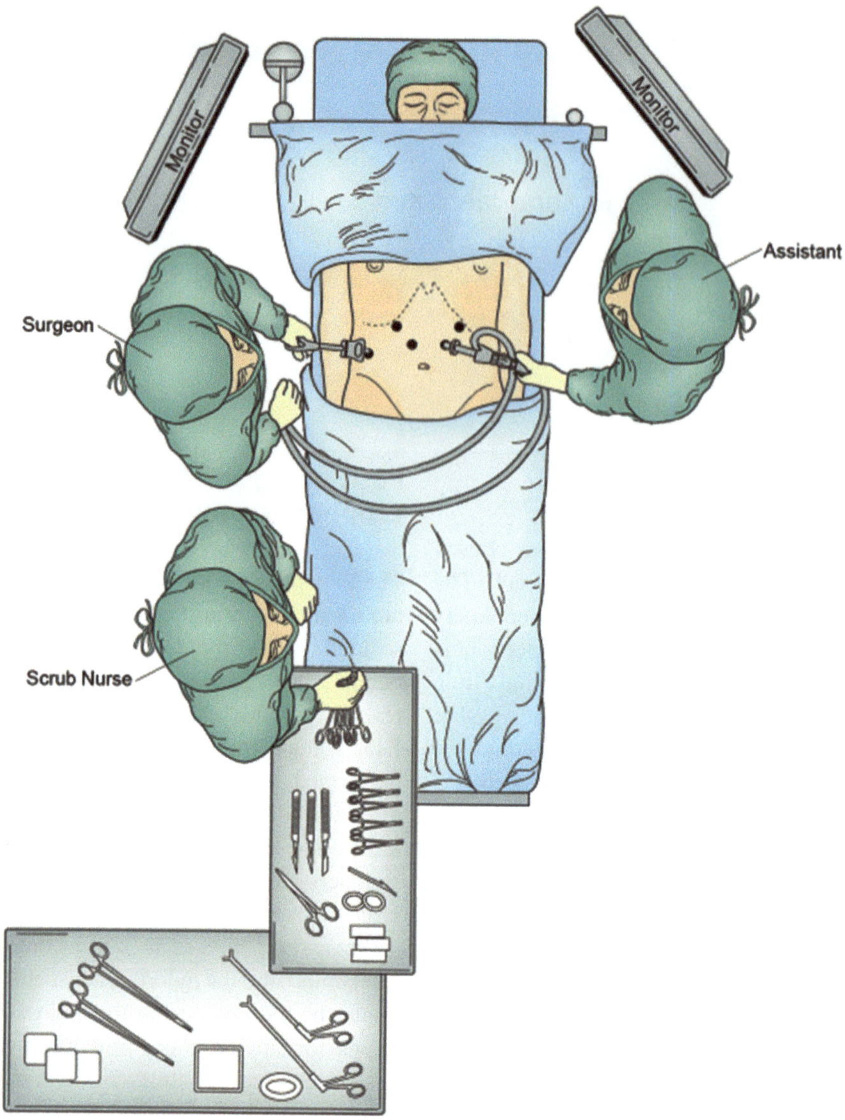


**Fig. 2.1** Operative positioning for laparoscopic mobilization of the stomach

way between the xiphoid process and umbilicus to the right of the midline. We use a 5-mm 30° laparoscope. The peritoneum and omentum are inspected for carcinomatosis and the liver is inspected for metastases. An additional 5-mm port is placed to the left of the midline in the same line as the other port. The patient is then placed in reverse Trendelenburg. A 5-mm port is placed along the costal margin in the right mid-clavicular line and another 5-mm port is placed in the left mid-clavicular line (Fig. 2.2). The bed is turned right side up to facilitate placement of the liver retractor port. A 5-mm port is placed laterally and close to the costal margin. A 5-mm liver retractor is then inserted and the left lobe of the liver is retracted to expose the esophageal hiatus.

## Gastric Mobilization

The dissection is started in the hiatus. The right crus is exposed using an energy device and blunt dissection. The LigaSure (Covidien) and Harmonic Scalpel (Ethicon) are both adequate

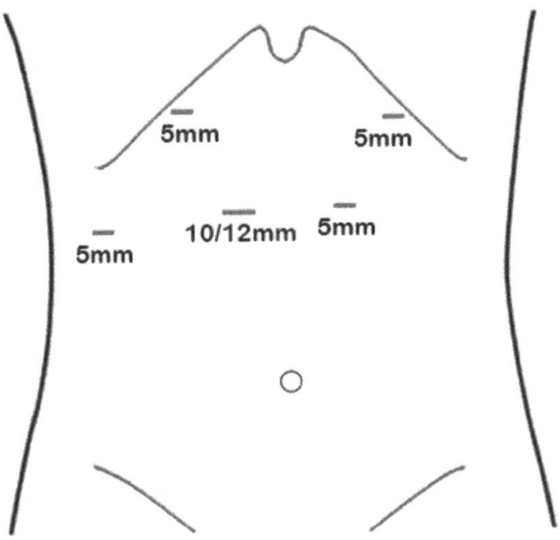


**Fig. 2.2** Trocar placement for laparoscopic mobilization of the stomach

for these steps. We typically remove the peritoneal lining around the crus, but do not routinely excise muscle fibers unless the tumor is adherent. The dissection from the crus is followed anteriorly and over to the left crus. If there is a hiatal hernia, it is helpful to reduce the sac and completely separate the sac from the crura. For patients who do not have a hiatal hernia or only a small hernia, we divide some of the right crural fibers to enlarge the hiatus so that it will easily accommodate the gastric conduit.

Next, the right gastroepiploic artery is visually identified. The stomach is separated from the omentum and mesocolon by retracting the omentum caudal to the point of transection and dividing it away from the gastroepiploic artery. We avoid trauma to the gastric conduit by minimizing retraction of the stomach or avoiding retraction altogether. We usually harvest an omental flap by leaving a pedicled portion of the omentum attached to the conduit perfused by two to three branches of the gastroepiploic arcade; any more than that would be too bulky. This tongue of omentum is dissected directly off the colon. The dissection continues parallel to the left gastroepiploic artery until the short gastric vessels are identified. The short gastric arteries are all serially transected using a vessel sealing device and the stomach is completely mobilized off the spleen and left crus. Additional attachments to the mesocolon are then freed medially. To prevent paraesophageal hernia and to allow maximum mobility of the stomach, the mesocolon should be completely separated from the stomach. Extreme caution must be taken in the vicinity of the takeoff of the right gastroepiploic artery from the gastroduodenal artery to avoid accidental injury of either artery. The lesser sac is then dissected, freeing the stomach from the pancreas. While the assistant retracts the gastric conduit up, the left gastric artery pedicle is dissected from the celiac axis. Nodal tissue is carefully dissected and swept towards the stomach (Fig. 2.3). Once this is complete, the left gastric pedicle is transected using an endovascular stapler cartridge.

Before the gastric conduit is created, we check to ensure that the stomach is circumferentially freed, and that the pylorus easily reaches the hiatus. A Kocher maneuver is not necessary for an Ivor Lewis esophagectomy. The posterior gastroesophageal (GE) junction is then dissected and the mediastinal esophagus is circumferentially dissected as cephalad as possible. It is easy to enter one or both pleural cavities during the mediastinal dissection, so it is best to wait until the latter part of the laparoscopic procedure to perform this dissection. A pleural defect can be a nuisance during laparoscopy and impair the surgeon's ability to insufflate the abdomen adequately.

## Creating the Gastric Conduit

The NGT is then pulled back into the pharynx. A point on the lesser curvature of the stomach between the right and left gastric arteries is identified just proximal to the incisura. Collateral vessels overlying this point are divided. Medium/thick tissue staple cartridges are then used to create the conduit, firing multiple stapler loads up until a point on the gastric fundus. We do not oversew the staple line. Ideally the gastric conduit is no smaller than 4 cm in width. The stomach is then sewn back to the specimen with a single mattress stitch. Alternatively, the last 2 cm of the stomach can be left undivided while creating the gastric conduit and then later divided within the chest. We leave a quarter inch penrose drain around the GE junction, secured by a suture to facilitate retrieval and dissection within the chest.

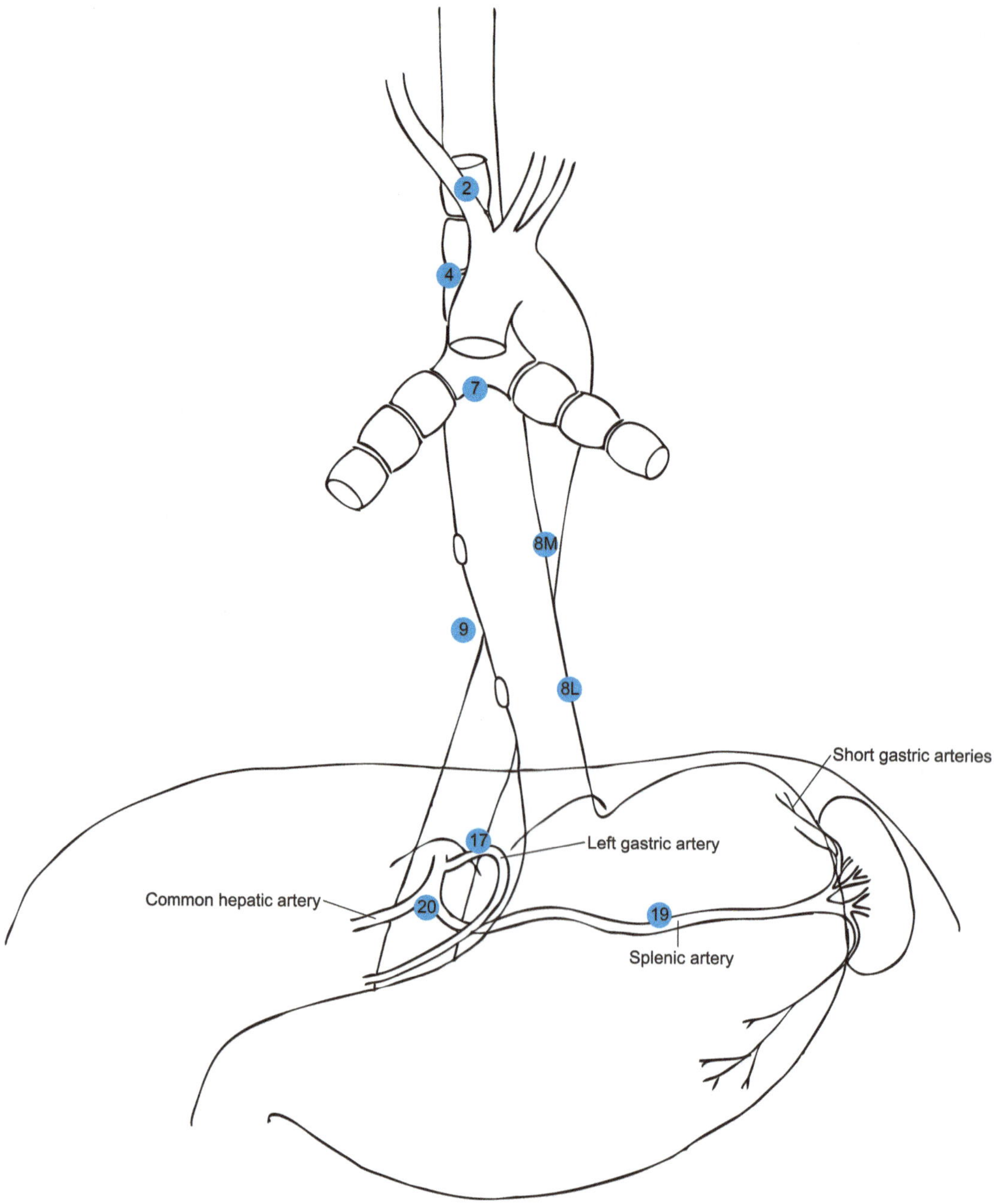


**Fig. 2.3** Key lymph node stations during Ivor Lewis esophagogastrectomy

## Feeding Jejunostomy

Finally, the feeding jejunostomy is placed. A loop of jejunum 30 cm distal to the ligament of Treitz is identified and the proximal bowel is tacked to the abdominal wall at the site of the jejunostomy using a 2-0 silk. We insert a jejunostomy catheter using Seldinger technique and a peel-away catheter kit. An additional stitch is placed on the opposite side of the first stitch to secure the jejunum to the abdominal wall. One additional stitch is placed 2–3 cm distally, tacking the jejunum to the abdominal wall, to prevent twisting of the jejunum around the jejunostomy insertion site.

### Closure

The fascia of the 12-mm port is closed with a figure-of-eight 0-vicryl suture. All the skin incisions are then closed and sterile dressings applied. A left-sided chest tube may be placed with the patient in supine position.

## Thoracic Dissection and Anastomosis

### Esophageal Mobilization

After the abdominal incisions are closed, the patient is placed in left lateral decubitus position. With the right lung collapsed, a 5-mm port is initially introduced in the anterior axillary line, at approximately the seventh intercostal space. The chest is insufflated to 8 cm of water pressure with a low flow rate to prevent hypotension. A 12-mm port is placed approximately 1 cm posterior to the posterior axillary line at the level of the major fissure to be used for the robotic camera. This is typically in the same interspace as the first port. An 8-mm robotic port is placed one hand breadth posterior to the camera port in the same intercostal space. A 5-mm robotic port is placed one intercostal space caudally, just lateral to the transverse process. A 12-mm assistant port is placed in the tenth intercostal space, just above the insertion of the diaphragm. The initial 5-mm port is then replaced with an 8-mm robotic port (Fig. 2.4). The robot should be docked over the patient's right shoulder and parallel with the table (Fig. 2.5).

We begin with a 30°, down-viewing camera. With the aid of insufflation, additional retraction on the diaphragm is rarely necessary. The inferior pulmonary ligament is divided and any lymph nodes at that station should be removed. A thoracic grasper placed through the 5-mm

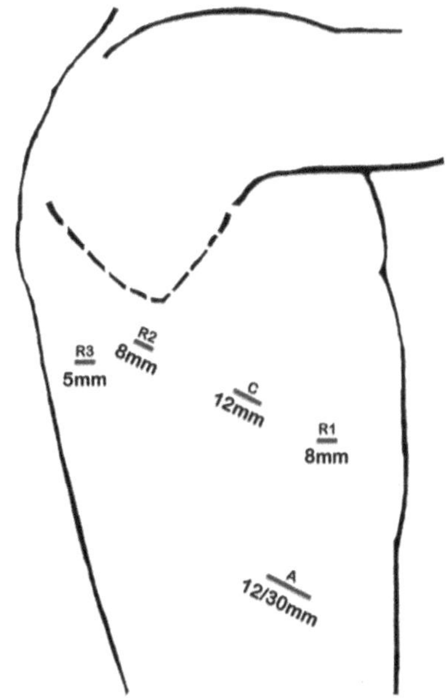


**Fig. 2.4** Trocar placement for robotic and thoracoscopic dissection and anastomosis

posterior port is used to retract the lung anteriorly, exposing the esophagus. We then divide the azygos vein with a vascular stapler cartridge. The mediastinal pleura overlying the esophagus is then opened anteriorly and posteriorly, allowing a layer of mediastinal pleura to stay attached to the esophagus.

The esophagus is mobilized circumferentially, using the Harmonic Scalpel (Ethicon) or Vessel Sealer (Intuitive) to ligate small perforating vessels from the aorta. This maneuver is typically done using the energy device in the right hand and a Cadiere forceps (Intuitive) in the left hand. A penrose drain is placed around the esophagus. The borders of dissection are the pericardium anteriorly, the aorta and spine posteriorly, and the edges of the mediastinal pleura laterally. All tissues within these borders should be mobilized and removed en bloc with the esophagus.

The network of lymphatics overlying the aorta should be removed en bloc as well. Using the Cadiere forceps (Intuitive) to grasp the penrose drain and provide traction on the esophagus greatly facilitates this part of the dissection (Fig. 2.6). For our standard Ivor Lewis operation,

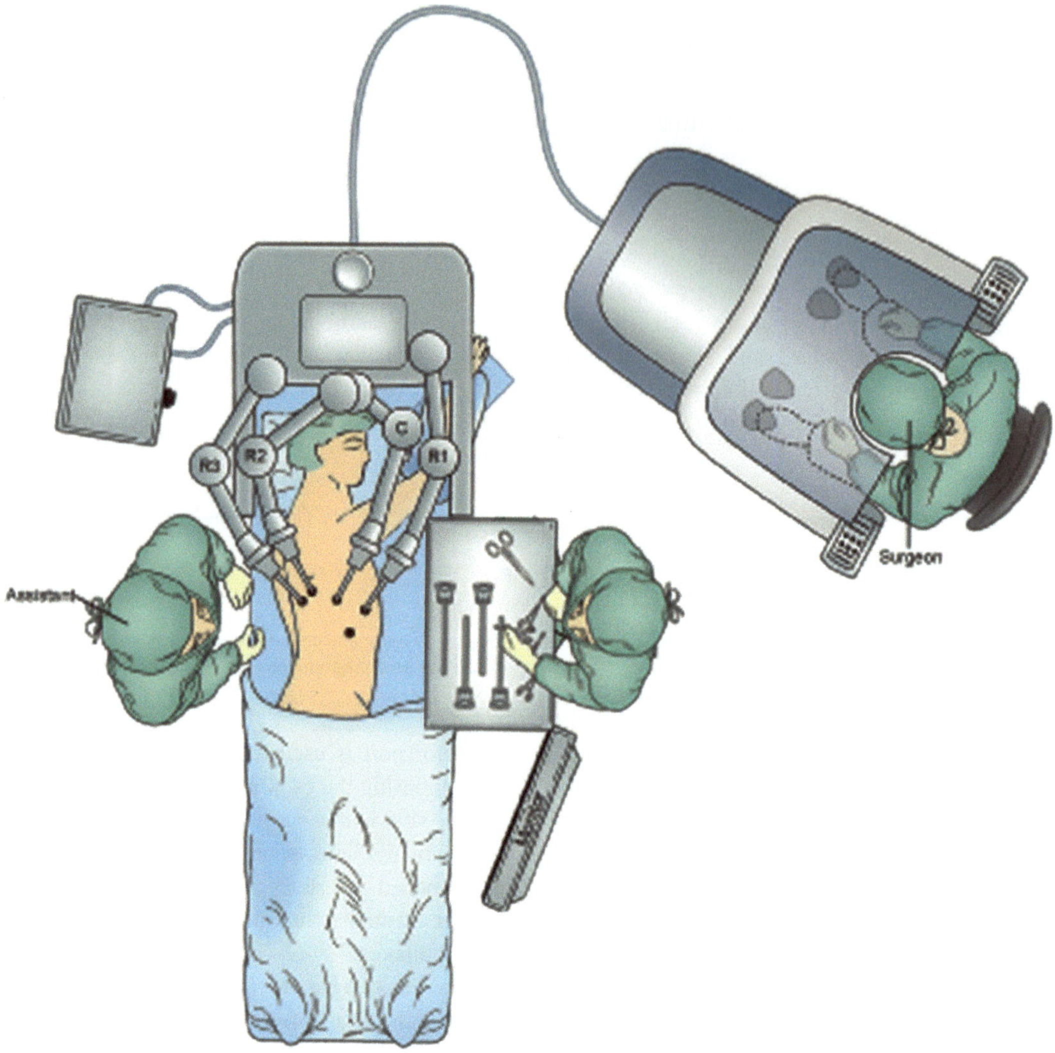


**Fig. 2.5** Operative positioning for robotic dissection and esophagogastric anastomosis

the esophagus is mobilized from just above the azygous vein to the diaphragmatic hiatus. Above the level of the aortic arch, use of electrocautery should be minimized, as the left recurrent laryngeal nerve is at risk for injury.

The subcarinal lymph node station should be completely excised. To facilitate exposure, we typically divide the bronchial branches of the vagus nerve and the main bronchial artery to the right mainstem bronchus. The thoracic duct is easily ligated using the robot to ligate all the tissue between the azygos vein and the aorta at the level of the diaphragmatic hiatus using a 0-silk tie.

## Anastomosis

After the mobilization is complete, the gastric conduit is gently pulled into the chest along with the omental flap. The esophagus is divided sharply at the level of the azygos vein. If the conduit has not yet been divided completely, it is done so at this point. Otherwise, the suture attaching the conduit to the proximal stomach and specimen is cut. The assistant port is enlarged to accommodate the specimen and an extra-small wound protector is placed. Frozen section is obtained on the proximal and distal margins. The proximal esophagus is sized using a Foley

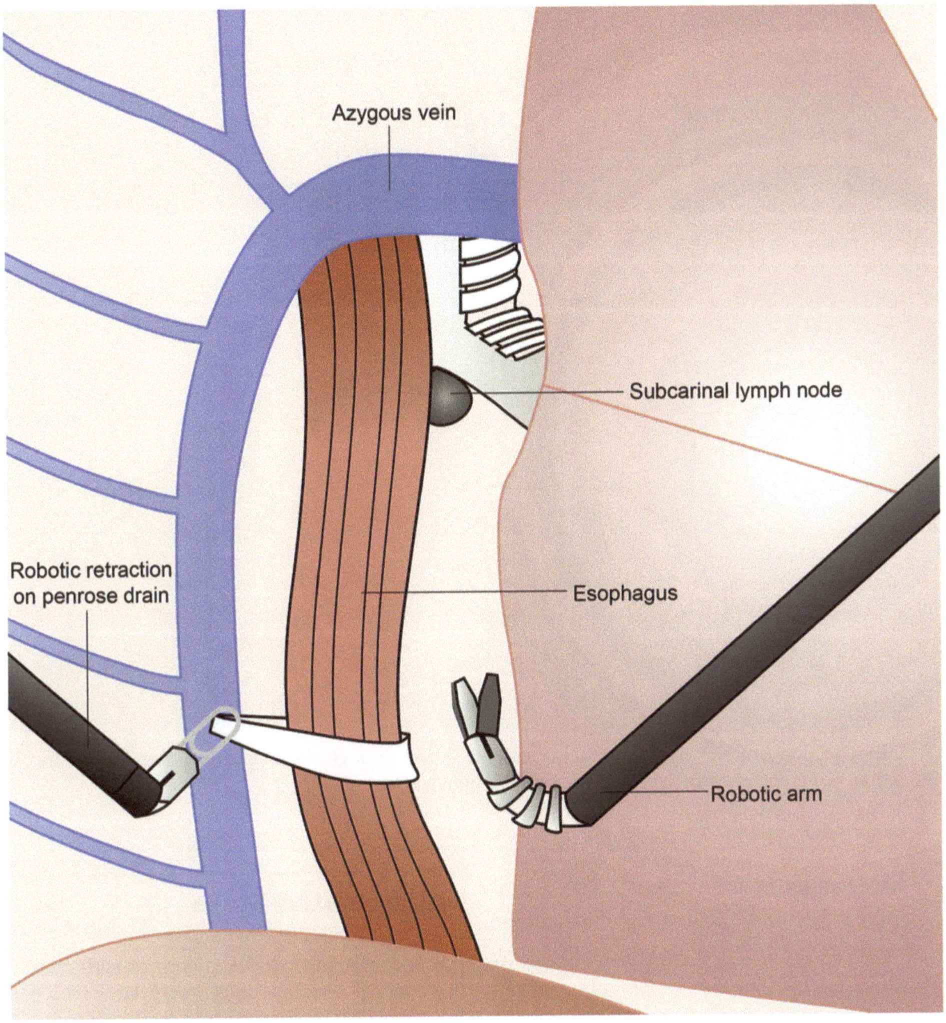


**Fig. 2.6** Operative diagram showing lateral retraction of a penrose drain encircling the esophagus

catheter balloon to gauge the appropriate sized stapler. The anvil of a circular stapler is placed through the assistant port/utility incision and then placed in the proximal esophagus. Using a needle holder in the right robotic arm, a double purse-string 2-0 absorbable suture is placed around the anvil. A zero degree camera usually provides a better image for this portion of the operation. After confirming the absence of cancer at the margins, the robot is undocked.

The remainder of the operation is carried out thoracoscopically using a 5-mm 30° camera placed through the anterior port. A gastrotomy is made in the proximal conduit by opening up the lesser curve staple line. The stapler is placed through the gastrotomy and the spike is brought out in a well-perfused portion of the greater curve (Fig. 2.7). The anastomosis should be made at the lowest point possible on the greater curve that will not create tension. Making the anastomosis too high on the conduit can create a redundant conduit within the chest, allowing the conduit to take on a sigmoid shape above the diaphragm and impeding conduit emptying. After firing the stapler, the donuts are inspected for completeness. The NGT is advanced beyond the anastomosis. A linear stapler is then used to close the gastrotomy and remove the excess portion of conduit

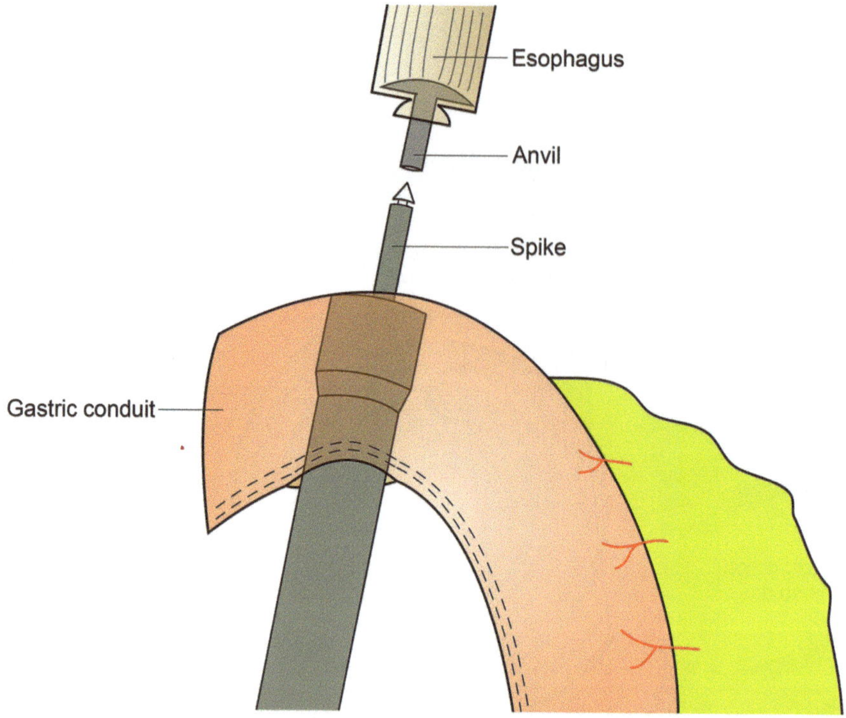


**Fig. 2.7** Operative diagram showing a circular stapler inserted through the staple line into the gastric conduit. The spike is attached to the anvil in the distal end of the esophagus

that lies proximal to the anastomosis. The omental flap is placed between the anastomosis and the posterior wall of the trachea and secured to the pleura with sutures.

## Closure

A 24-french chest tube and 19-french blake drain are placed in the posterior mediastinum. Local anesthetic is infiltrated into the intercostal spaces. The lung is reinflated and the remaining port sites are closed with absorbable sutures.

## Suggested Reading

Sarkaria IS, Rizk NP. Robotic-assisted minimally invasive esophagectomy: the Ivor Lewis approach. Thorac Surg Clin. 2014;24(2):211–22. doi:10.1016/j.thorsurg.2014.02.010. vii.

## Key Operative Steps

1. Esophagogastroduodenoscopy is performed prior to surgical resection. Inject the pylorus with botulinum toxin (200 units) and perform dilatation.
2. Ports are placed for laparoscopic mobilization of the stomach.
3. Dissection is started at the hiatus with exposure of the right and then left crus.
4. The right gastroepiploic artery is identified and the stomach is separated from the omentum and transverse mesocolon.
5. Harvest an omental flap by leaving a pedicled portion of the omentum perfused by 2–3 branches of the right gastroepiploic artery.
6. Divide the short gastric arteries.
7. Lift the stomach in the air to expose the left gastric artery. Sweep the lymphatic tissues towards the specimen. Divide the left gastric pedicle with an endo-vascular stapler.
8. Dissect the posterior gastroesophageal junction.
9. Pull the nasogastric tube back into the pharynx. Divide the stomach in between the right and left gastric arteries on the lesser curvature of the stomach just

proximal to the incisura. Create a gastric conduit at least 4 cm in width up to the fundus.
10. Place a feeding jejunostomy catheter.
11. Position the patient for the chest portion of the operation.
12. Divide the inferior pulmonary ligament and remove lymph nodes at that station.
13. Retract the lung and divide the azygos vein with a vascular stapler.
14. Open the mediastinal pleura overlying the esophagus (anteriorly and posteriorly).
15. Mobilize the esophagus circumferentially and ligate small perforating vessels.
16. Encircle the esophagus with a penrose drain for retraction.
17. Resect the network of lymphatics overlying the aorta.
18. Excise the lymphatic tissues in the subcarinal lymph node station. Divide the bronchial branches of the vagus nerve and the main bronchial artery to the right mainstem bronchus.
19. Ligate the thoracic duct.
20. Pull the gastric conduit into the chest and divide the esophagus at the level of the azygos vein.
21. Create an esophagogastrostomy with a circular stapler.
22. Place a chest tube and blake drain in the posterior mediastinum.

# 3 Open Technique for Transhiatal Esophagectomy

John C. Keech and Mark D. Iannettoni

## Historical Perspective

The first report of trans-mediastinal esophagectomy in 1913 came from Denk, who performed the procedure on cadavers and animals [1]. It was not until 1933 that the first successful transhiatal esophagectomy was performed by Turner, who reestablished gastrointestinal continuity by creating an ante-thoracic skin tube during a second operation [2]. Following the adoption of endotracheal anesthesia, transthoracic esophagectomy essentially replaced transhiatal esophagectomy except during concomitant pharyngectomy where the stomach was used for gastrointestinal continuity. Orringer and colleagues adopted a three-field esophagectomy approach in the 1970s through laparotomy, thoracotomy, and neck incision with the anastomosis performed in the neck. Their initial experience demonstrated a significant reduction in death from anastomotic leak. Orringer performed his first transhiatal esophagectomy without thoracotomy in 1974, utilizing blunt dissection of the esophagus and positioning the gastric conduit in the resected esophageal bed with the anastomosis in the neck. In 1978 Orringer reported his initial experience with this approach in 28 patients after which several reports from other authors followed; and some were not supportive [3]. The first meta-analysis of this technique was reported in 1994 by Katariya and colleagues, who observed 30-day mortality of 7.1 %, recurrent laryngeal nerve injury of 11.3 %, and anastomotic leak rate of 15.1 % [4]. In 1997 Ghandi and Naunheim published another meta-analysis of 1,192 patients, reporting a mortality rate of 6.7 %, recurrent laryngeal nerve injury rate of 9 %, and anastomotic leak rate of 12 % [5]. In 1999 Orringer and colleagues reported their 22-year experience on 1085 transhiatal esophagectomies at the University of Michigan [6]. Only 15 (5 %) patients required conversion to a thoracotomy, 3 % required splenectomy due to intraoperative injury; and there were 3 intraoperative deaths due to hemorrhage. Recurrent laryngeal nerve injury occurred in 7 % of patients and resolved spontaneously in 66 %; chylothorax occurred in <1 % of patients; the anastomotic leak rate was 13 %; gastric conduit necrosis occurred in 0.8 % of patients; and in-hospital mortality rate was 4 %. Later in 2007 Orringer and colleagues reported their updated experience [7]. The transhiatal approach was possible in 98 % of patients where the stomach was used as the conduit. Their more recent cohort of 944 patients from 1998 to 2006 was compared to their own cohort from 1976 to

J.C. Keech, M.D.
Department of Cardiothoracic Surgery, University of Iowa Hospitals and Clinics, Iowa City, IA, USA

M.D. Iannettoni, M.D., M.B.A. (✉)
Department of Cardiovascular Sciences, East Carolina Heart Institute, Brody School of Medicine at East Carolina University, 115 Heart Drive, Greenville, NC 27834, USA
e-mail: iannettonim14@ecu.edu

J. Kim and J. Garcia-Aguilar (eds.), *Surgery for Cancers of the Gastrointestinal Tract: A Step-by-Step Approach*, DOI 10.1007/978-1-4939-1893-5_3, 

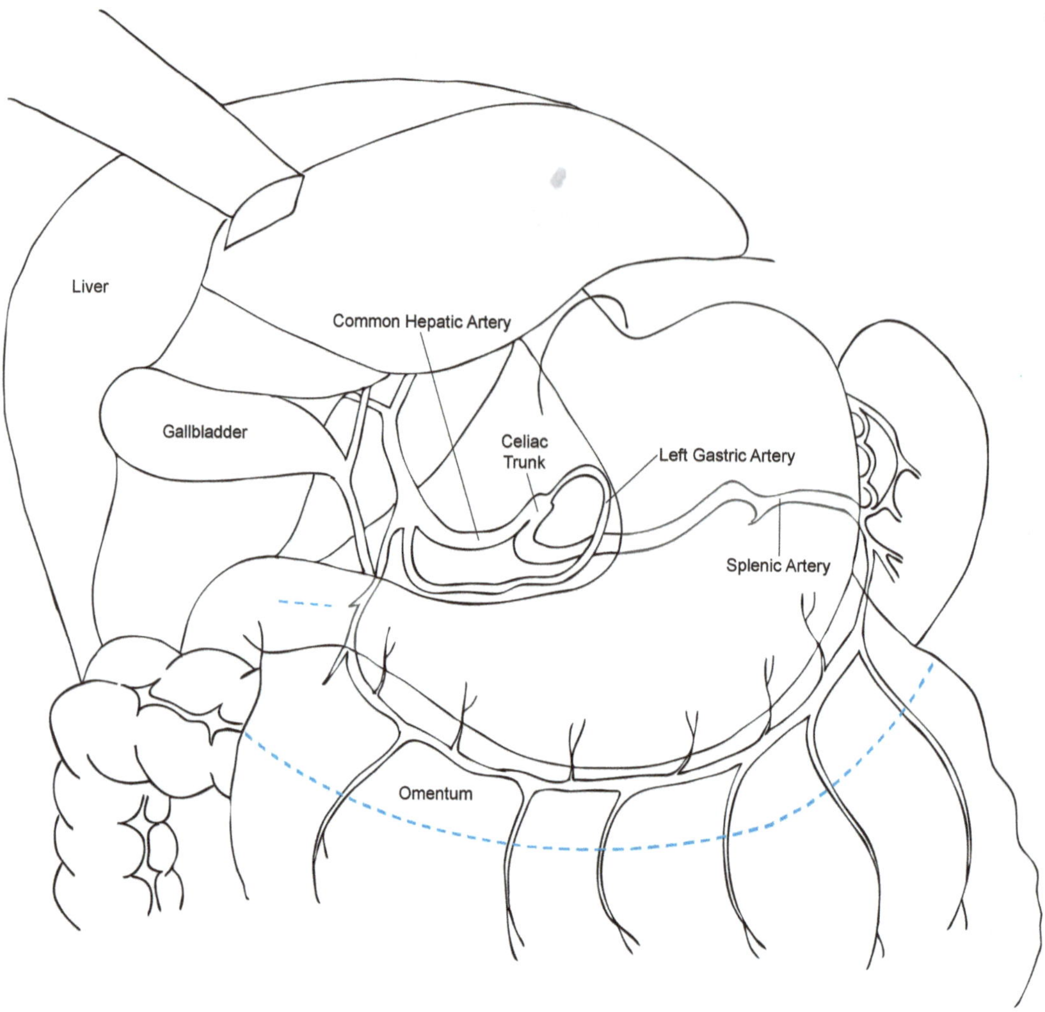


**Fig. 3.1** Gastric blood supply and preparation of the stomach for resection and gastric conduit creation

1998; and they observed that their in-hospital mortality rate decreased from 4 to 1 % and the anastomotic leak rate decreased from 14 to 9 % in the more recent time period.

## Anatomic Highlights

The blood supply of the mobilized stomach is based on the right gastric and right gastroepiploic vascular pedicles after division or ligation of the left gastric artery, the short gastric arteries, and the left gastroepiploic artery (Fig. 3.1). A gastric emptying procedure, such as a standard pyloromyotomy, should be performed and this should generally be accompanied by a Kocher maneuver to allow the pylorus to reach the level of the xiphoid. The mediastinal dissection is performed as much as possible under direct visualization with the blunt dissection completed with the volar aspect of the hand toward the esophagus. During the cervical portion of the operation, rigid retractors should be avoided on the trachea and tracheo-esophageal groove to minimize injury to the recurrent laryngeal nerve. The gastric resection should leave a gastric tube approximately 4–5 cm wide, and this is typically started at the second vascular arcade from the cardia on the lesser curvature of the stomach. Proper orientation of the stomach in the mediastinum is essential with the gastric staple line facing the patient's right, which can be confirmed visually and by palpation of the anterior stomach to avoid malrotation. The cervical anastomosis is performed with the esophagus anterior to the stomach and uses a linear stapler to create the anastomosis. The esophagus must overly the stomach by at least 3 cm.

## Indications for Transhiatal Esophagectomy

Indications for transhiatal esophagectomy have been previously reported by Orringer et al. [7]. Esophagectomy may be performed for benign disease, including Barrett's mucosa with high-grade dysplasia, achalasia, reflux stricture, recurrent hiatal hernia, recurrent gastroesophageal reflux, spasm/dysmotility, acute perforation, and caustic stricture. Esophagectomy for carcinoma may also be performed for any histology and also for disease at any level of the esophagus.

## Preoperative Details

The patient is instructed to perform aggressive outpatient pulmonary physiotherapy with an incentive spirometer and daily exercise. Smoking must be stopped at least 2 weeks before surgery. In patients with documented or suspected chronic pulmonary disease we obtain formal pulmonary function testing and arterial blood gas measurements. When adequate oral intake is not possible, a nasogastric feeding tube is placed and outpatient enteral nutrition is administered. If the stomach may not be a suitable conduit then a barium enema is performed to evaluate the colon as a potential conduit, and standard bowel prep is administered for possible colon interposition. In patients receiving neoadjuvant chemotherapy and radiation, we schedule the operation 4 weeks after the last treatment, but any time between 3 and 5 weeks after completion of neoadjuvant therapy is reasonable. The development of severe and possibly prohibitive radiation fibrosis occurs as early as 6 weeks post-radiation treatment.

## Surgical Technique

### Patient Positioning

The patient is positioned supine with arms tucked and padded at the sides and a shoulder roll under the scapula to extend the neck. If the patient had a feeding gastrostomy or jejunostomy tube placed preoperatively, this is removed and the skin is sutured closed. The head is turned to the patient's right and the entire neck, chest, and abdomen are prepped from the mandible to the symphysis pubis (Fig. 3.2).

### Mobilization of the Gastric Conduit

The abdominal portion of the operation is started first through a supra-umbilical laparotomy. The triangular ligament of the liver is taken down and an assessment of the abdominal cavity is performed to rule out metastatic disease and to ascertain the suitability of the stomach as a conduit. The right gastroepiploic vessels are identified and protected and the lesser sac is entered through an avascular portion of the greater omentum. The short gastric vessels high up on the greater curvature are divided close to the stomach (Fig. 3.1). The omentum is separated from the right gastroepiploic artery with a 1.5 cm distance away from the vessel to the level of the pylorus. The peritoneum over the esophageal hiatus is divided and the esophagus and its overlying fat pad are dissected free from the hiatus. The gastrohepatic omentum is divided and the left gastric vessels are isolated and divided, which can be accomplished by suture ligation or vascular staplers (Fig. 3.1). If an aberrant left hepatic artery is encountered in the gastrohepatic omentum, efforts should be made to preserve this vessel if possible. Gastrohepatic and left gastric artery lymph nodes should be included with the gastric specimen. Separate celiac axis lymph nodes should be sent in the setting of cancer resection. It is not typically necessary to divide the right gastric vessels and attempts should be made to preserve them.

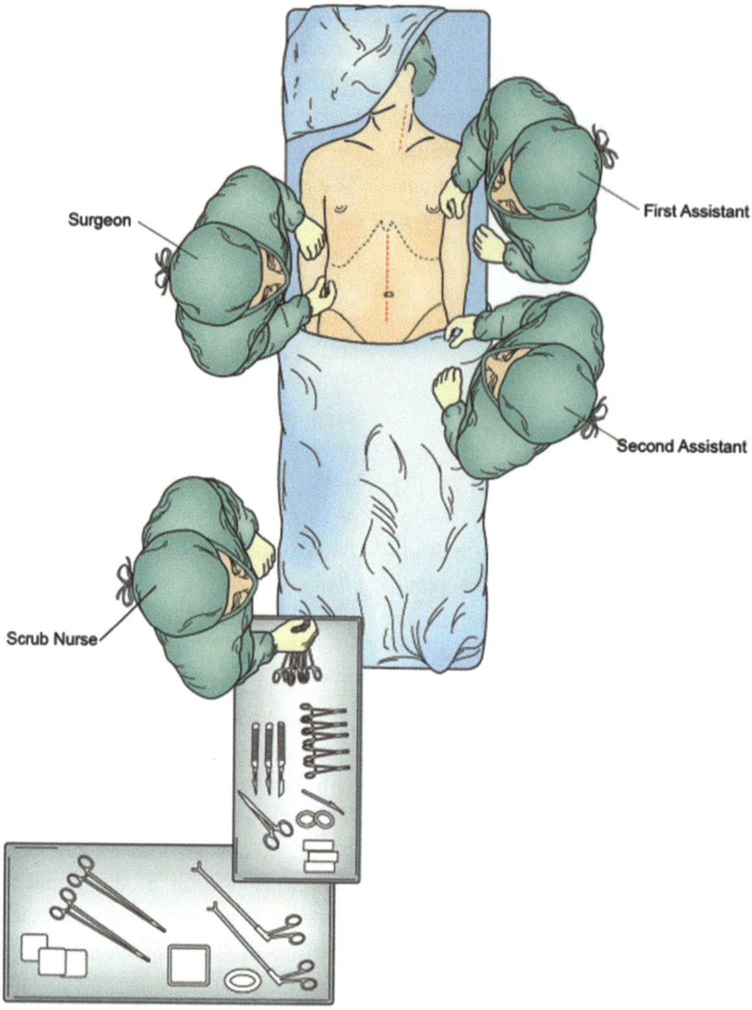


**Fig. 3.2** Patient positioning and operating room setup

## Drainage Procedure

A Kocher maneuver is performed to allow the pylorus to reach approximately the level of the xiphoid process. Occasionally, the pylorus can reach the xiphoid process without a Kocher maneuver. A gastric emptying procedure is then performed, classically a pyloromyotomy beginning 1.5 cm on the gastric side and continuing for approximately 1 cm onto the duodenum. Needle-tip electrocautery is particularly useful for this maneuver with care taken to avoid tears in the mucosa. Mucosal injuries should be repaired using 4-0 or smaller suture. Clips can be placed near the pylorus for future radiographic identification of the location of the pylorus during gastric emptying studies. Alternatively, several authors have reported excellent results using botulinum toxin injected into the pylorus instead of performing pyloromyotomy. However, long-term results and comparative results against other drainage techniques are not yet available for the botulinum toxin approach [8, 9].

## Initial Mediastinal Dissection

At the diaphragmatic hiatus, a narrow Deaver retractor is placed into the hiatus for additional exposure. The lymph nodes in the peri-esophageal fat around the distal esophagus are dissected towards the esophagus to be included with the specimen. Entry into one or both pleural spaces frequently occurs during this step. We routinely place bilateral chest tubes at the beginning of surgery due to the potential for unrecognized entry into the pleural spaces and subsequent development of symptomatic pleural effusions. Aorto-esophageal branches are divided by clamping and dividing or by using an energy sealant device. This maneuver is performed under direct visualization and is facilitated by encircling the distal esophagus with a penrose drain to retract the gastroesophageal junction into the abdomen. The distal half of the esophagus can often be dissected free from the surrounding tissues under direct visualization to the level of the carina using the above techniques and varying sizes of Deaver retractors. In the setting of carcinoma, the mobility of the esophagus is assessed by grasping the tumor and a gentle rocking motion to determine whether the esophagus is fixed to the prevertebral fascia, aorta, pericardium, or trachea/bronchi. Fixation to any of these structures would preclude safe transhiatal resection. A 14-French flexible jejunostomy tube can be inserted at this point, approximately 15 cm distal to the ligament of Treitz and secured with purse-string sutures and a Witzel maneuver. We typically do not bring the jejunostomy tube through the abdominal wall until the completion of the esophagectomy.

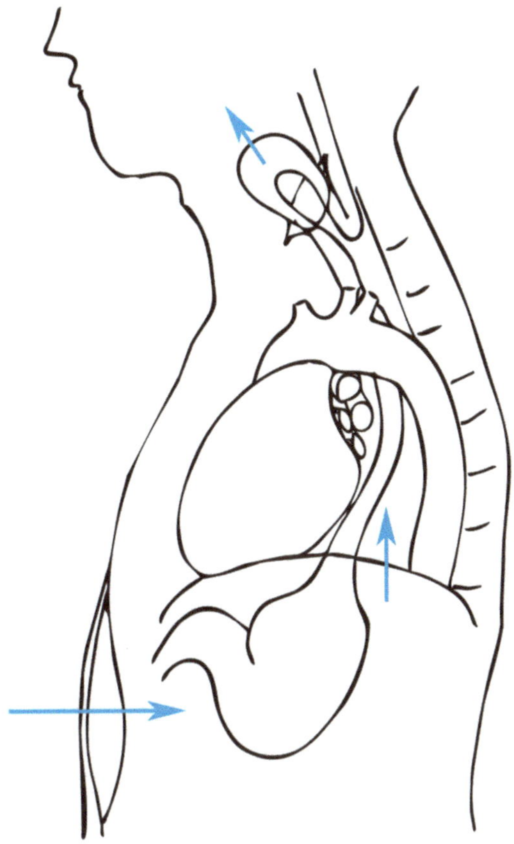

**Fig. 3.3** Posterior mediastinal and posterior esophageal mobilization through the abdominal and cervical neck incisions

## Cervical Mobilization

In the absence of mediastinal fixation, the cervical portion of the operation proceeds next. An oblique cervical neck incision is then made parallel to the anterior border of the sternocleidomastoid muscle, typically 6–7 cm from the suprasternal notch to the level of the cricoid cartilage. The platysma muscle is divided and the sternocleidomastoid muscle is retracted laterally with the contents of the carotid sheath. The trachea is carefully retracted medially without the use of retractors to avoid injury to the recurrent laryngeal nerve in the tracheo-esophageal groove. Frequently, the middle thyroid vein and the inferior thyroid artery need to be divided for better exposure. If adequate neck extension is not possible and adequate cervical esophagus is not accessible, then a partial upper sternal split may be necessary for additional exposure to access the retrosternal esophagus [10]. The esophagus is bluntly mobilized off the prevertebral fascia posteriorly and circumferentially dissected free from the surrounding soft tissues using blunt and sharp dissection, avoiding injury to the recurrent laryngeal nerve. The cervical esophagus is elevated out of the mediastinum and encircled with a penrose drain. With superior retraction the upper thoracic esophagus is bluntly dissected free from the superior mediastinum (Fig. 3.3). The esophagus can usually be mobilized to the level of the carina with this approach avoiding injury to the membranous wall of the trachea.

## Detailed Mediastinal and Cervical Dissection

One hand is placed into the abdominal cavity and through the hiatus posterior to the esophagus along the right aspect of the spine to avoid aortic injury while a sponge-on-a-stick is inserted into the cervical incision posterior to the esophagus in the prevertebral plane. The posterior esophagus is bluntly dissected away from the prevertebral fascia until the hand is able to palpate the sponge stick (Fig. 3.3). It is critical to note intra-arterial blood pressure monitoring during this phase of the dissection, since hypotension is likely to occur to some degree, often necessitating removal of the hand and sponge stick from the mediastinum temporarily. At this point, a sump drain is placed into the posterior mediastinum to assess bleeding and it is left in place for the duration of the dissection. With inferior retraction of the gastroesophageal junction, the surgeon's hand is then placed palm down on the anterior surface of the esophagus and the esophagus is dissected free from the posterior pericardium and carina. With simultaneous gentle blunt finger dissection through the cervical incision along the anterior border of the esophagus, the esophagus is completely freed from all anterior and posterior mediastinal attachments. Similar attention must be paid to systemic blood pressure during this dissection. Any remaining lateral esophageal attachments can be bluntly divided as the esophagus is elevated out of the neck incision. After this maneuver, any remaining lower esophageal attachments can be divided bluntly by inserting a hand anterior to the esophagus and placing the index and middle finger on either side of the esophagus and gently pulling these fingers inferiorly along the esophagus. Dense adhesions may need to be managed with blunt finger fracture techniques, however in most cases these can be brought down from the mediastinum for division under direct visualization. Alternatively, the adhesions can be managed by dividing the cervical esophagus and removing the esophagus and adhesions in retrograde fashion.

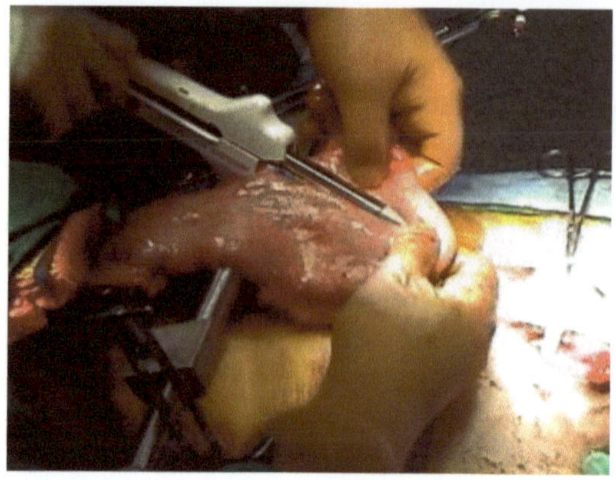

**Fig. 3.4** Gastric tube creation by placing the stomach on the anterior chest wall and creating a 4–5 cm wide gastric tube using several firings of the GIA stapler. This is begun at approximately the second vascular arcade on the lesser curve

## Esophageal and Gastric Transection and Esophagogastric Anastomosis

After circumferential mobilization of the entire intrathoracic esophagus, 8–10 cm of esophagus is delivered into the neck wound, the nasogastric tube is removed, and the esophagus divided using a linear stapler in an anterior-posterior orientation. There should be a slight oblique angle to the stapler with the tip slightly more distal than the heel. After division of the esophagus, the stomach and lower esophagus are withdrawn through the hiatus and placed on the anterior chest. A Deaver or Harrington retractor is then placed into the hiatus to inspect for mediastinal hemorrhage and entry into the pleural spaces. Bleeding vessels can be individually ligated or controlled with an energy sealant device. A laparotomy sponge is packed into the mediastinum through the hiatus at this point to help control minor bleeding.

The stomach is positioned with the fundus directed cephalad. The peri-gastric fat and vessels along the lesser curve at the second vascular arcade from the cardia are divided. This marks the starting point of the gastric resection using a linear stapler. The gastric conduit should be approximately 4–5 cm wide, which typically corresponds to a gastric resection line 4–6 cm away from the gastroesophageal junction (Fig. 3.4). Following completion of the partial

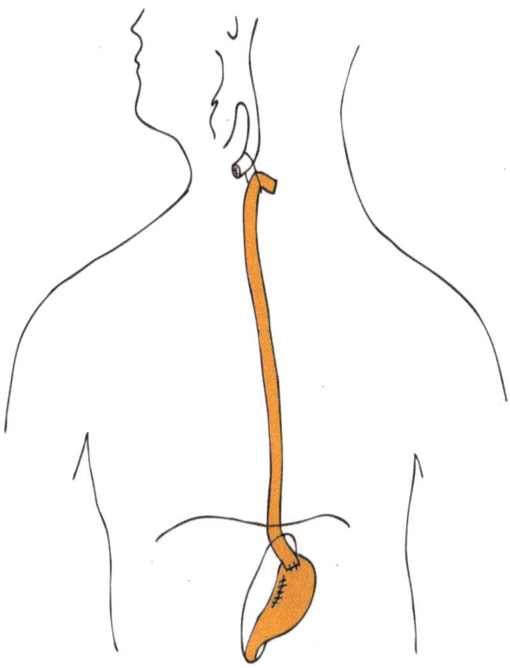

**Fig. 3.5** Preparation for conduit delivery into the mediastinum using a 1-in. penrose drain sutured to the anterior wall of the gastric fundus

gastrectomy, the specimen is removed from the field and the gastric staple line is oversewn with a running 4-0 Lembert suture. The purpose of this suture is twofold: (1) to prevent staple ingrowth into surrounding structures such as the aorta or trachea and (2) to control risk of leak from the gastric staple line.

The mediastinal sponges are removed and hemostasis is ensured. The most cephalad point of the greater curve is identified and a 1-in. penrose drain is sutured to the anterior fundus and gently pushed into the mediastinum through the hiatus until it can be palpated by fingers placed into superior mediastinum (Fig. 3.5). The fundus can be gently grasped with a Babcock clamp or gently pulled with fingers while a hand in the hiatus simultaneously pushes the stomach cephalad. Proper orientation of the stomach is essential during this maneuver, and the oversewn staple line should be facing the patient's right side. Palpation of the anterior surface of the stomach can also aid in determining proper orientation of the stomach. When the posterior mediastinal space is unsuitable for conduit placement, possibly from radiation or chronic inflammatory changes, the substernal route may be needed for placement of the stomach. This should be entertained when the posterior mediastinum does not easily allow passage of the surgeon's hand and forearm. With substernal conduit placement, the medial clavicle and sternoclavicular joint are typically resected to allow room for passage of the conduit. Alternatively a partial resection of the manubrium, with preservation of the sternoclavicular joint, may allow enough space for the conduit. Regardless of where the conduit lies, the visible portion of the gastric tip should appear pink and viable.

The diaphragmatic hiatus should be closed with interrupted 0 silk or larger sutures allowing 3 fingers to be placed alongside the stomach. The anterior stomach is secured to the hiatus with 3-0 silk sutures to prevent herniation of abdominal contents. The pyloromyotomy is covered with available omentum and the left lobe of the liver is repositioned. A left upper quadrant stab incision is made to allow the previously placed jejunostomy tube to be brought out through the abdominal wall, and the jejunum is fixed to the abdominal wall with several interrupted 4-0 silk sutures. The laparotomy is closed and covered with a sterile towel.

The cervical esophagogastric anastomosis is performed in a stapled side-to-side manner as described by Orringer et al. [11]. This method has been shown to reduce the rate of anastomotic leak over the hand-sewn anastomosis. The end of the divided esophagus is grasped with an Allis clamp and elevated out of the wound towards the head, and approximately 4–5 cm of the gastric fundus should be visible above the clavicles. The surgeon determines the point on the stomach where the esophagus will easily reach; and then makes a 1.5 cm vertical gastrotomy ensuring that the incision is low enough on the stomach to allow insertion of the 3 cm stapler. The esophageal staple line is now removed obliquely, allowing a longer anterior tip compared to the posterior corner. A stay suture is placed through the posterior corner of the esophagus to the superior aspect of the gastrotomy, and another stay suture

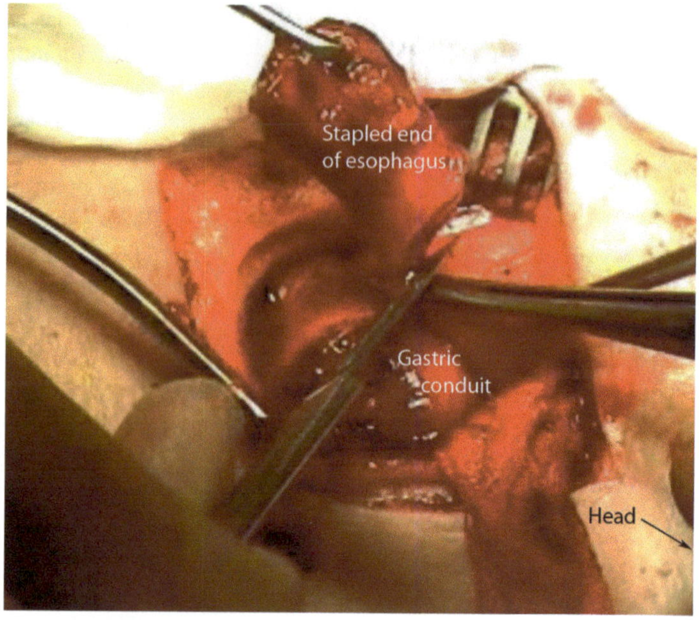


**Fig. 3.6** Preparation of cervical esophagus and stomach for cervical anastomosis by removing the staple line on the divided cervical esophagus, as shown here, and placing stay sutures in the anterior and posterior esophagus

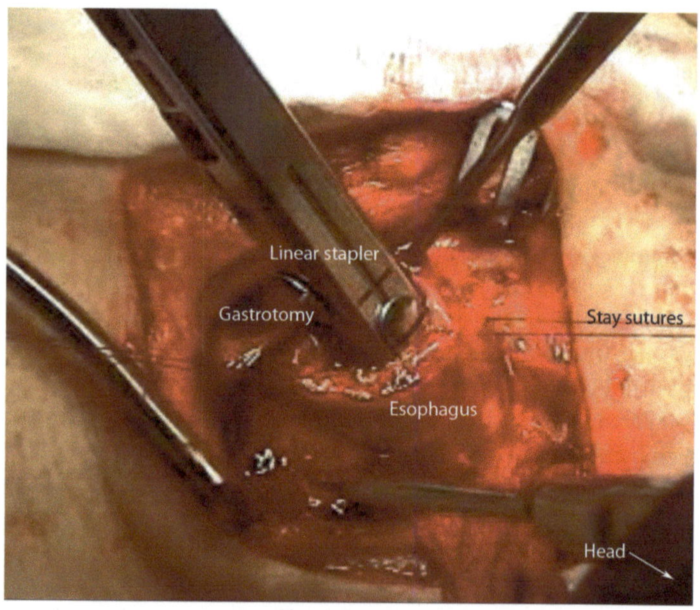


**Fig. 3.7** The cervical anastomosis is created using a 3.5 by 30 mm GIA stapler placed into the esophagus and gastrotomy

is placed in the anterior esophagus (Fig. 3.6). A linear stapler is inserted into the esophagus and stomach and advanced for its full length, aligning the midpoint of the esophagus with the anterior wall of the stomach. The stapler jaws are closed, but before firing the stapler, two 4-0 vicryl sutures are placed on either side of the anastomosis connecting the esophagus and stomach (Fig. 3.7). Then the stapler is fired. The anesthesia team carefully advances a 16-French nasogastric tube and under direct visualization the surgeon guides the tube into the stomach. The anastomosis is closed in two layers: the first layer is a full-thickness running layer of 4-0 absorbable suture (Fig. 3.8) and the second layer is an interrupted layer of 4-0 absorbable suture from the anterior

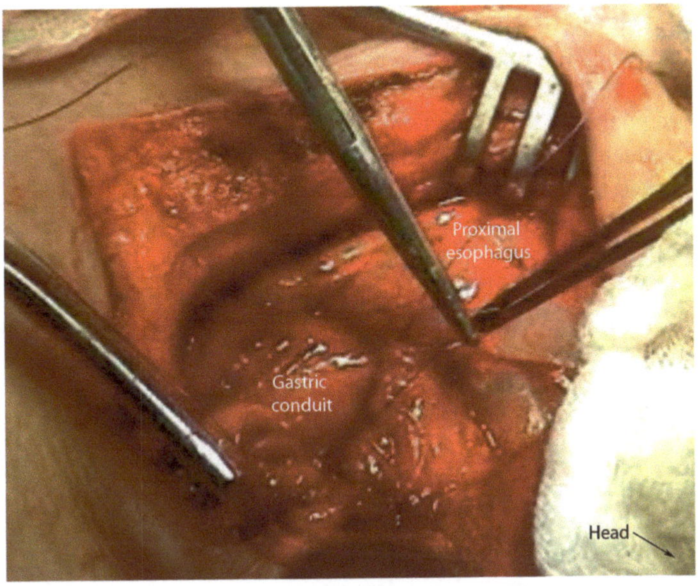


**Fig. 3.8** Completion of anastomosis involves a 2-layer hand-sewn closure following removal of the stapler. The first layer is a running layer of 4-0 absorbable suture as shown here

esophagus to the adjacent stomach. A 1/2-in. penrose drain is split so that either side of the drain can be placed near the anastomosis and brought out the lower portion of the incision and the wound closed in layers with absorbable suture.

## Postoperative Care

The patient is extubated in the operating room and does not typically require intensive care unit monitoring. Ambulation is begun on postoperative day (POD) #1 and aggressive pulmonary toilet is started immediately, which can be enhanced by the use of epidural anesthesia. Tube feedings are started on POD #3, as ileus does not typically last beyond 72 h. Tube feedings are advanced to their goal rate by POD #5, at which time the nasogastric tube is removed and a barium swallow is performed. Once the anastomosis has been confirmed to be intact, the penrose drain and chest tubes are removed. The patient is discharged home typically on POD #5. The patients remain *nil per os* (NPO) at the time of discharge until POD #15, at which time oral intake is begun. The jejunostomy tube is used until satisfactory oral intake is maintained and then is removed, typically by 4 weeks postoperatively. We have reported on our experience standardizing the phases of care during and after esophagectomy using a continuous process improvement methodology. This has resulted in a 43 % reduction in cost per case, length of stay reduction from 14 to 5 days, and a leak rate of less than 3 % [12].

## Complications

Tracheal tears are usually recognized by a rush of air during mediastinal dissection and typically occur in the membranous trachea but can also occur in the mainstem bronchi. When this complication is recognized, the endotracheal tube should be advanced with the aid of the surgeon's hand, beyond the level of the tear either into the distal trachea or left mainstem bronchus. Depending on the level of the tear, it can be repaired either through an upper sternal split (for mid to upper tracheal tears) or through a right thoracotomy for lower tracheal, carinal, or mainstem tears. If a thoracotomy is required, the abdomen should be closed first with 3–4 large 1-0 nylon sutures and covered with a sterile adhesive drape. The esophagectomy is completed through the thoracotomy and after repair of the airway, the abdomen is reopened and gastric conduit mobilization completed. It is important that the anesthesia team not shorten the endotracheal tube at the start of the operative case to accommodate this type of emergency.

Much of the esophageal mobilization is performed under direct visualization, often to the level of the carina, and major intraoperative bleeding is unusual. If fixation of the esophagus to the aorta or other mediastinal structures is identified, the transhiatal approach is not recommended and the transthoracic approach should be entertained to determine resectability. When major bleeding does occur, placement of a large bore catheter through the cervical incision may aid in evacuating blood while Deaver retractors in the hiatus facilitate exposure of the mediastinum. If hemostasis cannot be achieved, then the mediastinum is packed with laparotomy sponges and the abdomen rapidly closed and a thoracotomy is performed. If the bleeding is from the lower third of the esophagus, then a left thoracotomy may provide better exposure; otherwise, a right thoracotomy should be utilized.

Recurrent laryngeal nerve injury is a recognized complication of transhiatal esophagectomy and likely occurs during the cervical portion of the operation. Beyond a hoarse voice, this complication can result in dysphagia and aspiration with resulting pneumonia. The nerve is at risk for injury during retraction and dissection of the neck structures and is a preventable complication. Great care should be taken to avoid metal retractors placed on the trachea and instead, gentle finger retraction should be used.

Anastomotic leak should be suspected in anyone with a fever developing 48 h after surgery. It is confirmed either by observing leakage of swallowed liquid from the neck wound or by a barium contrast study. Once a leak is confirmed, then the neck wound should be immediately and entirely opened, which can usually be performed at the bedside. The wound is opened to the prevertebral fascia and packed with moist gauze, which is changed several times a day. Two to three days after opening the wound, the patient is asked to swallow water while observing the unpacked wound for drainage. This can provide an assessment of the size of the leak. We have also followed a practice of early and aggressive dilation once leak occurs which enhances wound healing and closure of the leak [13].

High or excessive chest tube output after esophagectomy can indicate injury to the thoracic duct or its branches. When chest tube output is more than 1,000 mL/day more than 48 h after surgery, this injury should be considered regardless of whether the output is milky. Administration of cream through the jejunostomy tube at a rate of 90 mL/h for 6 h is usually sufficient to turn serous thoracic duct output milky. It is typically not necessary to measure chylomicrons, triglycerides, or lymphocyte counts in the fluid to determine that a thoracic duct injury has occurred. Brief conservative management may be entertained with elemental jejunostomy tube feeds or total parenteral nutrition, but if significant and dramatic reductions in drainage have not occurred after several days, then operative repair is indicated [14]. Preoperative administration of cream may aid in the identification of the leak during thoracotomy for thoracic duct ligation. This repair can almost always be performed thoracoscopically and almost exclusively on the right side, regardless of the side of the leak.

## References


1. Denk W. Zur Radikaloperation des Osophaguskarfzentralbl. Chirurg. 1913;40:1065.
2. Turner GG. Excision of thoracic esophagus for carcinoma with construction of extrathoracic gullet. Lancet. 1933;2:1315.
3. Orringer MB, Sloan H. Esophagectomy without thoracotomy. J Thorac Cardiovasc Surg. 1978;76(5):643–54.
4. Katariya K, Harvey JC, Pina E, Beattie EJ. Complications of transhiatal esophagectomy. J Surg Oncol. 1994;57(3):157–63.
5. Gandhi SK, Naunheim KS. Complications of transhiatal esophagectomy. Chest Surg Clin N Am. 1997;7(3):601–10; discussion 11–2.
6. Orringer MB, Marshall B, Iannettoni MD. Transhiatal esophagectomy: clinical experience and refinements. Ann Surg. 1999;230(3):392–400; discussion 3.
7. Orringer MB, Marshall B, Chang AC, Lee J, Pickens A, Lau CL. Two thousand transhiatal esophagectomies: changing trends, lessons learned. Ann Surg. 2007;246(3):363–72. doi:10.1097/SLA.0b013e31814697f2; discussion 72–4.

8. Cerfolio RJ, Bryant AS, Canon CL, Dhawan R, Eloubeidi MA. Is botulinum toxin injection of the pylorus during Ivor Lewis [corrected] esophagogastrectomy the optimal drainage strategy? J Thorac Cardiovasc Surg. 2009;137(3):565–72. doi:10.1016/j.jtcvs.2008.08.049.
9. Martin JT, Federico JA, McKelvey AA, Kent MS, Fabian T. Prevention of delayed gastric emptying after esophagectomy: a single center's experience with botulinum toxin. Ann Thorac Surg. 2009;87(6):1708–13. doi:10.1016/j.athoracsur.2009.01.075; discussion 13–4.
10. Orringer MB. Partial median sternotomy: anterior approach to the upper thoracic esophagus. J Thorac Cardiovasc Surg. 1984;87(1):124–9.
11. Orringer MB, Marshall B, Iannettoni MD. Eliminating the cervical esophagogastric anastomotic leak with a side-to-side stapled anastomosis. J Thorac Cardiovasc Surg. 2000;119(2):277–88.
12. Iannettoni MD, Lynch WR, Parekh KR, McLaughlin KA. Kaizen method for esophagectomy patients: improved quality control, outcomes, and decreased costs. Ann Thorac Surg. 2011;91(4):1011–7. doi:10.1016/j.athoracsur.2011.01.001; discussion 7–8.
13. Orringer MB, Lemmer JH. Early dilation in the treatment of esophageal disruption. Ann Thorac Surg. 1986;42(5):536–9.
14. Orringer MB, Bluett M, Deeb GM. Aggressive treatment of chylothorax complicating transhiatal esophagectomy without thoracotomy. Surgery. 1988;104(4):720–6.

## Key Operative Steps

1. Begin the operation with supra-umbilical laparotomy and rule out metastatic disease.
2. Enter lesser sac through the avascular portion of the greater omentum.
3. Divide the short gastric vessels close to the stomach.
4. Separate the omentum 1.5 cm away from the right gastroepiploic artery to the level of the pylorus.
5. Divide the peritoneum over the esophageal hiatus and dissect the esophagus and its fat pad free from the hiatus.
6. Divide the gastrohepatic omentum and isolate and ligate the left gastric vessels.
7. Gastrohepatic, left gastric artery, and celiac axis lymph nodes should be included with the gastric specimen.
8. Preserve the right gastric artery.
9. Perform Kocher maneuver and pylorus drainage procedure.
10. Use Deaver retractor at hiatus for improved exposure.
11. Dissect lymph nodes around distal esophagus to be included with the specimen.
12. The pleural spaces may be entered. Bilateral chest tubes are usually necessary.
13. Divide aorto-esophageal branches. Encircling the distal esophagus with a penrose drain may facilitate this maneuver.
14. Place feeding jejunostomy tube.
15. Create oblique cervical neck incision.
16. Divide platysma and retract sternocleidomastoid and trachea. The middle thyroid vein and inferior thyroid artery may need to be divided.
17. Mobilize the esophagus off the prevertebral fascia posteriorly and dissect free from the soft tissues using blunt and sharp dissection. Avoid injury to the recurrent laryngeal nerve.
18. Elevate the cervical esophagus out of the mediastinum with a penrose drain and bluntly dissect the upper thoracic esophagus to the level of the carina.
19. Place hand up through the hiatus to the right of the spine. Place sponge stick in neck posterior to the esophagus and bluntly dissect until hand in abdomen is reached.
20. Dissect esophagus free from posterior pericardium and carina. Free remaining attachments.
21. Divide esophagus in neck with linear stapler.
22. Create gastric conduit that is 4–5 cm wide and oversew gastric staple line.
23. Advance gastric conduit through the hiatus up to the neck.
24. Close the diaphragmatic hiatus allowing 3 fingers to pass alongside the gastric conduit and secure the conduit to the hiatus with sutures.
25. Perform cervical esophagogastric anastomosis.

# Open Radical En Bloc Esophagectomy

4

Paul C. Lee and Nasser K. Altorki

## Introduction

The prognosis of esophageal cancer remains poor despite improvements in perioperative care, surgical techniques, and neoadjuvant therapy over the last decade, and more than 95 % of patients will succumb to their disease in the US. Among the patients resected with curative intent by transthoracic esophagectomy or transhiatal esophagectomy, the 5-year survival of patients rarely exceeds 30 % [1–4]. The majority of the patients develop metastatic disease, suggesting that the disease may already have disseminated at the time of diagnosis. While undoubtedly this is the case in most patients, an analysis of the patterns of failure after surgical resection also suggests inadequate loco-regional control. The locoregional failure rates are unacceptably high after conventional surgical resection, ranging from 30 to 60 % [5–8]. Interestingly, the addition of preoperative therapy of any kind does not have any significant impact on this high local failure rate. It is reasonable to postulate that a successful strategy in maximizing loco-regional control may translate into meaningful improvement in the survival of patients with esophageal cancer.

Logan in 1963 first described en bloc resection for tumors of the lower esophagus and cardia [9]. The reported 5-year survival was unparalleled at the time; however, it was achieved at the cost of high operative mortality. In 1983, Skinner reported extension of the en bloc approach to tumors of the middle and proximal esophagus [10]. A few years earlier in 1978, Orringer and Sloan had published their first report on the transhiatal approach for esophagectomy without thoracotomy [11]. The efficacy of the radical en bloc esophagectomy has been controversial up to the present time, with the majority of surgeons favoring conventional techniques of esophageal resection through either transthoracic or transhiatal approaches. However, we and other groups continue to advocate for radical en bloc esophageal resection as the optimal procedure to maximize locoregional control and improve long-term survival in patients with esophageal cancer.

The basic concept of en bloc esophagectomy is resection of the tumor-bearing esophagus within a wide envelope of surrounding tissues. For tumors of the middle or lower thoracic esophagus, the tumor-bearing esophagus is resected within an envelope of surrounding tissues that includes the pericardium anteriorly,

P.C. Lee, M.D.
Department of Cardiothoracic Surgery, New York Presbyterian Hospital, Weill Cornell Medical Center, 525 East 68th Street, New York, NY 10021, USA
e-mail: pcl9001@med.cornell.edu

N.K. Altorki, M.D. (✉)
Department of Cardiothoracic Surgery, New York Presbyterian Hospital, Weill Cornell Medical Center, 525 East 68th Street, M-404, New York, NY 10021, USA
e-mail: nkaltork@med.cornell.edu

J. Kim and J. Garcia-Aguilar (eds.), *Surgery for Cancers of the Gastrointestinal Tract: A Step-by-Step Approach*, DOI 10.1007/978-1-4939-1893-5_4, © Springer Science+Business Media New York 2015

both pleural surfaces laterally, as well as the thoracic duct and all other lympho-areolar tissue wedged posteriorly between the esophagus and the spine. The en bloc two-field lymphadenectomy necessarily includes removal of all nodal groups in the middle and lower mediastinum as well as the upper abdomen.

For a subset of patients, the lymphadenectomy is extended to include the superior mediastinal and cervical lymph nodes (three-field lymphadenectomy). The three-field concept was first introduced by Japanese surgeons, prompted by the observation that as many as 40 % of patients resected by radical two-field esophagectomy developed isolated recurrences in the cervical nodes [12]. Isono and colleagues reported in 1991 the results of three-field lymph node dissection and showed that occult cervical node metastases occurred in one-third of patients [13]. Even for lower-third tumors, up to 20 % of patients had occult cervical metastases. Most Western surgeons have been reluctant to adopt the three-field dissection technique mostly due to skepticism that long-term survival is achievable when nodal disease is present. A second reason for this reluctance is the reported high morbidity associated with the operation, particularly injury to one or both recurrent laryngeal nerves reported in as many as 50 % of patients [14, 15].

## Preoperative Assessment

Preoperative assessment is directed towards establishing the clinical stage of the tumor as well as assessing the patient's ability to tolerate the planned resection. Our standard diagnostic and staging workup includes an upper endoscopy with biopsy, computed tomography (CT) of the chest and upper abdomen, endoscopic ultrasonography (EUS), and positron emission tomography (PET). EUS is useful in selecting patients for clinical trials of preoperative induction therapy while PET is a generally more sensitive test for detection of distant visceral and skeletal metastases. Patients are considered for primary surgical resection if preoperative evaluation revealed no evidence of distant visceral metastases or clear evidence of direct neoplastic invasion of the airway or major vascular structures. The presence of extensive nodal disease is not considered a contraindication to resection unless it clearly extends beyond the proposed fields of dissection. Patients with locally advanced clinical stage disease are evaluated for induction chemotherapy or chemoradiotherapy by a multidisciplinary team prior to resection. Finally, all patients undergo thorough evaluation of pulmonary and cardiac function to determine their ability to withstand esophagectomy.

## Operative Technique

The basic concept underlying en bloc esophagectomy is resecting the tumor-bearing esophagus within a wide envelope of periesophageal tissue, which includes both pleural surfaces laterally, lymphovascular tissue and the thoracic duct posteriorly, a patch of pericardium anteriorly, and all the mediastinal nodes from the tracheal bifurcation to the hiatus. An upper abdominal lymphadenectomy is performed that includes the celiac, common hepatic, left gastric, parahiatal and lesser curvature lymph nodes (Fig. 4.1). A three-field nodal dissection can be incorporated by extending the lymphadenectomy to include the superior mediastinal lymph nodes and deep internal and external cervical lymph nodes (Fig. 4.2). The procedure is generally carried out through three incisions: right thoracotomy, laparotomy, and collar neck incision.

### The Thorax

A right fifth interspace thoracotomy is performed regardless of the location of the tumor (Fig. 4.3). The en bloc dissection of the middle and lower mediastinum (first field) begins by incising the mediastinal pleura over the anterior aspect of the azygos vein from the level of the azygos arch superiorly to the aortic hiatus inferiorly. The dissection proceeds leftwards anterior to the aorta and across the mediastinum to the opposite pleura,

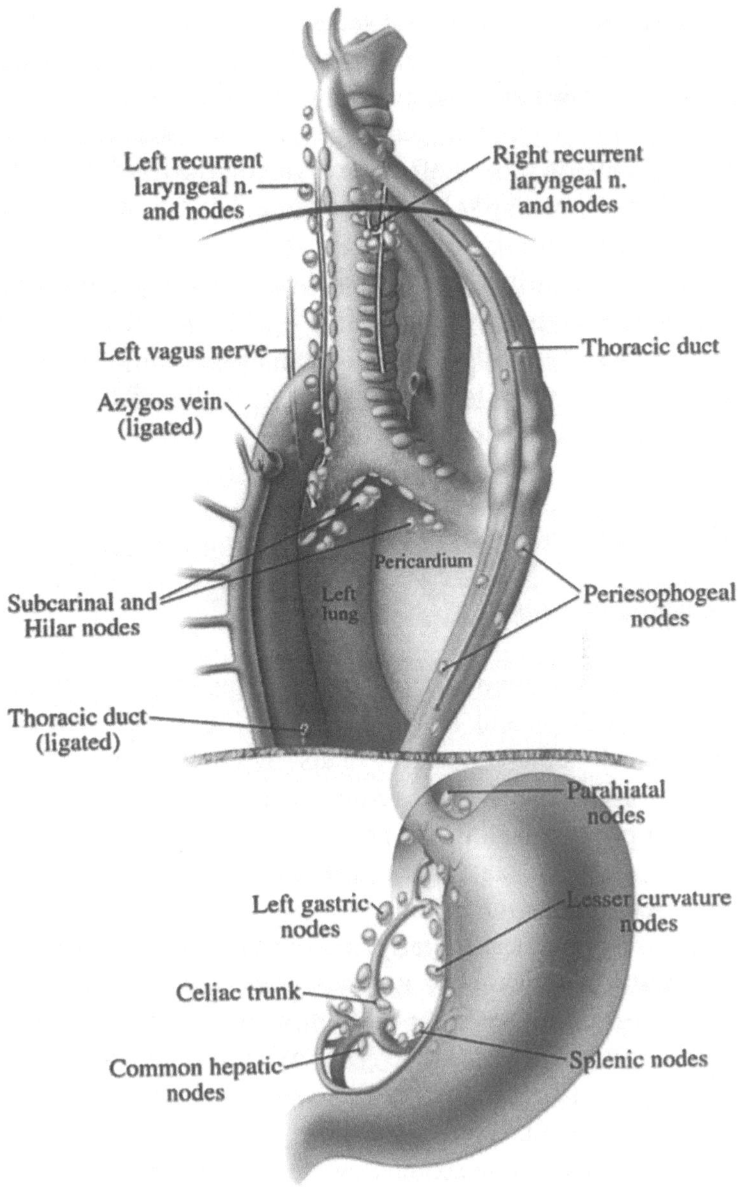


**Fig. 4.1** Mediastinal and upper abdominal lymph node fields in the en bloc resection. (Shields et al. General Thoracic Surgery vol 2, Philadelphia: Lippincott Williams & Wilkins, 2005, Fig. 131-21). With permission

which is entered along the entire length of the incision. The thoracic duct is thus mobilized anteriorly towards the specimen and is ligated inferiorly as it enters at the aortic hiatus and superiorly as it crosses over to the left side of the mediastinum (Fig. 4.4). All lymphatic channels are clipped or ligated between the thoracic duct and the spine to minimize the risk of a chylothorax. The arch of the azygos vein is resected en bloc with the specimen. The anterior dissection is commenced by division of the azygos vein at its caval junction and by carrying the dissection along the right main bronchus and the posterior aspect of the hilum of the right lung. The hilar and subcarinal nodes are cleared and a patch of pericardium is resected en bloc with the tumor-bearing esophagus for all but submucosal tumors ($T_1$) of the middle and lower thirds of the esophagus. Division of

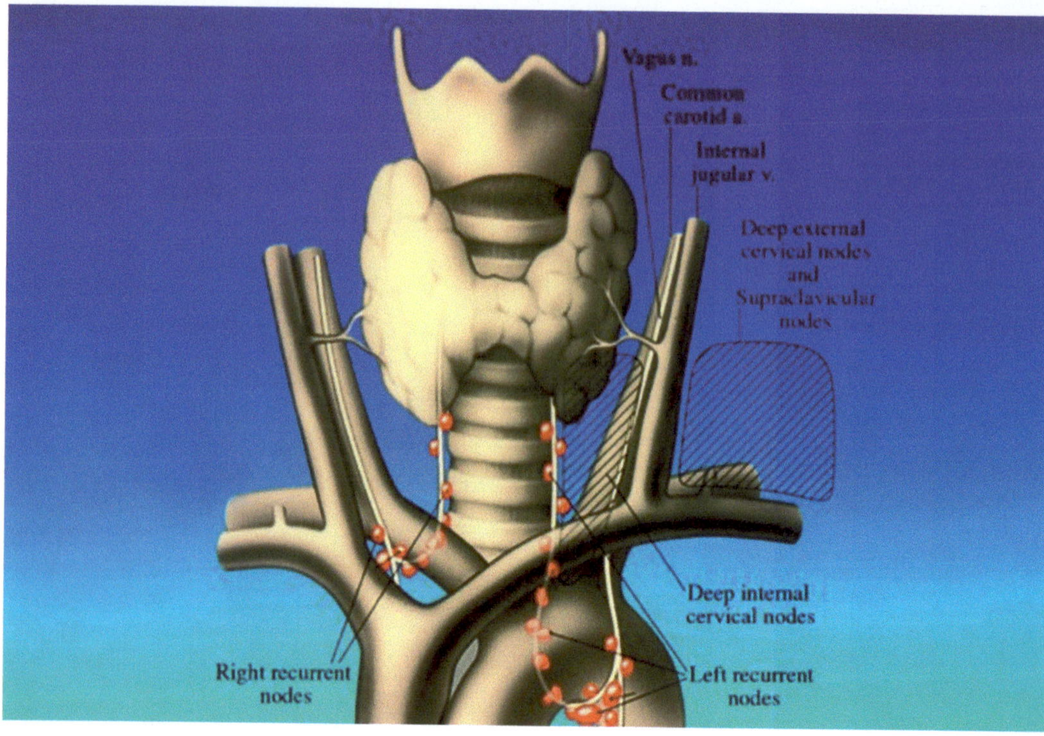


**Fig. 4.2** Recurrent and cervical nodal fields in the three-field dissection. (Shields et al. General Thoracic Surgery vol 2, Philadelphia: Lippincott Williams & Wilkins, 2005. Fig. 131-20). With permission

the bilateral pulmonary ligaments completes the esophageal mobilization (Fig. 4.5).

For tumors traversing the hiatus, a 1-in. cuff of diaphragm is circumferentially excised en bloc with the specimen. The completed first-field dissection clears all nodal tissue in the middle and lower mediastinum including the right and left paraesophageal, parahiatal, para-aortic, subcarinal, and bilateral hilar lymph nodes. This first-field is bounded superiorly by the tracheal bifurcation, inferiorly by the esophageal hiatus, anteriorly by the hilum of the lung and pericardium, and posteriorly by the descending thoracic aorta and the spine.

Dissection of the third field commences during the thoracic portion of the procedure and is later completed through a collar neck incision. Dissection of the superior mediastinal lymph nodes includes the nodes along the right and left recurrent laryngeal nerves throughout their mediastinal course. The left recurrent nerve is dissected using a no-touch technique and nodes along its anterior aspect are carefully excised. The right recurrent nerve is carefully exposed near its origin at the base of the right subclavian artery. The right vagus nerve serves as a good landmark in locating the right recurrent nerve. The right recurrent nodal chain begins at that level and extends through the thoracic inlet to the neck. The right recurrent nerve is dissected again using a strict no-touch technique. Through the subsequent cervical incision (Fig. 4.6), the remaining recurrent nodes are dissected along with the lower deep cervical nodes located posterior and lateral to the carotid sheath. Thus the third field comprises a continuous chain of nodes that extends from the superior mediastinum to the lower neck. These nodes may be more appropriately termed cervico-thoracic nodes rather than cervical nodes.

## The Abdomen

An upper midline incision is used to enter the abdomen (Fig. 4.6). After the omentum is separated

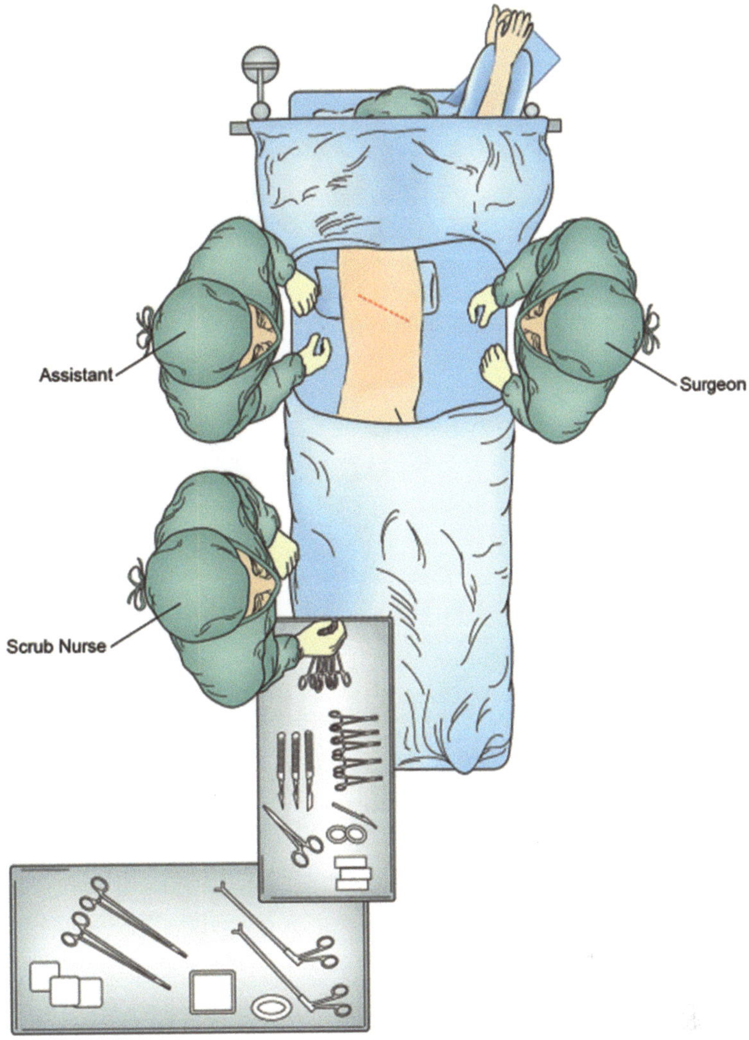


**Fig. 4.3** Operative positioning for right fifth interspace thoracotomy

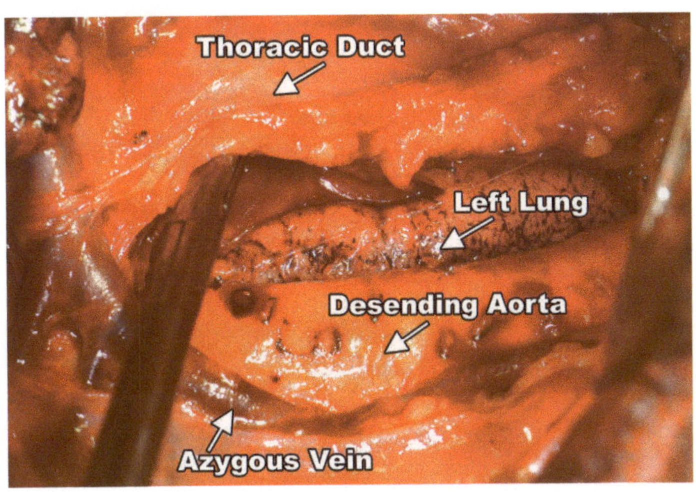


**Fig. 4.4** View from a right thoracotomy. Specimen with tumor-bearing esophagus is mobilized anteriorly along the descending thoracic aorta including the thoracic duct

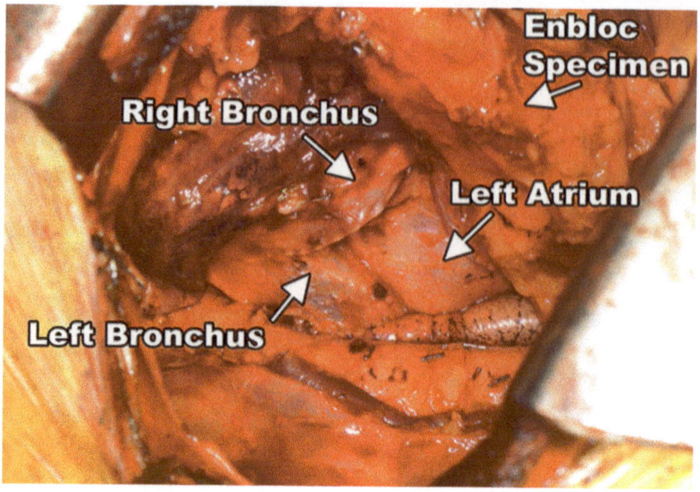


**Fig. 4.5** The en bloc specimen is completely mobilized, revealing the left lung, descending thoracic aorta, the tracheal bifurcation, and the pericardium

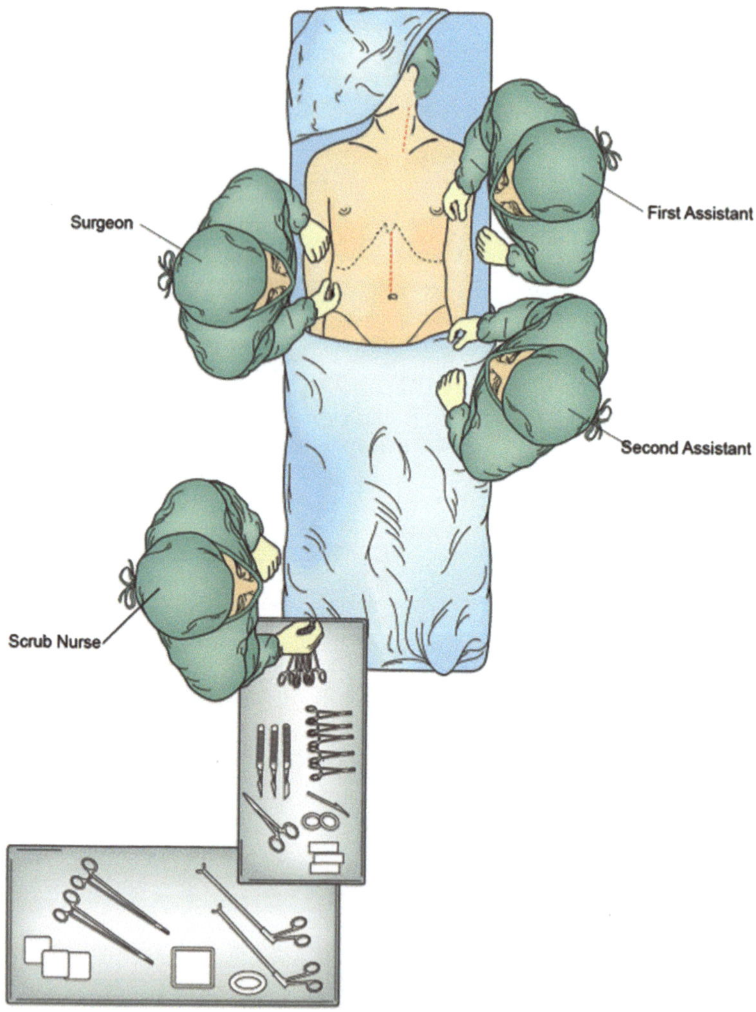


**Fig. 4.6** Operative positioning for upper midline abdominal incision and left neck incision

from the colon in the avascular plane, the lesser sac is entered. The omentum is resected as a separate specimen at least 1 in. outside the gastroepiploic arcade. The short gastric vessels are divided. The retroperitoneum is then incised along the superior border of the pancreas and the retroperitoneal lymphatic and areolar tissues are swept superiorly towards the esophageal hiatus and medially along the splenic artery to the celiac trifurcation. The left gastric artery is then identified and divided flush with its celiac origin. Common hepatic artery lymph nodes are dissected and swept towards the specimen. This retroperitoneal dissection is bounded by the dissected esophageal hiatus superiorly, the hilum of the spleen laterally, and the common hepatic artery and inferior vena cava medially (Fig. 4.7). Lastly, the lesser curvature and left gastric nodes are included with the specimen when the gastric tube is prepared.

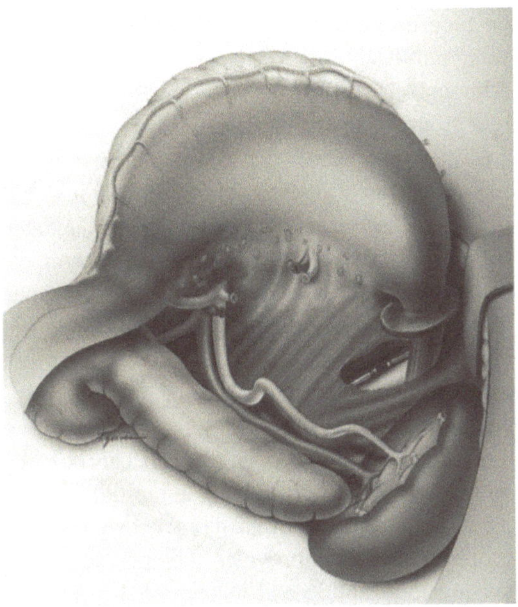

**Fig. 4.7** Abdominal en bloc dissection. (Shields et al. General Thoracic Surgery vol 2, Philadelphia: Lippincott Williams & Wilkins, 2005. Figure 4-131-14). With permission

## The Neck

A low collar incision is performed and subplatysmal flaps are raised superiorly and inferiorly. The strap muscles are divided. The esophagus, which was previously mobilized intrathoracically, is retrieved from the prevertebral space. The esophagus is then divided distally and the specimen is retrieved in the abdomen. The previously dissected recurrent nerves are easy to visualize (especially the right recurrent) and any residual nodal tissue is excised. The nodes posterior and lateral to the carotid sheath are then removed along with the supraclavicular nodes. This is particularly important for tumors of the middle and upper thirds of the esophagus. The dissection is limited superiorly by the inferior belly of the omohyoid. Within the abdomen the gastric tube is prepared and the specimen is removed (Fig. 4.8). Gastrointestinal continuity is established by a cervical esophagogastrostomy.

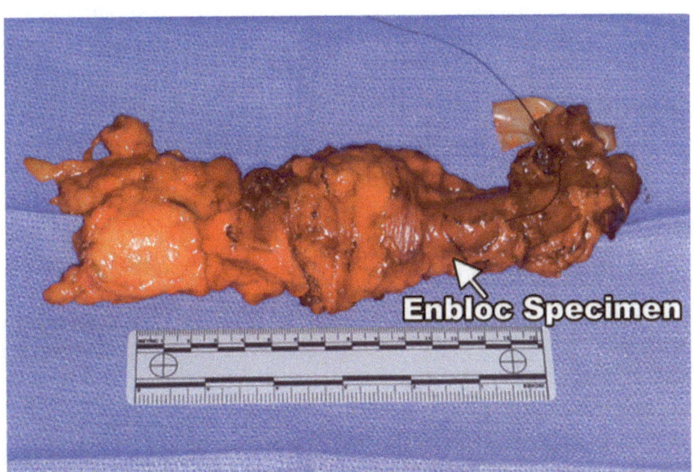


**Fig. 4.8** The en bloc specimen; note that the esophagus is resected within a wide envelope of surrounding tissues

A feeding jejunostomy tube is placed for early postoperative enteral feeding.

## Postoperative Care

In the past, all patients were cared for in an intensive care unit for 24 h for mechanical ventilation and fluid management. Currently, with improved epidural pain control and aggressive pulmonary physiotherapy, patients who undergo two-field resection are extubated in the operating room. Patients who undergo three-field resection often require 24 h of mechanical ventilation. After three-field dissection, some patients develop bronchorrhea and require more frequent pulmonary hygiene, often with repeated bronchoscopy for the first 48 h after extubation. The bronchorrhea generally resolves on the third or fourth postoperative day. Patients often have significant fluid requirement postoperatively, with spontaneous diuresis by the third postoperative day. Aggressive physical therapy is critical in getting patients out of bed and ambulating. Enteral jejunostomy feeding is started by the third or fourth postoperative day. Chest tubes are removed when drainage is less than 250 mL/day. Oral intake commences once anastomotic integrity is confirmed by a barium study on the sixth or seventh postoperative day. Patients are discharged eating a regular diet, but most require supplemental jejunostomy feeding at night. The feeding tube is usually removed 4 weeks following hospital discharge if oral intake is considered adequate.

## Summary

In 2001, we reported a series of 111 patients who underwent en bloc esophagectomy for esophageal cancer between 1988 and 1998 with either two-field or three-field dissection [16]. The overall hospital mortality was 5.4 %, similar to mortality rates of conventional esophagectomy. Complications occurred in 54 patients and were considered minor ($n=11$) and major ($n=43$, including 6 postoperative deaths). Anastomotic leaks occurred in 13.5 % of patients and all healed with simple drainage. Recurrent nerve injuries occurred in four patients and were unilateral not requiring tracheostomy. Five-year overall survival was 40 % with a median survival of 38 months. Of note, the 5-year survival for stage III patients was 39 % comparing favorably to 11 % after conventional transthoracic esophagectomy as reported by others [17]. This outcome is important since most of the patients presenting with esophageal cancer have stage III disease. Our overall local recurrence rate was 8 %.

A randomized trial comparing transthoracic en bloc esophagectomy to transhiatal resection was published by Hulscher in 2002 [18]. Although the difference in survival between the two groups was not statistically significant, there was a trend towards a survival benefit with en bloc resection at 5 years. More recently in 2011, our group published the results of the updated series of 465 patients who underwent complete resection esophageal carcinoma [19]. Multivariate regression analysis identified that en bloc surgical approach was an independent predictor of freedom from recurrence and for prolonged disease-free survival.

Radical en bloc esophagectomy can be done with low mortality and similar morbidity compared to conventional transthoracic or transhiatal esophagectomy. It provides the most thorough staging information and locoregional recurrence rates are substantially reduced. Our 5-year survival rate suggests that prolongation of survival is possible and extensive lymphadenectomy appears to have a favorable impact on survival, especially in patients with nodal metastases. Recent results suggest that en bloc esophagectomy should be recommended for patients with stage II or greater disease with good performance status and adequate cardiopulmonary reserve.

## References

1. Orringer MB, Marshall B, Iannettoni MD. Transhiatal esophagectomy: clinical experience and refinements. Ann Surg. 1999;230(3):392–400; discussion 3.
2. Ellis Jr FH, Heatley GJ, Krasna MJ, Williamson WA, Balogh K. Esophagogastrectomy for carcinoma of the esophagus and cardia: a comparison of findings and results after standard resection in three consecutive eight-year intervals with improved staging criteria.

J Thorac Cardiovasc Surg. 1997;113(5):836–46; discussion 46–8.
3. Lieberman MD, Shriver CD, Bleckner S, Burt M. Carcinoma of the esophagus. Prognostic significance of histologic type. J Thorac Cardiovasc Surg. 1995;109(1):130–8; discussion 9.
4. Putnam Jr JB, Suell DM, McMurtrey MJ, Ryan MB, Walsh GL, Natarajan G, et al. Comparison of three techniques of esophagectomy within a residency training program. Ann Thorac Surg. 1994;57(2):319–25.
5. Altorki NK. The rationale for radical resection. Surg Oncol Clin N Am. 1999;8(2):295–305.
6. Herskovic A, Martz K, al-Sarraf M, Leichman L, Brindle J, Vaitkevicius V, et al. Combined chemotherapy and radiotherapy compared with radiotherapy alone in patients with cancer of the esophagus. N Engl J Med. 1992;326(24):1593–8. doi:10.1056/nejm199206113262403.
7. Kelsen DP, Ginsberg R, Pajak TF, Sheahan DG, Gunderson L, Mortimer J, et al. Chemotherapy followed by surgery compared with surgery alone for localized esophageal cancer. N Engl J Med. 1998;339(27):1979–84. doi:10.1056/nejm199812313392704.
8. Law S, Fok M, Chow S, Chu KM, Wong J. Preoperative chemotherapy versus surgical therapy alone for squamous cell carcinoma of the esophagus: a prospective randomized trial. J Thorac Cardiovasc Surg. 1997;114(2):210–7.
9. Logan A. The surgical treatment of carcinoma of the esophagus and cardia. J Thorac Cardiovasc Surg. 1963;46:150–61.
10. Skinner DB. En bloc resection for neoplasms of the esophagus and cardia. J Thorac Cardiovasc Surg. 1983;85(1):59–71.
11. Orringer MB, Sloan H. Esophagectomy without thoracotomy. J Thorac Cardiovasc Surg. 1978;76(5):643–54.
12. Isono K, Onoda S, Okuyama K, Sato H. Recurrence of intrathoracic esophageal cancer. Jpn J Clin Oncol. 1985;15(1):49–60.
13. Isono K, Sato H, Nakayama K. Results of a nationwide study on the three-field lymph node dissection of esophageal cancer. Oncology. 1991;48(5):411–20.
14. Fujita H, Kakegawa T, Yamana H, Shima I, Toh Y, Tomita Y, et al. Mortality and morbidity rates, postoperative course, quality of life, and prognosis after extended radical lymphadenectomy for esophageal cancer. Comparison of three-field lymphadenectomy with two-field lymphadenectomy. Ann Surg. 1995;222(5):654–62.
15. Nishihira T, Hirayama K, Mori S. A prospective randomized trial of extended cervical and superior mediastinal lymphadenectomy for carcinoma of the thoracic esophagus. Am J Surg. 1998;175(1):47–51.
16. Altorki N, Skinner D. Should en bloc esophagectomy be the standard of care for esophageal carcinoma? Ann Surg. 2001;234(5):581–7.
17. Altorki NK, Girardi L, Skinner DB. En bloc esophagectomy improves survival for stage III esophageal cancer. J Thorac Cardiovasc Surg. 1997;114(6):948–55; discussion 55–6.
18. Hulscher JB, van Sandick JW, de Boer AG, Wijnhoven BP, Tijssen JG, Fockens P, et al. Extended transthoracic resection compared with limited transhiatal resection for adenocarcinoma of the esophagus. N Engl J Med. 2002;347(21):1662–9. doi:10.1056/NEJMoa022343.
19. Lee PC, Mirza FM, Port JL, Stiles BM, Paul S, Christos P, et al. Predictors of recurrence and disease-free survival in patients with completely resected esophageal carcinoma. J Thorac Cardiovasc Surg. 2011;141(5):1196–206. doi:10.1016/j.jtcvs.2011.01.053.

## Key Operative Steps

1. Perform right fifth interspace thoracotomy.
2. Incise mediastinal pleura over the anterior azygos vein from the azygos arch to the aortic hiatus and leftward across the aorta and to the opposite pleura.
3. Ligate the thoracic duct at the aortic hiatus and where it crosses over to the left side.
4. Resect azygos arch en bloc with the operative specimen.
5. Clear the hilar and subcarinal nodes.
6. Resect a patch of pericardium en bloc with esophagus if the tumor is adherent to the pericardium.
7. Divide bilateral pulmonary ligaments.
8. Thoracic lymphadenectomy with clearance of all nodal tissue including right and left paraesophageal, parahiatal, para-aortic, subcarinal, and bilateral hilar lymph nodes.
9. Dissection of the third field begins in the thorax including the superior mediastinal lymph nodes and the nodes along the right and left recurrent laryngeal nerves.
10. Complete the third-field dissection with a cervical incision removing the lower deep cervical lymph nodes.
11. Laparotomy requires an upper abdominal midline incision.
12. Enter the lesser sac through the avascular plane between the omentum and colon.
13. The omentum is resected and the short gastric vessels are divided.
14. Retroperitoneal tissues along the superior border of the pancreas are swept up to the esophageal hiatus.
15. The left gastric artery is divided.
16. The common hepatic artery lymph nodes are dissected and swept towards the specimen.
17. The lesser curvature lymph nodes are included with the specimen.
18. Retrieve the esophagus from the prevertebral space in the neck.
19. Divide the esophagus and retrieve the specimen in the abdomen.
20. Dissect the lymph nodes posterior and lateral to the carotid sheath along with the supraclavicular lymph nodes.
21. In the abdomen create the gastric conduit.
22. Perform cervical esophagogastrostomy, completed posteriorly with side-to-side stapled technique and anteriorly with 3–0 absorbable running suture.
23. Place feeding jejunostomy tube.

# 5 Minimally Invasive Three-Field Esophagectomy

Young Tae Kim

## Historical Perspective

Minimally invasive three-field esophagectomy with esophagogastrostomy is usually performed by thoracoscopic and laparoscopic approaches. Historically, this technique was developed to overcome the major limitations of laparoscopic transhiatal esophagectomy, which include poor visualization and technical difficulties of mediastinal lymph node dissection [1–3]. The minimally invasive three-field technique has enabled surgeons to mobilize intrathoracic esophageal segments and to dissect mediastinal lymph nodes under direct visualization [1].

## Anatomical Highlights

There are various methods of esophageal cancer surgery. The location of the tumor, choice of the organ for esophageal substitute, route of the conduit, and the level of planned anastomosis are important anatomic factors that surgeons should consider for successful surgery [4, 5]. If the tumor is located in the upper thoracic esophagus, usually the three-field (cervical, thoracic, and abdominal) approach is required to guarantee a sufficient resection margin [6]. If the mass is located either in the middle or lower thoracic esophagus, then the thoracic and abdominal approach (i.e., Ivor Lewis operation) is a preferred method [4]. However, with minimally invasive techniques, the three-field approach is the most frequently used method, mainly because of the technical difficulties of thoracic esophagogastric anastomosis [7]. Many surgeons prefer making an anastomosis through the cervical incision. Some surgeons, however, have reported a successful series of the thoracic and abdominal approach, where an anastomosis was made at the level of the thoracic esophagus using various minimally invasive techniques [8]. The stomach is by far the most frequently used organ as an esophageal replacement. By mobilizing and releasing its short gastric and left gastric vascular structures, the fundus of the stomach can readily advance to the cervical esophagus. Relocating the stomach requires only one anastomosis and it is the conduit with which most thoracic surgeons have the most experience. Usually the posterior mediastinal route is used to bring the gastric conduit to the neck in minimally invasive three-field esophagectomy [9].

Electronic supplementary material: Supplementary material is available in the online version of this chapter at 10.1007/978-1-4939-1893-5_5. Videos can also be accessed at http://www.springerimages.com/videos/978-1-4939-1892-8.

Y.T. Kim, M.D., Ph.D. (✉)
Department of Thoracic and Cardiovascular Surgery, Seoul National University Hospital, Seoul National University College of Medicine,
Suite #7303, 101 Daehak-ro Jongno-gu, Seoul 110-744, Republic of Korea
e-mail: ytkim@snu.ac.kr

J. Kim and J. Garcia-Aguilar (eds.), *Surgery for Cancers of the Gastrointestinal Tract: A Step-by-Step Approach*,
DOI 10.1007/978-1-4939-1893-5_5, © Springer Science+Business Media New York 2015

## Indications for Operation

Minimally invasive three-field esophagectomy is recommended for patients requiring total esophagectomy. As the esophagogastric anastomosis is performed in the neck, it can guarantee a longer margin from the upper border of the tumor to the proximal resection margin. Additionally, in the event that leakage from the cervical anastomosis should occur, it can be drained readily through the cervical incision [6]. However, in patients with prior right thoracotomy, the procedure may not be suitable because severe adhesions may be encountered during the thoracoscopic procedure.

## Preoperative Evaluation and Imaging

Initial evaluation for the patient with esophageal cancer includes the history and physical examination and fiberoptic esophagoscopy. The classic presenting symptom is dysphagia to solid food with weight loss in elderly male patients with history of heavy smoking and drinking. The physical examination may reveal enlargement of supraclavicular or neck lymph nodes. Although barium esophagography can be done as the first investigation, a flexible fiberoptic esophagoscopy is more frequently used in many centers. With flexible esophagoscopy a pathologic diagnosis can be made through cytologic brushings and tissue biopsies. Endoscopic ultrasonography (EUS) is usually recommended to evaluate the depth of the tumor as well as peri-esophageal lymph nodes. If there are lymph nodes suspicious for metastases, a needle biopsy can be performed safely and accurately under the guidance of EUS. If surgery is planned, a thorough examination of the entire stomach is recommended to ensure no pathology in the stomach, which will serve as the esophageal substitute. When the tumor obstructs the esophagus and flexible endoscopy cannot pass through it, upper gastrointestinal series can provide information of the gastric mucosa.

Computed tomography (CT) scan is usually indicated to evaluate the primary tumor, regional lymph nodes, as well as distant organs. The main value of CT in staging esophageal cancer lies in its ability to detect distant nodal or visceral metastases, such as liver or lung metastases.

If the tumor is located in the middle thoracic esophagus and if there are signs of involvement of the bronchus, including widened carina, external compression, tumor infiltration, and fistulization, then flexible fiberoptic bronchoscopy is mandatory. Because gross macroscopic bronchoscopic appearance may not be accurate, biopsy and brush cytology of suspicious areas should be performed. If patients have advanced disease, neck ultrasonography may provide additional accuracy for evaluation of cervical lymph node metastasis. The diagnostic yield of positron emission tomography (PET) for detection of unsuspected metastases in early-stage disease (i.e., Tis or T1) may be low and the risk of lymph node metastases increases with increasing T classification. Therefore, cost effectiveness in this setting is uncertain but we usually recommend PET/CT scan in the preoperative evaluation if available.

## Perioperative Preparation

### Bowel Preparation

A day before surgery, the patient follows a low-residue diet for dinner and then remains nil per os until surgery. Mechanical bowel preparation is not usually recommended if the stomach is to be used as an esophageal substitute. Preoperative mechanical and antibiotic bowel preparation are generally recommended only if colonic or jejunal conduit is anticipated [10].

### Anesthesia Needs

We prefer single-lung ventilation during thoracic esophageal dissection. Therefore, double-lumen endotracheal tubes or single-lumen endotracheal tubes combined with bronchial blocking devices are used. We also prefer to insufflate with $CO_2$ gas to facilitate esophageal dissection. It is important for the anesthesiologists to carefully monitor vital signs during $CO_2$ insufflation. If there is any sign of reduced cardiac venous return caused by high intrathoracic pressure, the thoracic cavity should be deflated immediately [11].

We prefer to place arterial and central venous lines and a Foley catheter. Accurate monitoring of the trends in central venous pressure and urine output is desirable. A significant amount of fluid can enter the interstitial space in the abdomen during surgery and intravascular volume loading is required to maintain intravascular volume. Therefore, liberal fluid administration is accepted, which is usually not recommended for pulmonary procedures. However, there is increasing evidence of earlier return of bowel function in abdominal surgery if intraoperative fluid is restricted and lower urine output is maintained in the tolerable range. Fluid restriction, therefore, may be credited for a reduction in pulmonary complications [12].

## Description of Operation

Minimally invasive three-field esophagectomy is performed in three stages, thoracoscopic esophageal dissection, laparoscopic gastric mobilization, and cervical esophagogastric anastomosis.

### Thoracoscopic Esophageal Dissection

The patient is positioned in left lateral decubitus with double-lumen endotracheal tube intubation. To facilitate the surgical procedure, it is recommended to tilt the patient to 30° prone position. The surgeon stands anterior to the patient. I prefer using four thoracic trocars (Fig. 5.1). The first trocar (10 mm) is placed at the sixth intercostal space anteriorly and is used for the camera. The 30° scope is used to inspect the pleural cavity and the surface of the lung for metastatic deposits. The second 12-mm port is placed at the most inferior portion of the right pleural cavity along the mid-axillary line. This port is used for the surgeon's left hand instruments. A 5-mm trocar is placed at the midpoint of the pleural cavity posteriorly. This port is for the assistant to pull the esophagus during the dissection. The last trocar (5 mm) is placed at the third intercostal space at the mid-axillary line. This port is for use by the surgeon's right hand (Fig. 5.2). Carbon dioxide insufflation (8–10 mmHg) is preferred because it pushes the right hemi-diaphragm downwards and collapses the lung to provide a nice view of the diaphragmatic crus.

It is usually not necessary to divide the inferior pulmonary ligament and dissection of the esophagus starts from the mid-esophagus below the subcarinal area and then extends downward. The incision is made along the anterior portion of the esophagus. Using energy devices, such as electrocautery or Harmonic Scalpel (Ethicon Endo-Surgery, Cincinnati, OH), the anterior surface of the esophagus is dissected from the posterior portion of the pericardium and the anterolateral surface of the aorta. After completion of the anterior dissection, I prefer to place a small sponge between the aorta and the esophagus. This will facilitate subsequent posterior dissection. If the esophagus is pulled anteriorly, the sponge will be located between the esophagus and the aorta, and the surgeon can carry out dissection without the danger of injuring the thoracic aorta (Fig. 5.3). Once the circumferential dissection of the esophagus is accomplished, a penrose drain is placed around the esophagus and it is used to retract the esophagus by the assistant surgeon (Fig. 5.4). Small perforators from the thoracic aorta should be controlled using either endoclips or energy devices. All the para-esophageal lymph nodes are dissected en bloc with the esophagus. It is usually not difficult to expose the diaphragmatic crus because $CO_2$ insufflation will push down the diaphragm and facilitate exposure.

I prefer to resect the thoracic duct en bloc with the esophagus. In case the thoracic duct is not resected and if there is any suspicion of injury, I recommend clipping it at the most proximal portion. It is noteworthy that the thoracic duct runs separately from the azygos vein at the level of the lower esophagus and its course varies. However, the thoracic duct is easily found at the level of the mid-esophagus because it is running

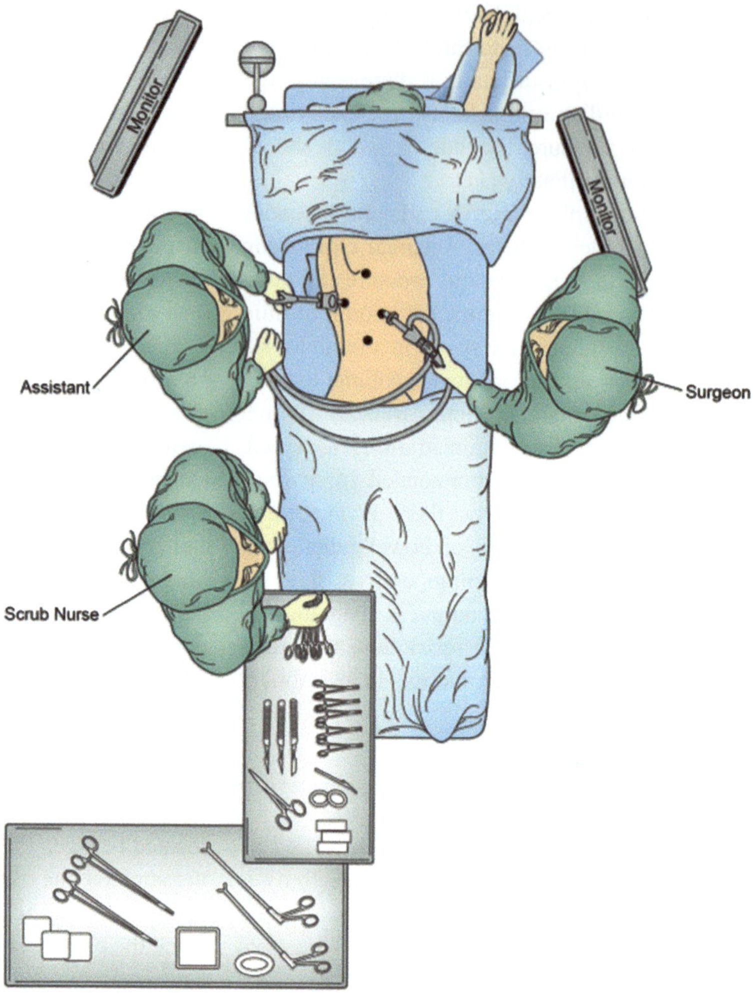


**Fig. 5.1** Operating room setup for thoracoscopic esophagectomy

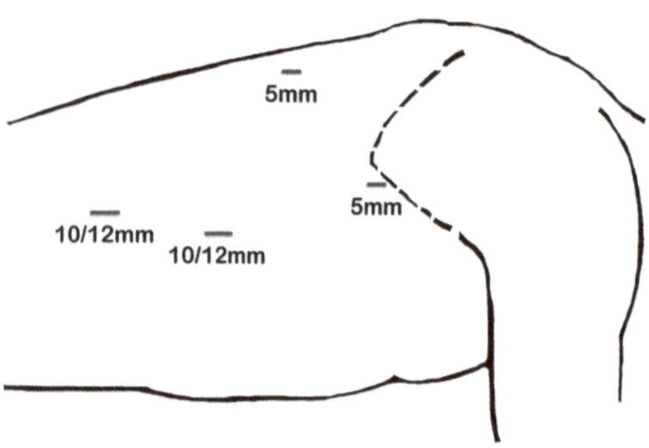


**Fig. 5.2** Port placement for thoracoscopic esophagectomy

parallel with the azygos vein along its medial border. Once the thoracic duct is found, it is easy to dissect it proximally downwards and the most proximal end can be easily clipped.

Attention is directed to the mid-esophagus and the subcarinal lymph nodes are dissected en bloc with the esophagus (Fig. 5.5). Depending on the situation, one can dissect the subcarinal lymph nodes separately from the esophagus. The dissection is continued upwards to the azygos vein. Usually, there are many blood vessels at this level, supplying the esophagus as well as the peri-esophageal lymph nodes. These blood vessels should be carefully controlled. The mediastinal pleura above the azygos vein is then opened and the azygos vein is divided with an endostapler. Further dissection is carried out so that the esophagus is circumferentially mobilized from the esophageal hiatus up to the thoracic inlet. Above the level of the azygos vein, the dissection is maintained close to the esophagus to

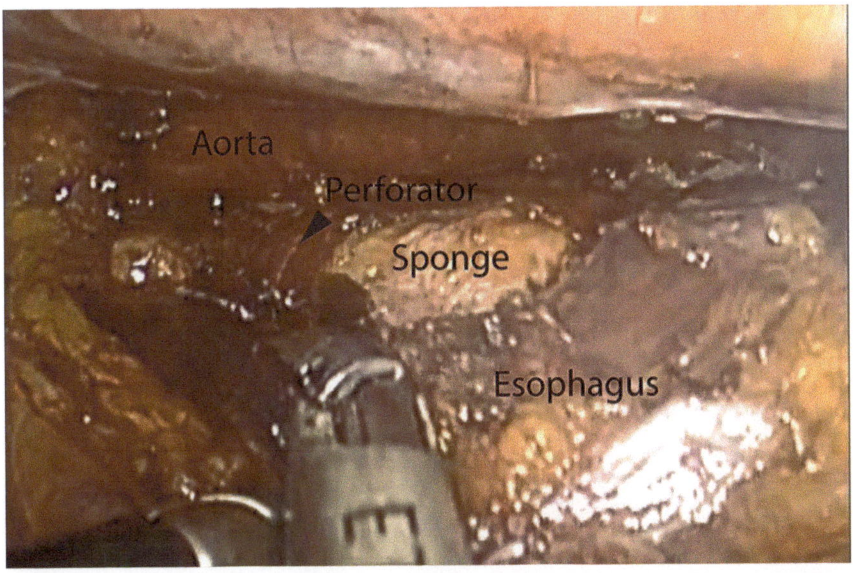


**Fig. 5.3** Dissection of the lower thoracic esophagus with a sponge placed between the esophagus and aorta

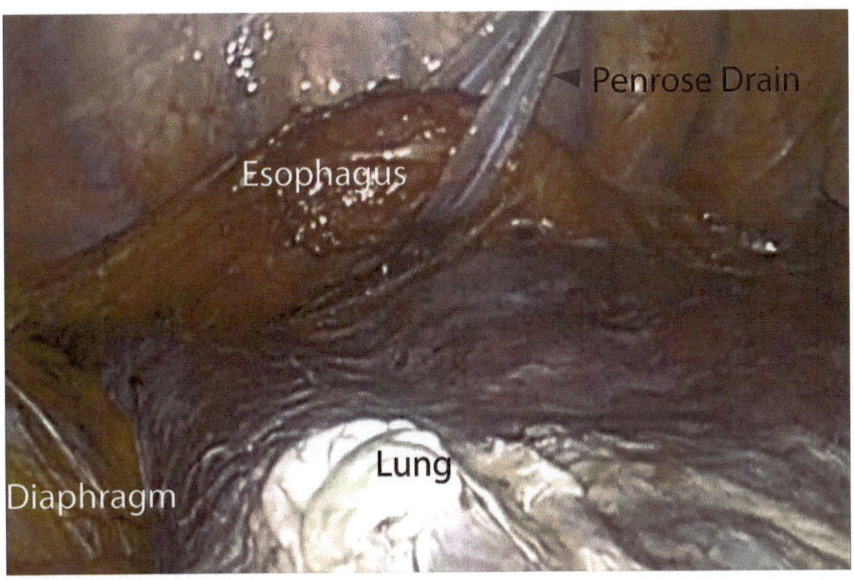


**Fig. 5.4** Retraction of the thoracic esophagus using a penrose drain

avoid potential injury to the left recurrent laryngeal nerve as well as the membranous portion of the trachea.

Mediastinal lymph node dissection is also performed. The left paratracheal lymph nodes are dissected with great care as not to injure the left recurrent laryngeal nerve. As it is difficult to dissect the left paratracheal lymph nodes, some surgeons suggest placing a single-lumen tube to facilitate exposure of the left paratracheal area. Personally, I prefer a double-lumen tube intubation. In case the left paratracheal lymph node dissection is difficult, I often make an upper partial sternotomy during the cervical procedure and dissect both paratracheal lymph nodes. It is especially beneficial because one can easily localize

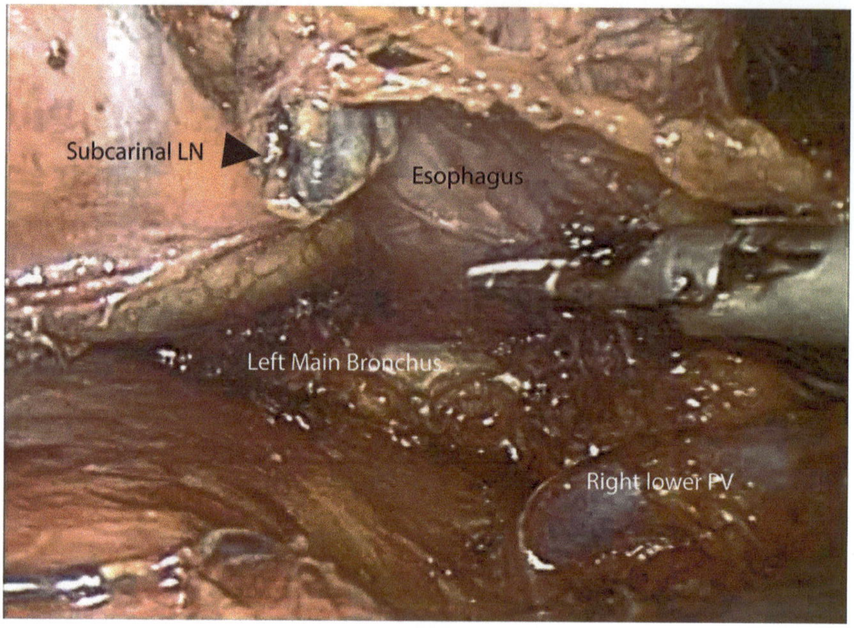


**Fig. 5.5** Dissection of the middle thoracic esophagus and subcarinal lymph nodes

both recurrent laryngeal nerves and lymph node dissection can be carried out under the direct vision.

Some surgeons prefer to leave a penrose drain attached to the uppermost portion of the esophagus so that they can easily find the esophagus at the time of neck dissection. However, I find that it is not necessary. At the completion of the thoracoscopic procedure, a 28-French chest tube is inserted through the inferior port for postoperative chest drainage. The lungs are inflated and the port sites are closed.

## Laparoscopic Gastric Conduit Preparation

The patient is placed in the supine lithotomy position. It is mandatory to take special care to avoid excessive abduction of the hip joint. The skin is prepped and draped from the neck to the pubic symphysis. The surgeon stands between the legs of the patient (Fig. 5.6). A 10-mm skin incision is placed in the midline above the umbilicus and abdominal insufflation is achieved by Veress needle. A 10-mm trocar is then placed through the same skin incision, and a 30° laparoscope is introduced. I prefer to use five abdominal trocars. Once the camera is placed, a thorough staging procedure is performed to determine if occult metastases are present. The second trocar (12 mm) is placed at the right anterior axillary line at the level of the umbilicus, for the liver retractor and stapler. A 5-mm trocar is placed at the right mid-clavicular line below the costal margin to be used by the surgeon's left hand. A 5-mm trocar is placed at the left mid-clavicular line below the costal margin and used for the surgeon's right hand. Another 5-mm trocar is placed at the left anterior axillary line at the level of the umbilicus for retraction by the assistant surgeon (Fig. 5.7). The patient is placed in reverse Trendelenburg position to help with exposure by displacing the stomach and colon caudally. The left lobe of the liver is retracted upward by placement of a liver retractor.

Using an endograsper in the left hand and an energy device in the right hand, the lesser sac is opened and divided up to the hiatus. To avoid losing pneumoperitoneum, I leave the dissection of

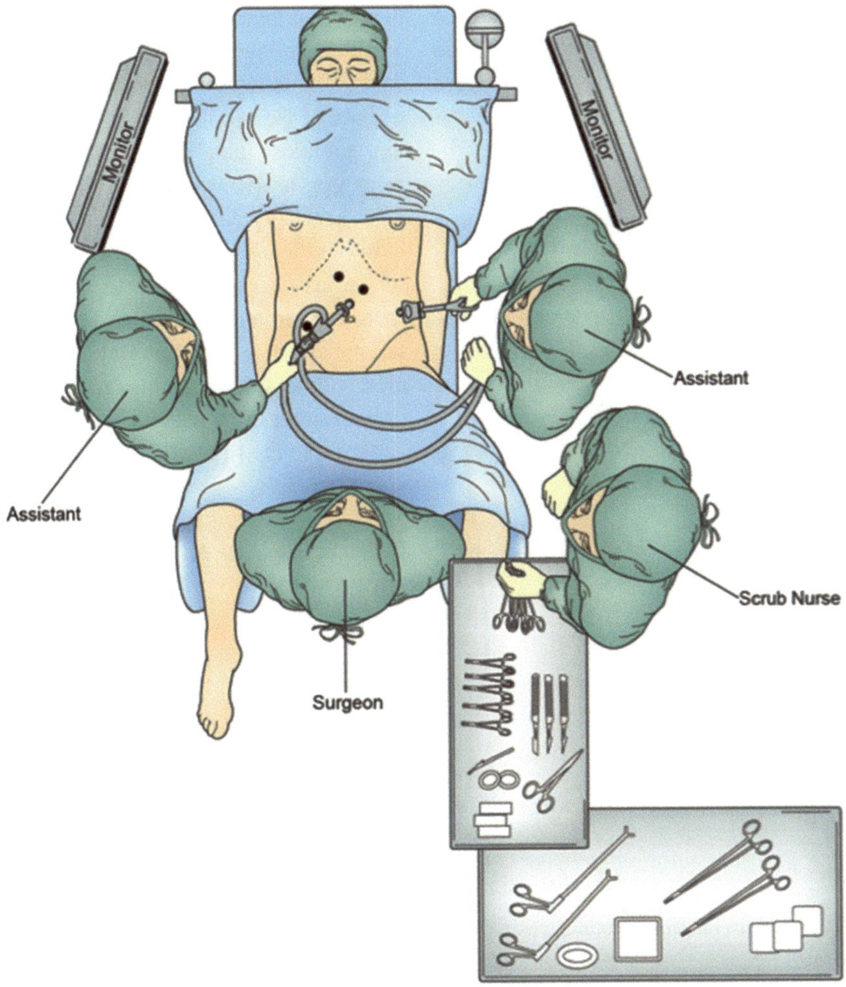


**Fig. 5.6** Operating room setting for laparoscopic gastric conduit preparation

the hiatus for last. The greater curvature of the stomach is prepared carefully to avoid injury to the right gastroepiploic vessels. The assistant surgeon pulls the greater omentum to the left. I prefer to start the dissection of the greater omentum at the 4 o'clock position because it is easy to find an area bare of omental vessels. I use an energy device for cauterization and division of the greater omentum. Further dissection is continued towards the gastrolienal ligament by dividing the short gastric vessels. During this procedure, the assistant surgeon may pull the stomach upwards and to the right to expose the space between the stomach and the spleen.

After completing preparation of the greater curvature, attention is directed to the left gastric vessels. The stomach is pulled upward and the surgeon approaches the left gastric vessels from the left in the space between the stomach and the pancreas. Alternatively, the stomach can be pulled to the left and the left gastric vessels can be approached from the right side of the lesser sac. The left gastric vessels are isolated and divided. One can either use vascular clips or a vascular endostapler for this procedure. The left gastric lymph nodes are resected en bloc with the surgical specimen. The posterior portion of the stomach is further dissected up to the hiatus. For the gastric drainage, some surgeons prefer pyloromyotomy or pyloroplasty. Some surgeons do not recommend a gastric drainage procedure [13]. However, I prefer injection of Botox (0.4 units) into the pylorus [14].

## Cervical Esophageal Dissection

An oblique left neck incision is made and the platysma is divided. The sternocleidomastoid muscle is retracted laterally. The middle thyroidal vessels and the omohyoid muscle are divided. The thyroid gland is retracted medially and the posterior portion of the esophagus is dissected. It is important not to use metal retractors for the medial side retraction to avoid injury of the recurrent laryngeal nerve. A careful dissection is carried out between the upper trachea and the anterior border of the cervical esophagus to avoid injury of the recurrent laryngeal nerve as well as the superior laryngeal nerve. The cervical esophagus is encircled with a penrose drain, and blunt dissection is carried inferiorly to join the dissection plane achieved in the right chest (Fig. 5.8) [6].

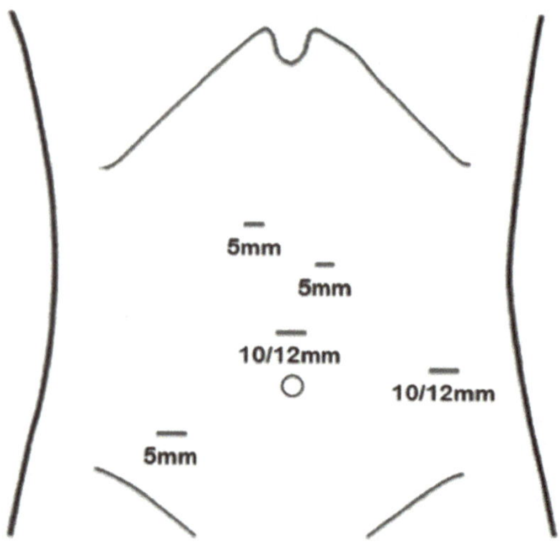


**Fig. 5.7** Port placement for laparoscopic preparation of the gastric conduit

## Gastric Pull-up and Esophagogastric Anastomosis

After completion of the cervical esophageal mobilization, attention is directed to the abdominal cavity. The lesser curvature fat pad is removed at the fourth branch point of the right gastric artery. Starting from that area, multiple linear staplers are used to construct the gastric conduit (4–5 cm in diameter) (Fig. 5.9). The conduit is separated from the specimen at the angle of His. The esophagus is circumferentially mobilized at the esophageal hiatus. If needed, a portion of the

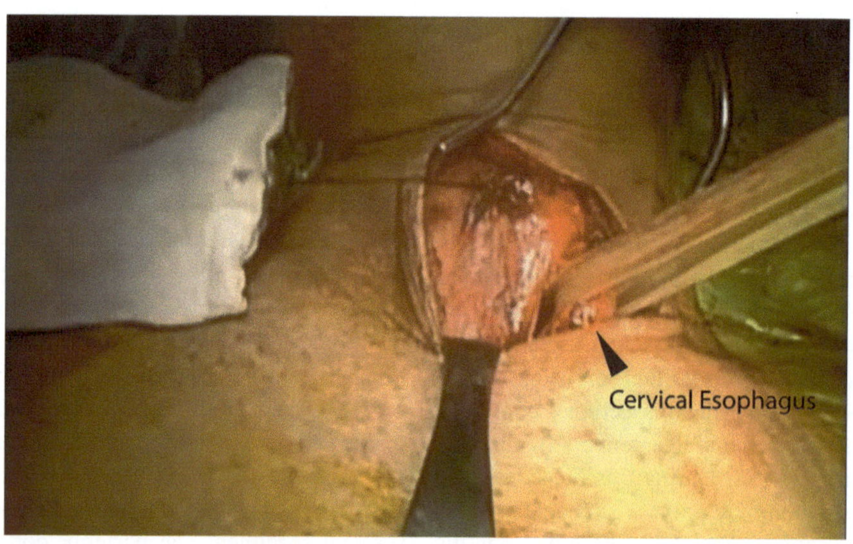


**Fig. 5.8** Dissection of the cervical esophagus

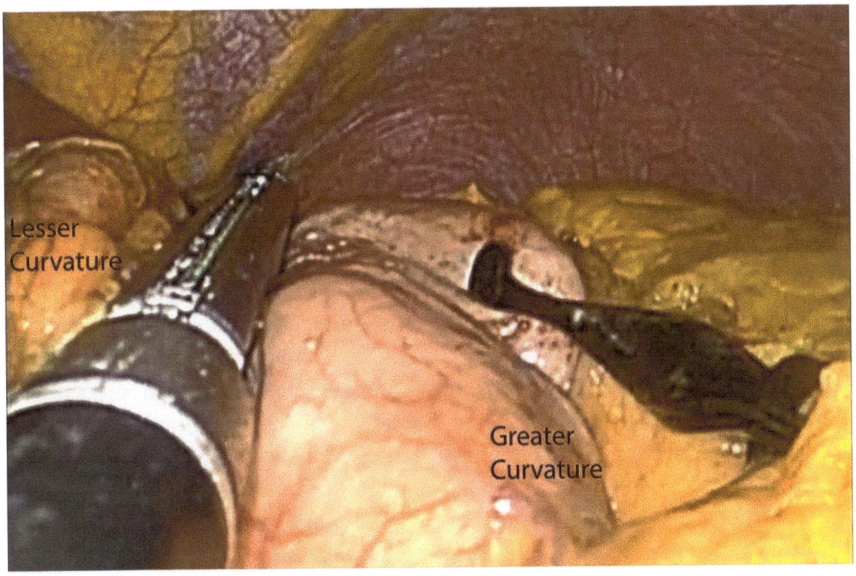


**Fig. 5.9** Preparation of the gastric tube using serial firings of the endostapler

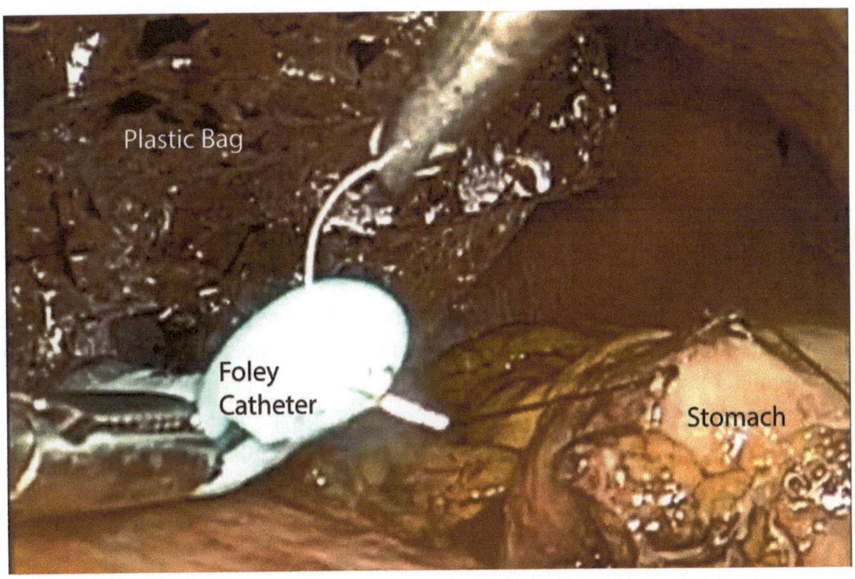


**Fig. 5.10** Preparation for gastric pull-up. The gastric tube is sutured onto the tip of a Foley catheter

right crus of the diaphragm is divided to enlarge the esophageal hiatus to facilitate exposure and transhiatal delivery of the surgical specimen. Under laparoscopic guidance, the surgical specimen is removed through the neck incision. A plastic bag is tied onto a Foley catheter. This Foley catheter is inserted to the neck wound through the posterior mediastinum and down to the hiatus. The distal portion of the gastric conduit is sutured onto the tip of the Foley catheter (Fig. 5.10). The gastric conduit is wrapped in the plastic bag and warm saline solution is poured into the bag. Wall suction is applied onto the Foley catheter and this results in vacuum wrapping of the gastric conduit.

Using this method, the gastric conduit can gently be pulled up without trauma to the ascending gastroepiploic arcade and without spiraling of the conduit.

The cervical esophagus is divided at an appropriate level, and the resection margin is sent for frozen section examination. An esophagogastric anastomosis is performed with either hand-sewn technique or with endostaplers. A nasogastric tube is passed through the anastomosis. The neck is irrigated with antibiotic solution, and the wound is closed. The laparoscope is reinserted to inspect the abdominal cavity for adequate hemostasis. The ports are removed and the port sites are repaired as usual.

## Postoperative Management

Many reports suggest that early extubation after esophagectomy is associated with reduced morbidity and decreased length of ICU stay [15, 16]. We prefer to extubate the patient either in the operating room or in the intensive care unit as soon as the patient is fully awake. It is often challenging to manage the fluid balance adequately after esophagectomy. Adequate circulating blood volume and systemic blood pressure is mandatory to maintain perfusion for the conduit. However, fluid overloading should also be avoided because it could lead to increased tissue edema and subsequent pulmonary edema, which may lead to pulmonary complications [17]. Urine output of 0.5 mL/kg/h during the first 24 h is acceptable [18]. Although pain is minimal after minimally invasive three-field esophagogastrectomy, intravenous patient-controlled analgesia is generally recommended in all patients.

It is our practice not to use total parenteral nutrition in early postoperative days. However, as we do not routinely place a feeding jejunostomy catheter in the laparoscopic procedure, we usually initiate total parenteral nutrition once the patient recovers from the surgical stress. It is usually the third or fourth postoperative day when the patient receives parenteral nutrition. On the seventh postoperative day, we give the patient a cup of grape juice to test for signs of anastomotic leakage. It is important to change the dressing of the drain site and completely empty the drainage bulb to clearly identify any subtle change in drainage color. If there is no sign of leakage, the patient starts with sips of water to make sure he or she has no sign of aspiration. Subsequently, the diet is advanced to clear liquids and then to a soft blended diet.

Injury of the recurrent laryngeal nerve results in significant postoperative morbidity. It happens more commonly after three-field resection compared to a two-field procedure [8]. Vocal cord paralysis compromises an effective cough and pulmonary toilet, which increase the risk of pneumonia. In addition to recurrent laryngeal nerve injury, cricopharyngeal motor dysfunction may result in dysphagia. Combined with the effect of an inability to completely close the vocal cords, the risk of aspiration increases. In my practice, if the patient's voice changes, there is liberal use of otolaryngology consultation to examine the vocal cords before the initiation of oral feeding. If there is vocal cord paralysis and the risk of aspiration exists, an injection laryngoplasty is performed to prevent aspiration during swallowing [19].

Because of lack of sphincter muscle, esophagectomy patients frequently experience reflux. H2-receptor blockers or proton pump inhibitors should be continued after discharge. Also, vagotomized patients may benefit from prokinetic agents such as erythromycin or dopamine antagonists. Low molecular weight heparin is continued until the patient is fully ambulatory to prevent deep vein thrombosis [20]. Prophylactic antibiotics, a first-generation cephalosporine, is administrated for 24 h after surgery [21].

## Complications

### Anticipated Complications

Operative mortality has been reported to be 0–7 % after esophagectomy, and it has been shown to be inversely related to surgeon experience and hospital volume [8, 9, 22–24]. It is well known that technique-related complications, such as anastomotic leak, paralyzed vocal cords, or chylothorax, are associated with increased length of hospital stay, increased in-hospital mortality, higher rate of medical complications, and poor overall survival [19]. Anastomotic dehiscence is the most serious complication associated with esophageal resection. The rate of anastomotic leak ranges from 7 to 22 %, depending on the surgeon's experience [8, 24, 25]. Its associated morbidity and mortality vary depending on the location of the esophagogastric anastomosis. The anastomotic leak rate for intrathoracic anastomosis is significantly lower compared to that for cervical anastomosis [26]. However, the mortality associated with an intrathoracic leak is three times higher than for cervical leak.

Anastomotic stricture will result in dysphagia, which often requires anastomotic dilation. Early stricture formation is likely related to inflammatory changes associated with wound healing. The treatment of early strictures consists of dilation. Most anastomoses require only one dilation, but if symptoms persist then repeated dilations may be necessary [27]. Delayed stricture is most commonly caused by recurrent carcinoma or reflux esophagitis. Thus, an aggressive search for anastomotic recurrence including barium swallow, contrast-enhanced CT of the chest, and esophagoscopy with biopsy is necessary before initiating anastomotic dilation. In the absence of recurrent cancer, most strictures can be easily dilated [28].

Patients often experience dumping syndrome, which includes sweating, palpitations, tachycardia, nausea, and epigastric distention after meals. These intestinal vasomotor symptoms are thought to occur because of the rapid transit of hyperosmolar gastric contents into the jejunum, which results in rapid hyperglycemia followed by reactive hypoglycemia. Dietary modifications including multiple small meals, avoidance of fluids during meals, avoidance of milk products or high-carbohydrate meals, and the occasional use of antidiarrheal medications allow the patient to overcome these symptoms.

Delayed gastric emptying occurs in a minority of patients after esophagogastrectomy and has been attributed to many factors, such as vagotomy, torsion of the stomach into the posterolateral gutter of the right chest, the size of the gastric conduit, the pressure gradient between the intrathoracic stomach and the abdominal duodenum, compression of the distal stomach at the level of the diaphragmatic hiatus, and lack of a drainage procedure. Furthermore, if patients have delayed gastric emptying, the risk of aspiration pneumonia increases [29].

Delayed gastric emptying early in the postoperative period is often caused by mucosal edema at the level of the pyloromyotomy or pyloroplasty and generally resolves within 10–14 days. It is important to keep the stomach decompressed to prevent aspiration and to decrease tension on the esophagogastric anastomosis. With the use of Botox injection technique, this complication is not common in my own practice. In patients with persistent delayed gastric emptying, erythromycin has been shown to improve emptying [30].

Postoperative chylothorax presents as persistently elevated chest tube output that increases with the initiation of oral intake. As the patient's diet is advanced to include a higher fat content, the chest tube output becomes milky white. Prevention of unrecognized thoracic duct injuries and subsequent chylothorax requires careful dissection along the course of the thoracic duct during esophagectomy. The thoracic duct begins at the confluence of the cisterna chyli and enters the thorax through the aortic hiatus posterior to the aorta and anterior to the vertebral bodies of T10-L2. It then ascends just to the right of the anterior surface of the vertebral bodies between the aorta and the azygos vein in the right hemithorax. At the level of the T4 and T5 vertebral bodies, the duct crosses over to the left side of the spine and passes behind the aortic arch and into the neck. In the neck, the duct passes posteriorly to the carotid sheath and drains into the junction of the left jugular and subclavian veins. Any injury to the thoracic duct identified intraoperatively should be managed with ligation of all tissues lying between the azygos vein and the descending aorta. Careful inspection of the thorax along the course of the duct should be performed to identify chylous leaks before closure of the thorax [31]. Personally, I prefer to resect the thoracic duct en bloc with the esophagus. In case the thoracic duct is not resected, I explore the thoracic duct and clip it at the most proximal portion. Usually, the thoracic duct is found at the level of mid-esophagus because it is running parallel with the azygos vein along its medial border. Once the thoracic duct is found, it is easy to dissect proximally downwards and the most proximal end can easily be clipped.

## References


1. Levy RM, Wizorek J, Shende M, Luketich JD. Laparoscopic and thoracoscopic esophagectomy. Adv Surg. 2010;44:101–16.
2. DePaula AL, Hashiba K, Ferreira EA, de Paula RA, Grecco E. Laparoscopic transhiatal esophagectomy with esophagogastroplasty. Surg Laparosc Endosc. 1995;5(1):1–5.
3. Swanstrom LL, Hansen P. Laparoscopic total esophagectomy. Arch Surg. 1997;132(9):943–7; discussion 7–9.
4. Nguyen NT, Follette DM, Lemoine PH, Roberts PF, Goodnight Jr JE. Minimally invasive Ivor Lewis esophagectomy. Ann Thorac Surg. 2001;72(2):593–6.
5. Orringer MB, Marshall B, Iannettoni MD. Transhiatal esophagectomy: clinical experience and refinements. Ann Surg. 1999;230(3):392–400; discussion 3.
6. Swanson SJ, Sugarbaker DJ. The three-hole esophagectomy. The Brigham and Women's Hospital approach (modified McKeown technique). Chest Surg Clin N Am. 2000;10(3):531–52.
7. Nguyen NT, Roberts P, Follette DM, Rivers R, Wolfe BM. Thoracoscopic and laparoscopic esophagectomy for benign and malignant disease: lessons learned from 46 consecutive procedures. J Am Coll Surg. 2003;197(6):902–13.
8. Luketich JD, Pennathur A, Awais O, Levy RM, Keeley S, Shende M, et al. Outcomes after minimally invasive esophagectomy: review of over 1000 patients. Ann Surg. 2012;256(1):95–103.
9. Palanivelu C, Prakash A, Senthilkumar R, Senthilnathan P, Parthasarathi R, Rajan PS, et al. Minimally invasive esophagectomy: thoracoscopic mobilization of the esophagus and mediastinal lymphadenectomy in prone position—experience of 130 patients. J Am Coll Surg. 2006;203(1):7–16.
10. Marks JL, Hofstetter WL. Esophageal reconstruction with alternative conduits. Surg Clin North Am. 2012;92(5):1287–97.
11. Sandbu R, Birgisdottir B, Arvidsson D, Sjostrand U, Rubertsson S. Optimal positive end-expiratory pressure (PEEP) settings in differential lung ventilation during simultaneous unilateral pneumothorax and laparoscopy: an experimental study in pigs. Surg Endosc. 2001;15(12):1478–83. doi:10.1007/s00464-001-9002-0.
12. Bundgaard-Nielsen M, Secher NH, Kehlet H. 'Liberal' vs. 'restrictive' perioperative fluid therapy—a critical assessment of the evidence. Acta Anaesthesiol Scand. 2009;53(7):843–51.
13. Nguyen NT, Dholakia C, Nguyen XM, Reavis K. Outcomes of minimally invasive esophagectomy without pyloroplasty: analysis of 109 cases. Am Surg. 2010;76(10):1135–8.
14. Bagheri R, Fattahi SH, Haghi SZ, Aryana K, Aryanniya A, Akhlaghi S, et al. Botulinum toxin for prevention of delayed gastric emptying after esophagectomy. Asian Cardiovasc Thorac Ann. 2013;21(6):689–92. doi:10.1177/0218492312468438.
15. Blom RL, van Heijl M, Bemelman WA, Hollmann MW, Klinkenbijl JH, Busch OR, et al. Initial experiences of an enhanced recovery protocol in esophageal surgery. World J Surg. 2013;37(10):2372–8. doi:10.1007/s00268-013-2135-1.
16. Caldwell MT, Murphy PG, Page R, Walsh TN, Hennessy TP. Timing of extubation after oesophagectomy. Br J Surg. 1993;80(12):1537–9.
17. Kita T, Mammoto T, Kishi Y. Fluid management and postoperative respiratory disturbances in patients with transthoracic esophagectomy for carcinoma. J Clin Anesth. 2002;14(4):252–6.
18. Slinger PD. Perioperative fluid management for thoracic surgery: the puzzle of postpneumonectomy pulmonary edema. J Cardiothorac Vasc Anesth. 1995; 9(4):442–51.
19. Swanson SJ, Batirel HF, Bueno R, Jaklitsch MT, Lukanich JM, Allred E, et al. Transthoracic esophagectomy with radical mediastinal and abdominal lymph node dissection and cervical esophagogastrostomy for esophageal carcinoma. Ann Thorac Surg. 2001;72(6):1918–24; discussion 24–5.
20. Gutt CN, Oniu T, Wolkener F, Mehrabi A, Mistry S, Buchler MW. Prophylaxis and treatment of deep vein thrombosis in general surgery. Am J Surg. 2005; 189(1):14–22. doi:10.1016/j.amjsurg.2004.04.009.
21. Bratzler DW, Houck PM. Antimicrobial prophylaxis for surgery: an advisory statement from the National Surgical Infection Prevention Project. Am J Surg. 2005; 189(4):395–404. doi:10.1016/j.amjsurg.2005.01.015.
22. Birkmeyer JD, Siewers AE, Finlayson EV, Stukel TA, Lucas FL, Batista I, et al. Hospital volume and surgical mortality in the United States. N Engl J Med. 2002;346(15):1128–37. doi:10.1056/NEJMsa012337.
23. Kelsen DP, Ginsberg R, Pajak TF, Sheahan DG, Gunderson L, Mortimer J, et al. Chemotherapy followed by surgery compared with surgery alone for localized esophageal cancer. N Engl J Med. 1998; 339(27):1979–84. doi:10.1056/nejm199812313392704.
24. Collins G, Johnson E, Kroshus T, Ganz R, Batts K, Seng J, et al. Experience with minimally invasive esophagectomy. Surg Endosc. 2006;20(2):298–301. doi:10.1007/s00464-005-0093-x.

25. Luketich JD, Schauer PR, Christie NA, Weigel TL, Raja S, Fernando HC, et al. Minimally invasive esophagectomy. Ann Thorac Surg. 2000;70(3):906–11; discussion 11–2.
26. Rindani R, Martin CJ, Cox MR. Transhiatal versus Ivor-Lewis oesophagectomy: is there a difference? Aust N Z J Surg. 1999;69(3):187–94.
27. Cassivi SD. Leaks, strictures, and necrosis: a review of anastomotic complications following esophagectomy. Semin Thorac Cardiovasc Surg. 2004;16(2):124–32.
28. Lerut T, Coosemans W, Decker G, De Leyn P, Nafteux P, van Raemdonck D. Anastomotic complications after esophagectomy. Dig Surg. 2002;19(2):92–8. doi:52018.
29. Fok M, Cheng SW, Wong J. Pyloroplasty versus no drainage in gastric replacement of the esophagus. Am J Surg. 1991;162(5):447–52.
30. Burt M, Scott A, Williard WC, Pommier R, Yeh S, Bains MS, et al. Erythromycin stimulates gastric emptying after esophagectomy with gastric replacement: a randomized clinical trial. J Thorac Cardiovasc Surg. 1996;111(3):649–54.
31. Lai FC, Chen L, Tu YR, Lin M, Li X. Prevention of chylothorax complicating extensive esophageal resection by mass ligation of thoracic duct: a random control study. Ann Thorac Surg. 2011;91(6):1770–4. doi:10.1016/j.athoracsur.2011.02.070.

## Key Operative Steps

### Thoracoscopic Dissection

1. Begin dissection below the carina.
2. Incise the mediastinal pleural along the anterior surface of the esophagus and dissect the esophagus on the pericardium and the aorta.
3. Incise the mediastinal pleura along the posterior surface of the esophagus. Place a sponge between the aorta and esophagus to facilitate posterior dissection.
4. Once circumferential dissection is completed, place a penrose drain to retract the esophagus.
5. Control small perforators from aorta with clips or energy device.
6. Dissect all para-esophageal lymph nodes en bloc with the esophagus.
7. Resect thoracic duct en bloc with the esophagus.
8. Subcarinal lymph nodes should be dissected en bloc with the esophagus.
9. Divide the azygos vein with an endostapler.
10. Dissect the upper thoracic esophagus. Ensure complete dissection of the esophagus from the esophageal hiatus to the thoracic inlet.
11. Perform upper mediastinal lymph node dissection.

### Preparation of Gastric Conduit

1. Open the lesser sac and divide up to the hiatus.
2. Start dissection of the greater omentum using an energy device.
3. Divide the short gastric vessels.
4. Divide the left gastric vessels with vascular clips or an endostapler.
5. Dissect the left gastric artery lymph nodes en bloc with the specimen.
6. Perform pyloric drainage procedure or inject Botox into the pylorus.

### Cervical Dissection and Anastomosis

1. Make oblique left neck incision, divide the platysma, and retract the sternocleidomastoid.
2. Divide the middle thyroidal vessels and omohyoid muscle.
3. Retract the thyroid gland medially and dissect the posterior esophagus.
4. Encircle the cervical esophagus with a penrose drain.
5. Perform blunt dissection inferiorly to join dissection plane in the right chest.
6. Construct the gastric conduit and bring up to the neck.
7. Divide the cervical esophagus and perform esophagogastric anastomosis.

# Part II

# Stomach and Duodenum

# Open Distal Gastrectomy

# 6

Callisia Clarke and Brian Badgwell

## Gastric Cancer Overview

Gastric cancer remains a major cause of cancer related death in the United States with adenocarcinoma accounting for 95 % of all cases. Though its overall incidence is decreasing, approximately 22,000 cases are diagnosed annually. Due to advanced disease at diagnosis, over 10,000 patients will die of their disease [1]. Worldwide, the incidence and histology of gastric carcinoma varies with geography. The disease is more prevalent in Eastern Asia and South America when compared to western populations [2].

Lauren described two histologic subtypes of gastric adenocarcinoma, intestinal (well differentiated) and diffuse (undifferentiated) [3]. Over time it has become clear that these subtypes represent separate biologic entities with differing etiologies, epidemiology, and prognosis. In general, the intestinal type is more common in epidemic areas such as Japan and is linked to environmental factors such as diet and chronic *Helicobacter pylori* infection. It is typically seen in older males and affects the distal stomach. Diffuse or infiltrative gastric adenocarcinoma is the predominant subtype seen in North America. It affects younger patients, confers a worse prognosis, and is believed to result primarily from genetic etiologies. In particular, *E-cadherin* germline mutations have been implicated as a major causative factor [3–5].

Surgical resection remains a mainstay in the multidisciplinary approach to the treatment of gastric cancer and remains the only curative option. Advances in chemotherapy and radiation therapy have improved outcomes in resectable patients. However, in patients with advanced disease not amenable to complete surgical resection, they offer only palliative benefits. Studies comparing total gastrectomy and subtotal gastrectomy for distal gastric cancers have demonstrated equivalent overall 5-year survival with a trend toward decreased morbidity and improved quality of life in patients undergoing subtotal resection [6]. As such, distal (i.e., subtotal) gastrectomy is the recommended surgical treatment for cancers of the distal stomach.

## Preoperative Planning

### Diagnosis

Once a diagnosis has been made, the National Comprehensive Cancer Network (NCCN) consensus guidelines for gastric cancer can be utilized as a resource to guide the appropriate workup and management [7]. All patients should undergo a thorough history and physical exam and laboratory evaluation including a complete blood count and chemistry profile. Upper

C. Clarke, M.D. • B. Badgwell, M.D., M.S. (✉)
Department of Surgical Oncology, The University of Texas MD Anderson Cancer Center, 1400 Pressler Street, Houston, TX 77030, USA
e-mail: bbadgwell@mdanderson.org

J. Kim and J. Garcia-Aguilar (eds.), *Surgery for Cancers of the Gastrointestinal Tract: A Step-by-Step Approach*,
DOI 10.1007/978-1-4939-1893-5_6, © Springer Science+Business Media New York 2015

gastrointestinal endoscopy (i.e. esophagogastroduodenoscopy, EGD) with biopsy is the modality of choice for the diagnosis of gastric cancer; it also provides important information regarding the location of the tumor within the stomach in relation to the gastroesophageal (GE) junction and pylorus.

## Staging

The American Joint Commission for Cancer TNM system is the most widely used staging system for gastric cancer; however this is based on final pathologic evaluation [8]. Clinical staging is important with the advent of neoadjuvant and perioperative therapies in the management of gastric cancer. In alignment with NCCN guidelines, radiographic evaluation should include a computed tomography (CT) of the chest, abdomen, and pelvis with oral and intravenous contrast [7]. The use of positron emission tomography (PET)/CT has increased significantly. PET/CT may provide additional information, especially in cases where there is no evidence of metastatic disease. In particular, studies have shown that PET may provide additional insight regarding distant nodal disease and may also prove helpful in the assessment of treatment response in the neoadjuvant setting [9, 10]. Endoscopic ultrasound (EUS) is another valuable tool in the assessment of locoregional disease and is being used routinely at tertiary institutions. While its accuracy may be operator dependent, EUS at high volume centers is able to determine T and N staging with 75–80 % accuracy [11, 12].

## Diagnostic Laparoscopy and Cytology

Despite advances in technology, the accuracy of radiographic evaluation in identifying hepatic metastasis and peritoneal disease in gastric cancer is limited. In one study the accuracy of ultrasound (US) and CT in detecting liver metastasis was only 76 % and 79 %, respectively [13]. Similarly, peritoneal carcinomatosis was only correctly identified by US and CT in 84 % and 81 % of cases, respectively [13]. For this reason, diagnostic laparoscopy plays an essential role in the preoperative workup of all patients with gastric cancer. It is estimated that 23–37 % of patients who are deemed to have localized gastric cancer by preoperative US or CT will be upstaged at the time of diagnostic laparoscopy, thereby sparing a significant number of patients the morbidity of laparotomy [13–16].

Diagnostic laparoscopy may be performed as a separate procedure or just prior to laparotomy. It is proposed that this procedure should follow an "inverted TNM mode" [17]. The first step in staging diagnostic laparoscopy is acquisition of a cytology specimen. It is critical that this be obtained prior to any manipulation of the tumor. If ascites is noted on entering the abdomen, the fluid should be aspirated and sent for cytologic evaluation. In the absence of obvious ascites, peritoneal lavage should be performed with normal saline [17]. The significance of positive peritoneal cytology has been investigated and even in the absence of macroscopic metastatic disease, patients with positive lavage cytology have a prognosis similar to those of patients with documented metastatic disease [18, 19]. Patients with positive cytology are classified as M1 according to the AJCC Cancer Staging Manual, seventh edition [17, 20, 21].

Next, the visceral and peritoneal surfaces should be closely inspected and suspicious areas biopsied and sent for pathology. Careful attention should be paid to the liver, omentum, diaphragms, and ovaries. Perigastric nodes should also be inspected along the lesser and greater curvatures, as well as along the gastrohepatic and hepatic ligaments. Lastly, the stomach should be examined as extraserosal involvement can sometimes be seen in T4 lesions.

## Indications for Distal Gastrectomy

- Diagnosis of gastric adenocarcinoma
- Disease limited to the distal stomach
- Satisfactory performance status
- No evidence of distant disease

## Contraindications to Distal Gastrectomy

- Detection of metastatic disease
- Detection of distant nodal disease
- Positive peritoneal cytology
- Diagnosis of *linitis plastica*

## Surgical Technique

The goals of surgical resection are to achieve negative microscopic margins (i.e., R0 resection) and to perform adequate lymphadenectomy. Gross examination of margins underestimates microscopic disease and studies have demonstrated that in patients with 2 cm of grossly negative gastric margins, almost one third of these patients will have positive microscopic margins [22]. In order to achieve an R0 resection, subtotal gastrectomy with 5–6 cm gastric margins grossly free of disease and a distal margin of at least 2 cm is recommended [22–24]. En bloc resection of involved adjacent organs may also be necessary to achieve complete surgical resection and should be performed whenever possible in the absence of distant metastasis. Finally, NCCN guidelines define adequate lymphadenectomy as ≥15 lymph nodes removed from the perigastric region and along the named vessels of the celiac axis.

### Positioning, Incision, and Exposure

For an open approach to distal gastrectomy, the patient should be placed in the supine position with arms abducted. Subcutaneous heparin should be administered prior to induction and sequential compression devices placed on both lower extremities for deep vein thrombosis prophylaxis. After induction of general anesthesia, a nasogastric tube should be passed into the stomach and placed to suction for decompression. The patient should be securely strapped to the table.

Multiple standard abdominal incisions can be used to access the abdomen. We prefer a generous upper midline incision extending from the xiphoid to below the umbilicus. This allows for excellent exposure of the left upper quadrant and the upper abdomen in general. Other options include a bilateral subcostal (Chevron) incision or left paramedian incision. A self-retaining retracting system is often utilized to facilitate visualization and is particularly helpful in retraction of the liver. In addition, reverse Trendelenburg positioning can further enhance exposure. Some surgeons will perform intraoperative upper endoscopy to help plan surgical resection and the equipment should be available if needed. In patients with metastatic or unresectable disease discovered at the time of surgery, consideration should be given to placement of feeding jejunostomy catheter if the patient has symptoms that indicate inability to tolerate oral intake and the issue of nutritional supplementation has been discussed preoperatively.

### Extent of Lymphadenectomy

There continues to be considerable debate regarding the extent of lymphadenectomy in the treatment of gastric cancer. Gastrectomy with extended (D2) lymphadenectomy is the standard treatment in Japan and many other eastern Asian countries [25]. Japanese centers have reported improved overall survival with extended lymphadenectomy [26, 27]. Western studies have demonstrated improved accuracy in staging and suggest that the added benefit from extensive lymph node dissection is likely due to stage migration [28, 29].

In the United States, a modified D2 lymph node dissection (without pancreatectomy and splenectomy) for gastric cancer is recommended but not required. It has been determined that removal of an adequate number of nodes (≥15) is beneficial for staging purposes. As such, the NCCN guidelines recommend gastrectomy with D1 or a modified D2 lymph node dissection, with the goal of examining at least 15 lymph nodes for patients with localized gastric cancer.

The authors favor a modified D2 lymph dissection and the technique is described below.

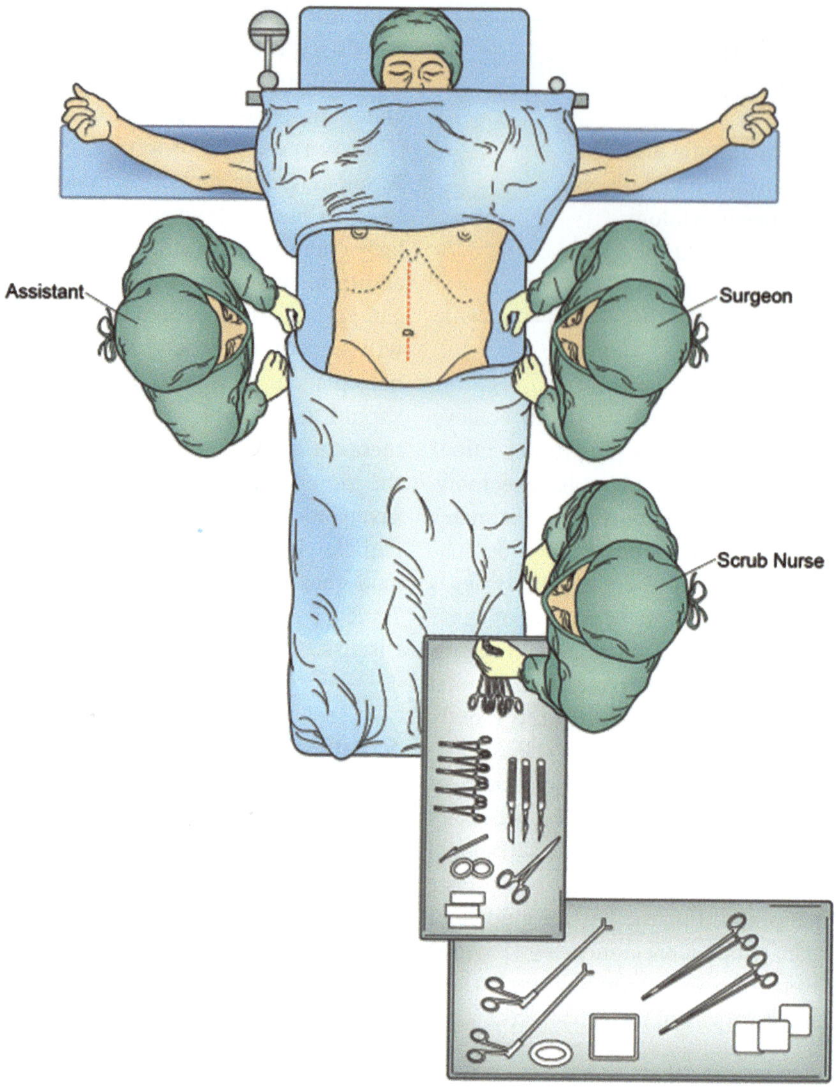


**Fig. 6.1** Operating room setup

## Anatomic Considerations

The extent of gastric resection is dependent on tumor location, but the surgeon should aim for a proximal margin of 5–6 cm that is grossly free of tumor. The surgeon should perform en bloc resection of the greater and lesser omentum and lyse the attachments of the peritoneal leaf of the transverse mesocolon, pancreatic capsule, and lesser sac. We recommend that surgeons perform modified D2 lymphadenectomy with examination of ≥15 nodes.

## Mobilization and Resection

The operating room layout for open distal gastrectomy is outlined in Fig. 6.1. Diagnostic laparoscopy should be performed prior to laparotomy if not already done as a separate procedure. We explore the abdomen for evidence of distant metastases, and assess the involvement of adjacent organs and structures not amenable to resection. Our first maneuver is to enter the lesser sac by dissection along the avascular plane between the greater omentum and the mesentery of the

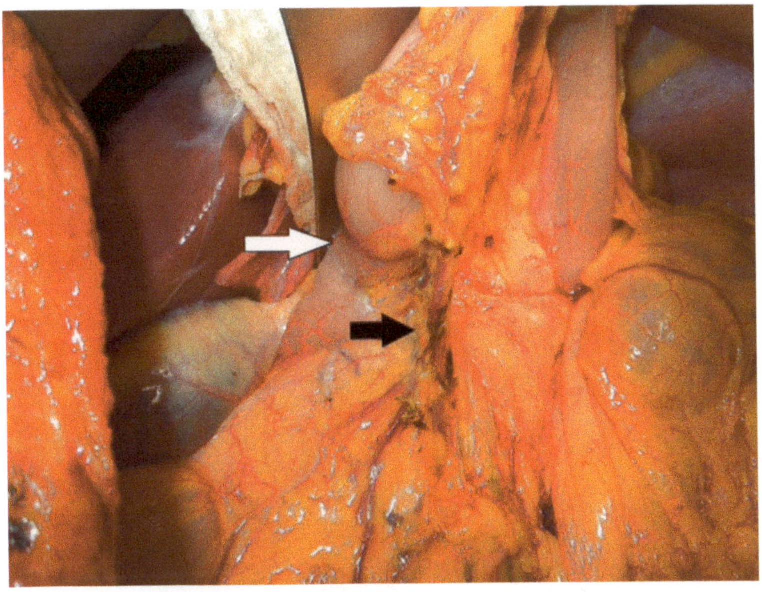

**Fig. 6.2** Right gastroepiploic vessel dissection. The *white arrow* indicates the location of the pylorus and the *black arrow* indicates the gastroepiploic vessels

transverse colon. The greater omentum should be completely mobilized from the transverse colon extending from the hepatic to splenic flexures.

Expose the anterior surface of the pancreas and delineate the superior pancreatic margin until the right gastroepiploic vessels are identified as shown in Fig. 6.2. The vessels should be individually clamped, divided, and ligated close to the gastroduodenal artery. Next, we mobilize the left hepatic lobe by dividing the triangular ligament and taking care to avoid injury of the left phrenic vein. Once the left lateral segment is retracted the lesser omentum will be visualized. We perform lesser omentectomy by removing all the tissue along the lesser curvature from the inferior edge of the hepatoduodenal ligament to the right crus of the diaphragm. The right gastric artery and vein are identified, clamped, transected, and ligated close to the takeoff from the hepatic artery (Fig. 6.3).

We palpate the gastroduodenal junction to assess tumor involvement. If no tumor is present, then the duodenum is divided approximately 2 cm from the pylorus. When the tumor involves the duodenal bulb, care must be taken not to compromise the ampulla of Vater, the common bile duct or the minor papilla. We prefer using a thoracoabdominal (TA) or gastrointestinal anastomosis (GIA) stapler to transect the duodenum as shown in Fig. 6.4. With the duodenum divided, exposure of the nodal tissues along the hepatic artery, celiac axis, and splenic artery is enhanced. We continue our dissection along the superior border of the pancreas taking all the nodal tissues along the common hepatic artery towards the celiac axis. Identify the left gastric vessels and ligate them at their origin (Fig. 6.5). The nodal tissues around the left gastric artery should be removed with the specimen. We identify the splenic artery near its origin and dissect towards the splenic hilum, removing all the nodal tissues with the specimen. The extent of D1 lymphadenectomy for distal gastrectomy includes stations 1, 3, 4 (excluding station 4 nodes along the short gastric vessels which are preserved), 5, 6, and 7; while D2 lymphadenectomy includes the D1 stations along with stations 8, 9, 11, and 12.

The greater omentum is removed from the greater curvature of the stomach taking care to preserve the proximal short gastric arteries that will supply the remnant stomach. A location on the stomach, proximal to the tumor, is identified with the goal of a 5–6 cm margin that is grossly free of tumor. The stomach is divided at this point using a GIA stapler. Frozen section assessment of the surgical margins should be performed to confirm histologically negative margins.

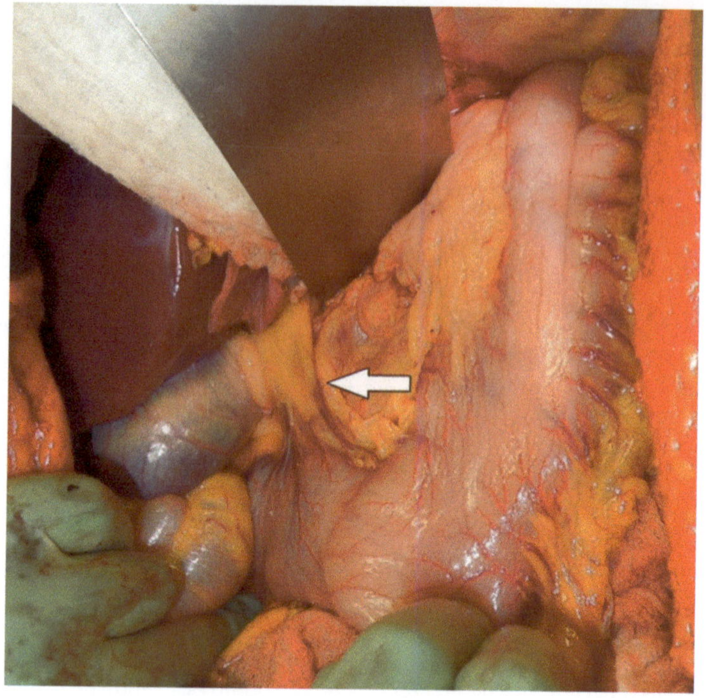

**Fig. 6.3** Right gastric vessels prior to dissection. The *white arrow* indicates the location for dissection of the right gastric vessels

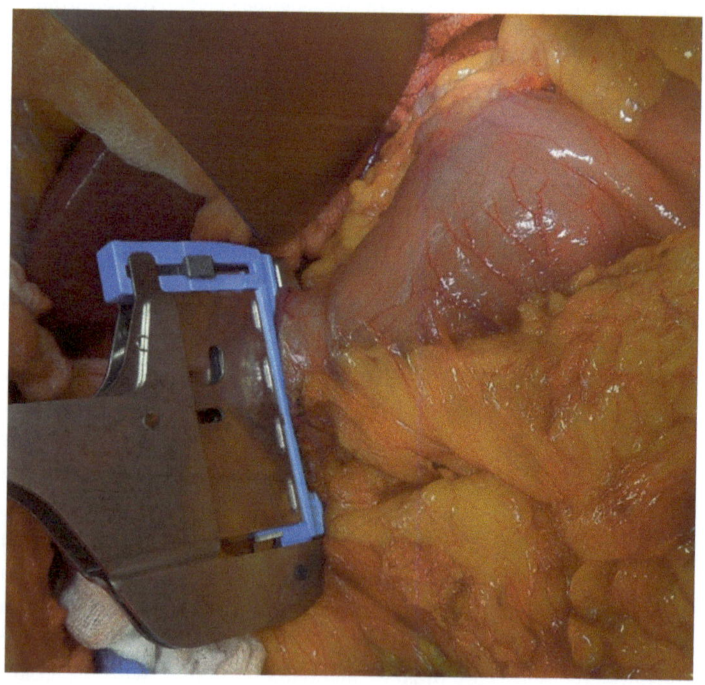

**Fig. 6.4** The image shows the duodenum being divided by a TA stapling device

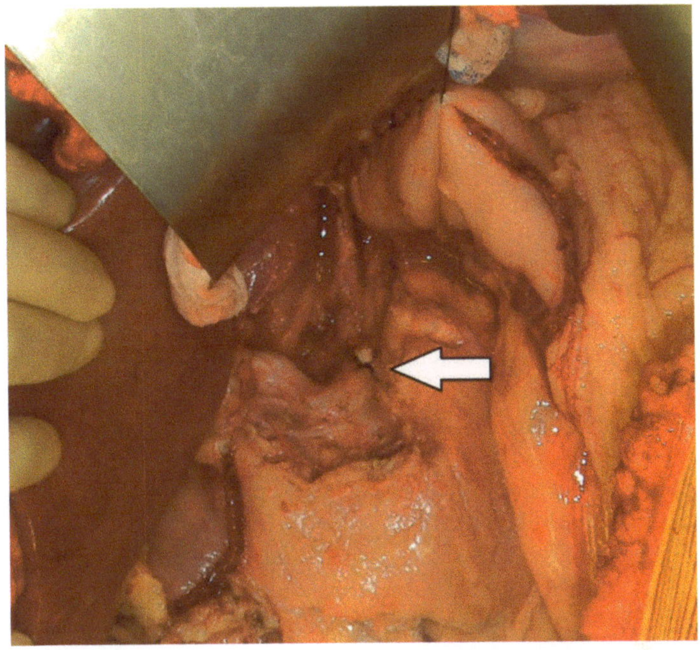

**Fig. 6.5** D2 lymph node dissection with left gastric vessel ligation. The *white arrow* indicates the celiac trunk with suture ligation of the left gastric artery

## Reconstruction with Roux-en-Y Gastrojejunostomy

Several reconstructive methods have been described after distal gastrectomy. Our preferred approach is retrocolic Roux-en-Y gastrojejunostomy. Another commonly used method is Billroth II anastomosis. Both methods are briefly described below.

For reconstruction with Roux-en-Y gastrojejunostomy, the jejunum is divided approximately 20 cm distal to the ligament of Treitz. The transverse colon is retracted up and out of the wound and an avascular window in the mesocolon is identified. A small 4-cm incision is made in the avascular area to the left of the middle colic vessels. The Roux limb is then delivered through the created defect so that the jejunum abuts the gastric remnant without tension. Although the gastrojejunostomy can be either stapled or hand-sewn, we prefer a hand-sewn two-layer anastomosis. The posterior serosal layer is made by placing seromuscular interrupted 3–0 silk sutures in Lembert fashion approximately 5 mm apart, affixing a 4-cm segment of jejunum to the posterior gastric wall. The two corner sutures are tagged with hemostats and used for traction while creating the anastomosis. The remaining silk sutures should be cut. Next, a 4-cm segment of the gastric staple line is removed close to the greater curvature. A similar defect approximately two-thirds the size of the gastric opening is made in the anti-mesenteric wall of the jejunum using electrocautery. The mucosal layer of the anastomosis is created using 3–0 absorbable sutures in a running fashion taking care to incorporate the full thickness of each wall. This inner layer is created by starting in the middle of the posterior mucosal wall and running the suture in both directions until they meet at the anterior surface to create a circumferential watertight anastomosis. A Connell technique can be used starting at each turning corner to ensure that the mucosa is inverted. Finally, an anterior serosal layer of 3–0 silk sutures with seromuscular bites taken in Lembert fashion imbricates the anterior mucosal layer and completes the anastomosis. To prevent internal hernias, the wall of the Roux limb is secured to the mesocolon at its point of entry into the retrocolic space and any remaining defect can be closed. A jejunojejunostomy is then created using the same two-layered hand-sewn technique described above. The proximal jejunum is anastomosed to the Roux limb approximately 60 cm from the gastrojejunostomy. Again, the mesenteric defects of the jejunal limbs are closed by reapproximating the cut edges of the mesentery.

## Reconstruction with Billroth II Gastrojejunostomy

Again our method of choice for a retrocolic Billroth II reconstruction is a two-layered hand-sewn anastomosis. A loop of jejunum is brought up through the created window in the avascular portion of the transverse mesocolon so that the gastric remnant is approximately 20 cm from the ligament of Treitz. A hand-sewn gastrojejunostomy can be created using the techniques described above for Roux-en-Y gastrojejunostomy. We do not advocate the routine placement of drains unless there is concern for possible pancreatic leak or injury. If necessary a 19-French Blake drain is exteriorized through a separate incision.

## Postoperative Management

- Day of surgery: Deep breathing exercises and aggressive pulmonary toilet are initiated.
- Postoperative day #1: Early ambulation is started. Intravenous fluids are changed to maintenance rate if the patient is euvolemic.
- Postoperative day #2: The nasogastric tube is discontinued. The patient remains nil per os (NPO). The sterile dressing is removed. Tube feedings are initiated if a jejunostomy tube was placed at the time of surgery. We recommend starting at a low rate of 10–20 mL/h and slowly increasing as tolerated over the next few days or once the patient has return of bowel function. Careful attention should be paid to complaints of abdominal cramping and/or distention.
- Postoperative day #3: The patient is started on a clear liquid diet.
- Postoperative day #4: The diet is advanced over the next 24–48 h to a postgastrectomy diet. Once tolerating full liquid or postgastrectomy diet, transition to oral medications is completed and intravenous fluids are discontinued.
- Postoperative day #5–6: The morning dose of heparin is held and the epidural is discontinued. The urinary catheter is discontinued 6 h later.
- The patient meets criteria for discharge when: (1) ambulating, (2) pain is controlled on oral pain medications, and (3) tolerating postgastrectomy diet while meeting caloric goals by eating or by supplemental enteral feeds.
- If a drainage catheter was placed at the time of surgery, a serum and drain amylase concentration should be obtained once the patient is tolerating a diet. If the output is non-bilious and there is no chemical evidence of pancreatic leak (drain amylase <3× serum amylase), then the drain can be removed.

## Complications

### Early Postoperative Complications

The most frequent complications encountered after distal gastrectomy are those seen in any patient undergoing major abdominal surgery. These include postoperative bleeding, wound infection, pneumonia, deep venous thrombosis, and urinary tract infection. Complications specific to distal gastrectomy include delayed gastric emptying, duodenal stump leak, gastrojejunostomy leak/obstruction, and jejunojejunal anastomotic leak/obstruction. Anastomotic leaks are associated with a high morbidity and mortality if left unrecognized. The key to management is early diagnosis and intervention. Symptoms may include fever, abdominal pain, distention, tachycardia, and laboratory abnormalities such as leukocytosis or acidosis. Most anastomotic leaks can be managed nonoperatively. However, duodenal stump leaks often require surgical intervention.

## Late Postoperative Complications

Late complications are usually due to reconstruction and may require surgical intervention for resolution of symptoms. They include anastomotic stricture, internal hernia, dumping syndrome, and afferent or efferent loop syndromes.

## Surveillance

NCCN guidelines state that all patients should be followed closely after surgical resection. They recommend a complete history and physical exam every 3–6 months for 1–2 years, every 6–12 months for 3–5 years, and then annually. There is no specific recommendation for frequency of imaging studies. Our practice is to repeat CT scan of the chest, abdomen, and pelvis every 6 months for 5 years.

## Conclusion

Distal/subtotal gastrectomy remains the surgery of choice for gastric cancers of the distal stomach. It can be safely performed with excellent outcomes if the principles of appropriate patient selection, sound preoperative planning, and good surgical technique are adhered.

## References


1. Siegel R, Naishadham D, Jemal A. Cancer statistics, 2013. CA Cancer J Clin. 2013;63(1):11–30. doi:10.3322/caac.21166.
2. Jemal A, Bray F, Center MM, Ferlay J, Ward E, Forman D. Global cancer statistics. CA Cancer J Clin. 2011;61(2):69–90. doi:10.3322/caac.20107.
3. Lauren P. The two histological main types of gastric carcinoma: diffuse and so-called intestinal-type carcinoma. An attempt at a histo-clinical classification. Acta Pathol Microbiol Scand. 1965;64:31–49.
4. Shah MA, Khanin R, Tang L, Janjigian YY, Klimstra DS, Gerdes H, et al. Molecular classification of gastric cancer: a new paradigm. Clin Cancer Res. 2011;17(9):2693–701. doi:10.1158/1078-0432.CCR-10-2203.
5. Carneiro F, Huntsman DG, Smyrk TC, Owen DA, Seruca R, Pharoah P, et al. Model of the early development of diffuse gastric cancer in E-cadherin mutation carriers and its implications for patient screening. J Pathol. 2004;203(2):681–7. doi:10.1002/path.1564.
6. Bozzetti F, Marubini E, Bonfanti G, Miceli R, Piano C, Gennari L. Subtotal versus total gastrectomy for gastric cancer: five-year survival rates in a multicenter randomized Italian trial. Italian Gastrointestinal Tumor Study Group. Ann Surg. 1999;230(2):170–8.
7. Ajani JA, Bentrem DJ, Besh S, D'Amico TA, Das P, Denlinger C, et al. Gastric cancer, version 2.2013: featured updates to the NCCN Guidelines. J Natl Compr Canc Netw. 2013;11(5):531–46.
8. Washington K. 7th edition of the AJCC cancer staging manual: stomach. Ann Surg Oncol. 2010;17(12):3077–9. doi:10.1245/s10434-010-1362-z.
9. Chen J, Cheong JH, Yun MJ, Kim J, Lim JS, Hyung WJ, et al. Improvement in preoperative staging of gastric adenocarcinoma with positron emission tomography. Cancer. 2005;103(11):2383–90. doi:10.1002/cncr.21074.
10. Kole AC, Plukker JT, Nieweg OE, Vaalburg W. Positron emission tomography for staging of oesophageal and gastroesophageal malignancy. Br J Cancer. 1998;78(4):521–7.
11. Willis S, Truong S, Gribnitz S, Fass J, Schumpelick V. Endoscopic ultrasonography in the preoperative staging of gastric cancer: accuracy and impact on surgical therapy. Surg Endosc. 2000;14(10):951–4.
12. Karpeh Jr MS, Brennan MF. Gastric carcinoma. Ann Surg Oncol. 1998;5(7):650–6.
13. Stell DA, Carter CR, Stewart I, Anderson JR. Prospective comparison of laparoscopy, ultrasonography and computed tomography in the staging of gastric cancer. Br J Surg. 1996;83(9):1260–2.
14. Lowy AM, Mansfield PF, Leach SD, Ajani J. Laparoscopic staging for gastric cancer. Surgery. 1996;119(6):611–4.
15. Kriplani AK, Kapur BM. Laparoscopy for preoperative staging and assessment of operability in gastric carcinoma. Gastrointest Endosc. 1991;37(4):441–3.
16. Burke EC, Karpeh MS, Conlon KC, Brennan MF. Laparoscopy in the management of gastric adenocarcinoma. Ann Surg. 1997;225(3):262–7.
17. D'Ugo DM, Pende V, Persiani R, Rausei S, Picciocchi A. Laparoscopic staging of gastric cancer: an overview. J Am Coll Surg. 2003;196(6):965–74. doi:10.1016/S1072-7515(03)00126-1.
18. Ribeiro Jr U, Safatle-Ribeiro AV, Zilberstein B, Mucerino D, Yagi OK, Bresciani CC, et al. Does the intraoperative peritoneal lavage cytology add prognostic information in patients with potentially curative gastric resection? J Gastrointest Surg. 2006;10(2):170–6. doi:10.1016/j.gassur.2005.11.001; discussion 6–7.
19. Ribeiro Jr U, Gama-Rodrigues JJ, Bitelman B, Ibrahim RE, Safatle-Ribeiro AV, Laudanna AA, et al. Value of peritoneal lavage cytology during laparoscopic staging of patients with gastric carcinoma. Surg Laparosc Endosc. 1998;8(2):132–5.
20. Ribeiro Jr U, Gama-Rodrigues JJ, Safatle-Ribeiro AV, Bitelman B, Ibrahim RE, Ferreira MB, et al. Prognostic significance of intraperitoneal free cancer

cells obtained by laparoscopic peritoneal lavage in patients with gastric cancer. J Gastrointest Surg. 1998;2(3):244–9.
21. Bryan RT, Cruickshank NR, Needham SJ, Moffitt DD, Young JA, Hallissey MT, et al. Laparoscopic peritoneal lavage in staging gastric and oesophageal cancer. Eur J Surg Oncol. 2001;27(3):291–7. doi:10.1053/ejso.2001.1113.
22. Papachristou DN, Agnanti N, D'Agostino H, Fortner JG. Histologically positive esophageal margin in the surgical treatment of gastric cancer. Am J Surg. 1980;139(5):711–3.
23. Bozzetti F, Bonfanti G, Bufalino R, Menotti V, Persano S, Andreola S, et al. Adequacy of margins of resection in gastrectomy for cancer. Ann Surg. 1982;196(6):685–90.
24. Bozzetti F. Principles of surgical radicality in the treatment of gastric cancer. Surg Oncol Clin N Am. 2001;10(4):833–54, ix.
25. Japanese Gastric Cancer Association. Japanese gastric cancer treatment guidelines 2010 (ver. 3). Gastric Cancer. 2011;14(2):113–23. doi:10.1007/s10120-011-0042-4.
26. Otsuji E, Kuriu Y, Ichikawa D, Okamoto K, Hagiwara A, Yamagishi H. Characteristics of gastric carcinoma invading the muscularis propria. J Surg Oncol. 2005;92(2):104–8. doi:10.1002/jso.20345.
27. Nakamura K, Ueyama T, Yao T, Xuan ZX, Ambe K, Adachi Y, et al. Pathology and prognosis of gastric carcinoma. Findings in 10,000 patients who underwent primary gastrectomy. Cancer. 1992;70(5):1030–7.
28. Schwarz RE, Smith DD. Clinical impact of lymphadenectomy extent in resectable gastric cancer of advanced stage. Ann Surg Oncol. 2007;14(2):317–28. doi:10.1245/s10434-006-9218-2.
29. Smith DD, Schwarz RR, Schwarz RE. Impact of total lymph node count on staging and survival after gastrectomy for gastric cancer: data from a large US-population database. J Clin Oncol. 2005;23(28):7114–24. doi:10.1200/JCO.2005.14.621.

## Key Operative Steps

1. Enter the lesser sac through the avascular plane between the omentum and transverse colon.
2. Mobilize the greater omentum from the transverse colon to the splenic flexure.
3. Expose the anterior surface of the pancreas.
4. Clamp and ligate the right gastroepiploic vessels.
5. Mobilize and retract the left hepatic lobe.
6. Perform lesser omentectomy up to the right crus.
7. Clamp and ligate the right gastric artery and vein.
8. Divide the duodenum with a TA stapler.
9. Dissect lymphatic tissues along the superior border of the pancreas from the common hepatic artery towards the celiac axis.
10. Clamp and ligate the left gastric vessels. Remove the nodal tissue around the artery.
11. Identify the splenic artery near its origin and dissect towards the splenic hilum, removing all the lymphatic tissue with the specimen.
12. Resect the greater omentum and ensure preservation of proximal short gastric arteries.
13. Divide the stomach with 5–6 cm gross margins.
14. Reconstruct with retrocolic Roux-en-Y or Billroth II gastrojejunostomy.
15. Close sites of potential internal hernia.

# 7 Laparoscopic Distal/Subtotal Gastrectomy

John B. Hamner and Joseph Kim

## Introduction

Worldwide, gastric cancer remains a deadly disease as the fourth most common malignancy [1, 2]. Approximately 95 % of these gastric cancers are adenocarcinomas and the remaining 5 % are a mix of gastrointestinal stromal tumors (GIST), neuroendocrine tumors, and lymphomas. These add up to a yearly incidence of gastric cancer of over one million cases [1]. Although this is a major health concern throughout the world, there is considerable worldwide variation in the incidence and outcomes of gastric cancer. It is the most commonly diagnosed malignancy in Asian countries such as South Korea and Japan, whereas it is far less common in the United States and European nations [3].

Regardless where gastric cancer is diagnosed, surgical intervention remains the only option for cure in patients with early stage disease. Standard surgical therapy (i.e., gastrectomy) entails complete en bloc resection of the tumor, adjacent organ that directly involved, and lymphadenectomy. Specifically, a 5-cm surgical margin and D2 lymph node dissection is the standard for curative intent surgical intervention [4]. For many years, the operation has been primarily performed via open laparotomy. With technical advances and evolving surgical techniques, more curative operations are now being performed by minimally invasive approaches. In this chapter, we describe a step-by-step approach to performing laparoscopic distal gastrectomy for adenocarcinoma of the stomach.

## Historical Perspective

The first reported laparoscopic approach to gastrectomy dates back to 1992, when surgeons from Singapore performed a laparoscopic distal gastrectomy with Billroth II reconstruction for a bleeding gastric ulcer in a 76-year-old patient [5]. The operation was successful, taking 4 h to complete and requiring 17 linear stapler loads [6]. The patient was uneventfully discharged home on the 5th postoperative day. The report of this initial operation was followed by Azagra and colleagues who performed the first laparoscopic gastrectomy for cancer; and they subsequently published the first series of laparoscopic gastrectomy for malignancy [7, 8]. Over the next decade, advances in laparoscopic techniques and equipment such as high definition video monitors, angled laparoscopes, and thermal energy dissecting/coagulating instruments have facilitated

Electronic supplementary material: Supplementary material is available in the online version of this chapter at 10.1007/978-1-4939-1893-5_7. Videos can also be accessed at http://www.springerimages.com/videos/978-1-4939-1892-8.

J.B. Hamner, M.D., F.A.C.S.
J. Kim, M.D., F.A.C.S. (✉)
Division of Surgical Oncology, City of Hope, 1500 East Duarte Road, Duarte, CA 91010, USA
e-mail: jokim@coh.org

J. Kim and J. Garcia-Aguilar (eds.), *Surgery for Cancers of the Gastrointestinal Tract: A Step-by-Step Approach*,
DOI 10.1007/978-1-4939-1893-5_7, © Springer Science+Business Media New York 2015

the safe performance of an increasing number of these procedures. However, one of the major limitations of minimal access surgery was the technically demanding performance of extended lymphadenectomy. The feasibility of laparoscopic lymphadenectomy was first reported in 1999 by Uyama et al. for cancers of the distal third of the stomach [9]. Currently, the number of laparoscopic operations for gastric cancer have increased dramatically, particularly in Asian countries such as Japan and South Korea. In Japan alone, more than 4,500 laparoscopic gastric cancer operations are performed yearly [10].

## Indications

The diagnosis of early gastric cancer in itself is an indication for surgery, but the decision to proceed with laparoscopic or open surgery should be weighed carefully. There are several considerations that must be given to each individual patient. First, it is well established that the laparoscopic approach requires longer operative time than the open operation. In our experience, open distal gastrectomy with extended lymphadenectomy can be completed in approximately 1½ h, whereas the corresponding laparoscopic procedure will typically require 3–3½ h to complete. Since patients with medical comorbidities may warrant short anesthesia times, an open procedure may be preferred. Second, minimally invasive surgical instruments, even when used with advanced skills, can damage fragile tissues. In patients >80 years old we have observed the tissues to be more fragile and susceptible to injury with laparoscopic instruments. In these patients, we favor using open surgical techniques. In most other patients with gastric cancer, our preference is to perform the procedure laparoscopically. Our approach is supported by data showing that laparoscopic operations are associated with less blood loss, quicker return of bowel function, and fewer overall complications [10].

## Anatomic Considerations

While detailed anatomic descriptions of the stomach are found elsewhere, a brief review of the arterial supply and lymphatic drainage of the stomach is important. The major arterial branches that supply the stomach are key landmarks for gastrectomy and lymphadenectomy. The stomach's rich arterial blood supply originates primarily from branches of the celiac axis/trunk (Fig. 7.1). The celiac axis arises directly from the aorta and immediately gives off its three branches: (1) the left gastric artery, (2) the common hepatic artery and (3) the splenic artery. The left gastric artery supplies primarily the lesser curvature of the stomach and the gastroesophageal junction. The splenic artery courses behind the superior border of the pancreas and its branches include the short gastric vessels and the left gastroepiploic artery, which supply much of the greater curvature of the stomach. Finally, the major branches of the common hepatic artery include the right gastric artery that supplies the lesser curvature and the pylorus and the gastroduodenal artery that joins the right gastroepiploic artery to supply the greater curvature of the stomach. Venous drainage of the stomach typically follows the arterial network, emptying into the portal venous system via the splenic, superior mesenteric, and portal veins. Identification of the coronary vein adjacent to the left gastric artery is critical to prevent inadvertent injury. This vein may empty directly into the portal vein and failure to identify and ligate this vessel appropriately can result in brisk and troublesome bleeding.

The stomach has an extensive network of lymphatic channels, which is the most common site of extra-gastric disease spread. According to the Japanese Classification of Gastric Carcinoma [11], there are 33 lymphatic stations providing drainage of the stomach (Fig. 7.1). The extent of lymphadenectomy or lack thereof (i.e., D0, D1, or D2) is defined by the nodal stations removed. A D0 lymphadenectomy involves "shelling out" the stomach without removal of the adjacent

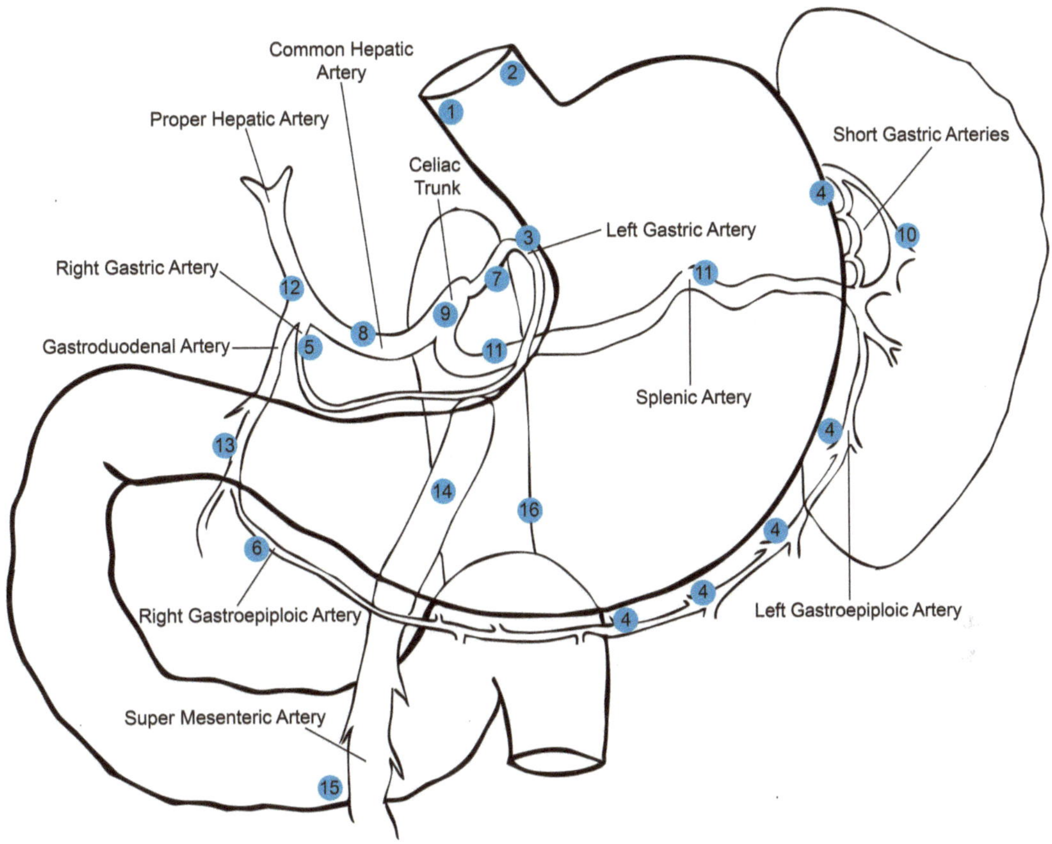


**Fig. 7.1** This figure demonstrates the major arteries that must be identified during laparoscopic distal gastrectomy as well as the lymph node stations according to the Japanese Classification of Gastric Carcinoma

lymphatic tissues. D1 lymphadenectomy involves harvesting all of the perigastric lymph node stations along the lesser and greater curvatures of the stomach. Specifically, these are the pericardial nodes (station 1), nodes along the lesser curvature (station 3), nodes along the short gastric and gastroepiploic vessels (stations 4a and 4b), the nodes along the pyloric channel (stations 5 and 6), and nodes at the left gastric artery (station 7). The D2 nodal stations include the D1 stations as well as the lymphatic tissues along the proximal common hepatic artery (station 8), the celiac trunk (station 9), the splenic artery (station 11), and hepatoduodenal ligament (station 12). Knowledge of these lymphatic stations is important for oncologically sound gastrectomy. In our practice, we routinely perform what is termed a D1 + β dissection for distal gastric cancers. This is a modification of the classic D2 lymphadenectomy that omits splenectomy and dissection of lymphatic tissues along the distal splenic artery or splenic hilum.

## Preoperative Considerations

After the diagnosis of gastric cancer has been obtained, several steps are necessary prior to surgery. This includes a staging workup consisting of endoscopic ultrasound and computed tomography of the chest, abdomen, and pelvis to evaluate the extent of disease and to rule out distant metastasis. Once early gastric cancer has been confirmed, cardiac clearance is obtained as indicated in the elderly and in patients with serious comorbidities. Other laboratory tests are performed as indicated based on each individual patient's needs. Once the preoperative evaluation has been completed, the patient is ready for surgery. We maintain the patient on *nil per os* after midnight on the evening prior to surgery with the daytime diet limited to clear liquids. No other bowel prep is administered.

## Surgical Technique

### Patient Positioning and Setup

After transport to the operating room, the patient is placed in the supine position on the operating table. We do not use lithotomy position for gastrectomy. Prior to induction of general endotracheal anesthesia, sequential compression devices are placed on the bilateral lower extremities and intravenous antibiotics are administered. After endotracheal intubation, a Foley catheter and orogastric tubes are placed. We do not place central venous catheters, although radial artery catheters are often placed to facilitate accurate hemodynamic monitoring. Once these initial steps have been completed, both arms are tucked and the abdomen is prepped and covered with an Ioban drape.

The attending surgeon with the assistance of the surgical oncology fellow typically performs the procedure. The operating surgeon stands on the patient's left side and the assistant and scrub technician stand on the right. Video monitors are placed above either side of the patient's head at the operating surgeon's eye level providing equal visualization to both the operating surgeon and the assistant (Fig. 7.2). Finally, the patient is placed at 30-degree reverse Trendelenburg position, which allows gravity to retract organs to better visualize key structures.

### Instruments

When performing laparoscopic distal gastrectomy, appropriate minimally invasive equipment is mandatory. Small and medium-sized Weck™ (Teleflex Inc., Research Triangle Park, NC) clips are used for ligation of relatively large blood vessels encountered during gastrectomy. Much of the dissection, however, can be performed with energy sealant devices. We frequently use an energy dissector that also features monopolar electrocautery. A laparoscopic liver retractor is routinely used to retract the left lateral segment of the liver, and laparoscopic linear stapling devices are used for division of the duodenum and stomach and for creation of the gastrojejunal anastomosis. We use the Endostitch™ (Covidien Inc. Mansfield, MA) device to close the common channel of the gastrojejunostomy. Finally, a sterile extraction bag is introduced through a 12-mm port and used to remove the specimen from the peritoneal cavity.

### Trocar Placement

Five trocars are used to perform the laparoscopic distal gastrectomy. They are placed in a semi-elliptical pattern with the base of the ellipse at the umbilicus (Fig. 7.3). We employ three 10/12-mm trocars and two 5-mm trocars. The first trocar is a 10/12-mm trocar in the midline just below the umbilicus that is placed via the Hasson technique. Occasionally, the peritoneal cavity is first accessed with a Veress needle at Palmer's point in the left upper quadrant. After the first trocar is placed, the abdomen is insufflated to 15 mmHg and the remaining bladed trocars are placed under direct visualization. The two 5-mm trocars are placed a hand's breadth apart to the right of the midline. One 5-mm trocar is placed directly to the right of the peri-umbilical trocar and the second 5-mm trocar is placed in the lateral aspect of the right upper quadrant. The remaining two 10/12-mm trocars are placed to the left of the umbilicus mirroring the positions of the trocars on the right side of the abdomen.

### Diagnostic Laparoscopy

Once the initial trocar is placed at the umbilicus, the abdomen is explored with a 10-mm, 30-degree angled laparoscope to confirm the absence of metastatic disease. Some centers routinely obtain peritoneal washings for cytologic examination.

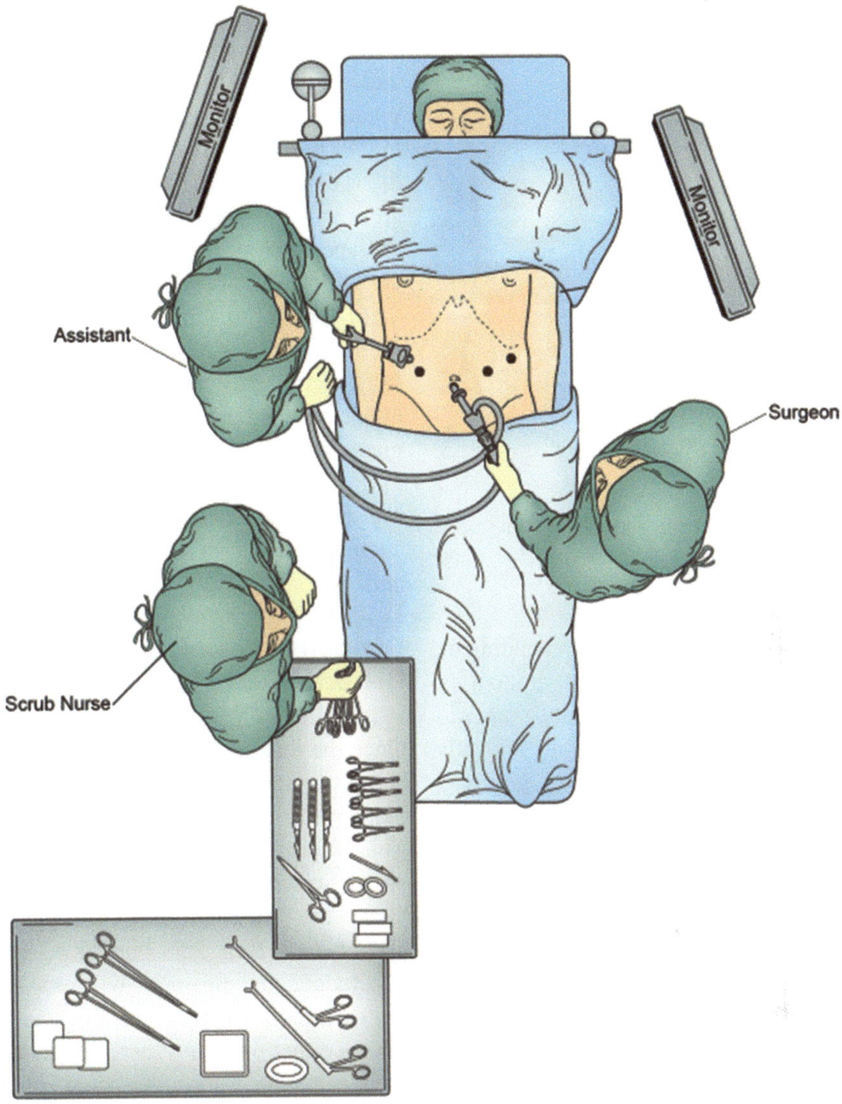


**Fig. 7.2** Patient positioning and operating room setup

Although these washings may be performed [4], we have observed an extremely low number of locoregional or peritoneal recurrences in our institutional experience that does not justify the routine performance of peritoneal washings. On initial inspection of the abdomen, the peritoneal surfaces are carefully examined. This allows the surgeon to rule out peritoneal seeding and carcinomatosis. The hemidiaphragms, liver, and pelvis are also inspected since these locations are common sites for metastasis to occur.

## Initial Mobilization of the Stomach and Division of the Duodenum

Mobilization of the stomach begins by dividing the gastrocolic ligament. The omentum is retracted cephalad and upward toward the anterior abdominal wall. The avascular embryonic fusion plane between the omentum and transverse colon is identified and divided to enter the lesser sac. Once the proper plane is identified, the omentum is completely mobilized off of the

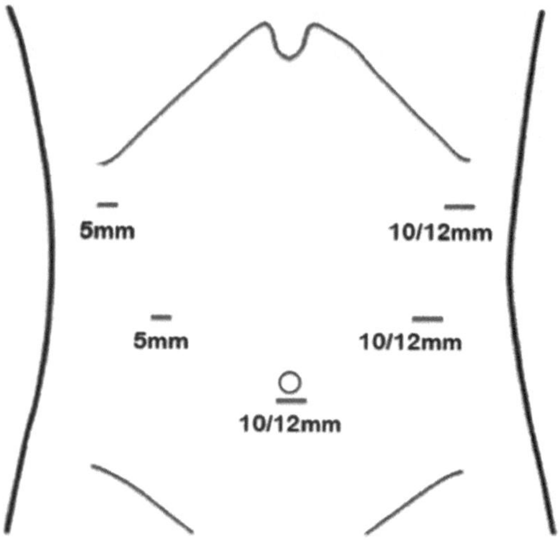


**Fig. 7.3** Trocar placement using three 10/12-mm trocars and two 5-mm trocars

transverse colon from right to left. Depending on the patient's body habitus and the amount of intra-abdominal fat, this first step can be particularly difficult, but it is critical for an oncologically sound operation. Of note, we use the Ligasure™ (Covidien Inc. Mansfield, MA) device for this step, but other energy devices may be used.

The stomach is then lifted upward and posterior attachments between the stomach and pancreas are divided. We do not routinely dissect the anterior leaflet of the transverse mesocolon nor do we resect the capsule of the pancreas (i.e., omental bursectomy). After disease in the lesser sac has been excluded, we then perform intraoperative esophagogastroduodenoscopy (EGD). This procedure, by the primary surgeon or assistant, is always performed to confirm the location of the tumor and to mark the point of transection of the stomach. An atraumatic bowel clamp is used to occlude the proximal jejunum near the ligament of Treitz and the endoscope is passed into the stomach. Once the tumor is identified endoscopically, the serosal surface of the stomach is marked with cautery 5 cm proximal to the tumor to allow adequate margins.

After EGD has been completed, mobilization of the stomach continues. The omentum along the greater curvature of the stomach is mobilized up to the level of the proposed line of transection. Then, our attention is turned to fully mobilizing the distal stomach. The right gastroepiploic artery and vein (Fig. 7.4) terminate near the distal greater curvature of the stomach at the inferior border of the pancreatic neck. This vascular bundle is dissected close to the substance of the pancreas and the lymphatic tissues are swept toward the specimen. The right gastroepiploic vessels are ligated using Weck clips. The division of these vessels leads to a plane for subsequent transection of the duodenum. The duodenum is carefully encircled by creating a plane posterior to the duodenum and opening the hepatoduodenal ligament. We use the vein of Mayo as the landmark to ensure that we are distal to the pylorus. We transect the duodenum using a linear stapler with a tan cartridge.

## Division of Vessels and Lymph Node Dissection

Once the duodenum has been divided, the stomach is retracted cephalad and to the left. These maneuvers expose the gastroduodenal artery. This landmark helps to identify the right gastric artery, which is located in the fatty tissues that tether the proximal duodenum/pylorus to the porta hepatis (Fig. 7.5). Further dissection of the hepatoduodenal ligament will expose the right gastric artery, which is typically small enough to divide either with an energy sealant device or with surgical clips. We then proceed with dissection of the gastrohepatic ligament, which exposes the common hepatic artery. The proximal segment of this artery is skeletonized and the nodal tissues are swept toward the specimen. The entire length of the gastrohepatic ligament is divided and often requires placement of the laparoscopic liver retractor. The ligament is divided up to the right crus of the diaphragm near the gastroesophageal junction. This ensures complete lymphadenectomy at station 1. The surgeon must be cognizant that a replaced or accessory left hepatic artery may course through the gastrohepatic ligament. When this anatomic variant is encountered in the setting of normal liver function, the artery and its associated nodal tissue

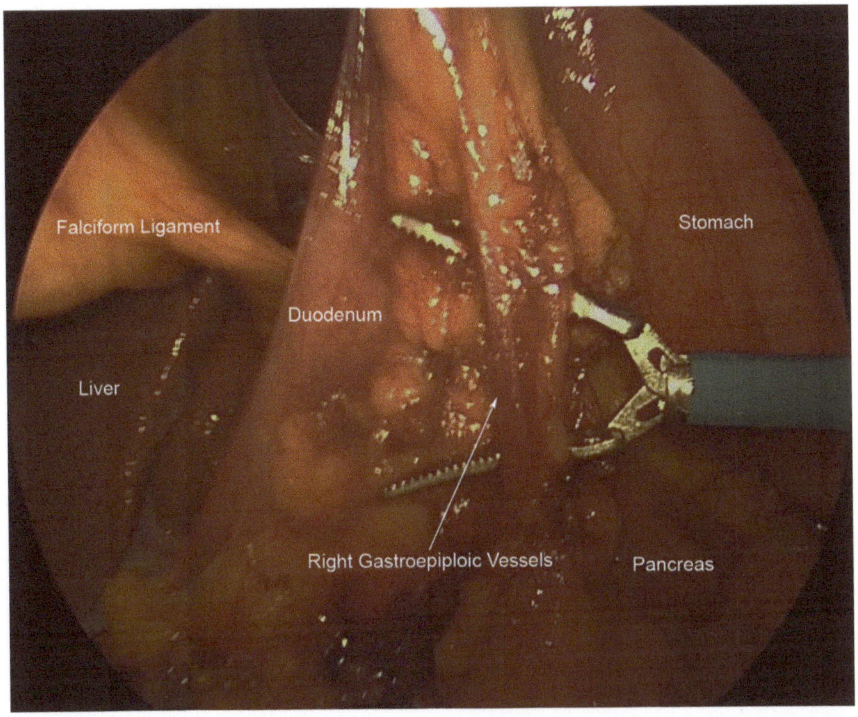


**Fig. 7.4** Laparoscopic view of the right gastroepiploic vascular bundle

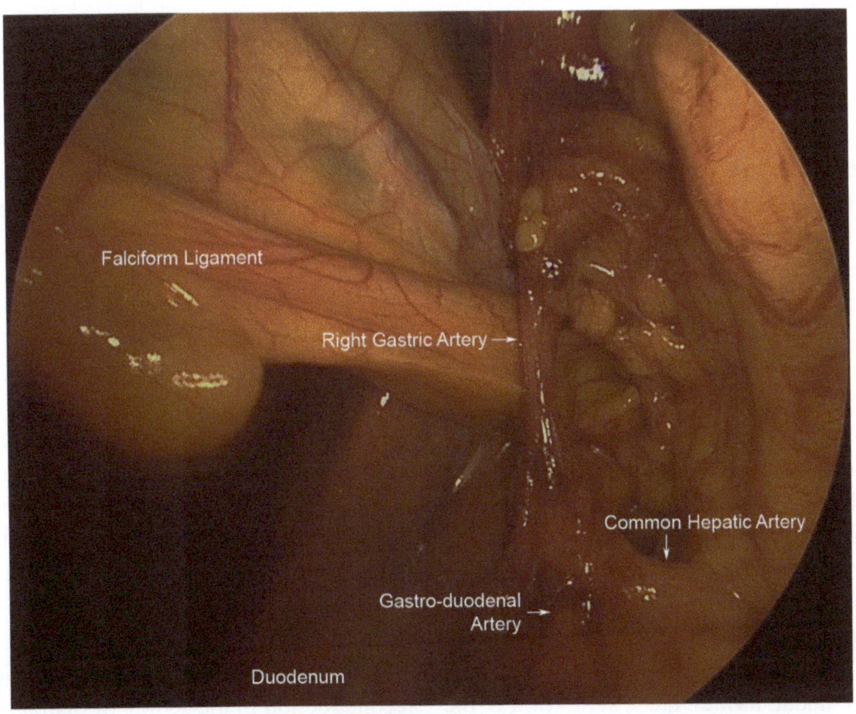


**Fig. 7.5** View of the right gastric artery. Also visualized are the stapled end of the duodenal stump, the common hepatic artery, and the take off of the gastroduodenal artery

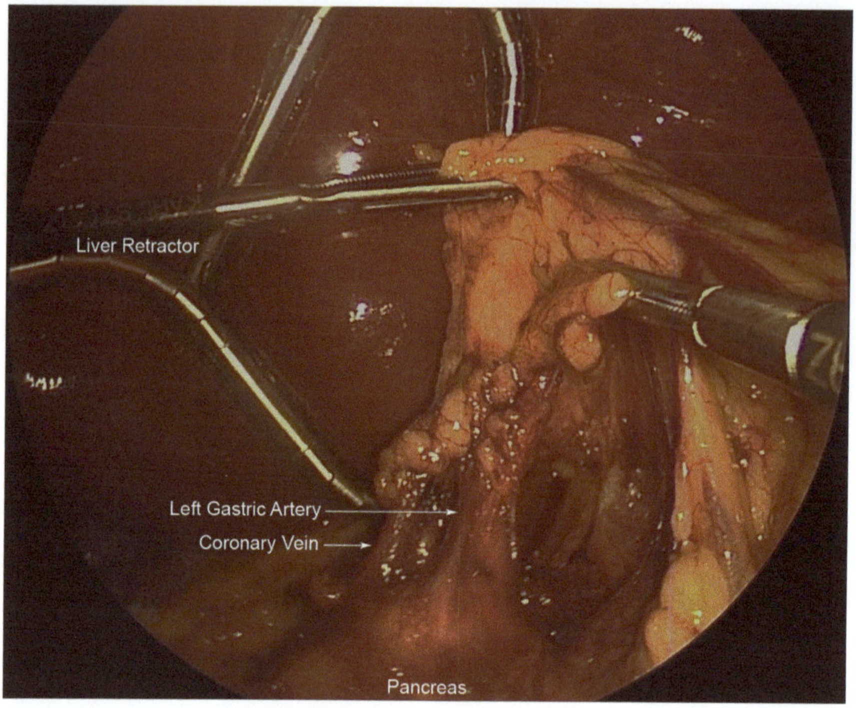


**Fig. 7.6** Laparoscopic view of the coronary vein (*small arrow*) and left gastric artery (*large arrow*)

must be sacrificed and taken with the specimen. Collateral blood flow via the portal system and right hepatic artery will provide adequate oxygenation to the left lobe of the liver. Failure to sacrifice this artery will compromise the oncologic integrity of the operation.

Next, we begin dissection at the superior border of the pancreas with gentle caudal retraction of the pancreas. The anterior to posterior identification of structures helps to expose the proximal common hepatic nodal tissues (station 8) and the celiac axis. It is during this dissection that the coronary vein is identified to the right of the left gastric vessels (Fig. 7.6). Attention should be paid to identify the takeoff of all three branches: the left gastric artery, the common hepatic artery, and the splenic artery. Proper identification of these branches will help avoid the catastrophic complication of ligating the celiac axis. Following this, the left gastric artery is encircled and its associated nodal tissues are swept toward the specimen. The vascular bundle is divided near its origin with Weck clips. We then dissect the lymphatic tissues along the superior border of the pancreatic body exposing the proximal splenic artery. This completes our lymphadenectomy.

## Proximal Transection of the Stomach and Anastomosis

The proposed line of transection for gastrectomy was marked during the intraoperative EGD procedure. We transect the stomach with serial firings of the linear stapler with thick tissue cartridges. This typically requires 2–3 cartridges to completely transect the stomach. Once completed, one of the 10/12-mm trocars is removed and a 15-mm sterile retrieval bag is placed into the abdomen. The specimen is placed into the bag which is temporarily left in the peritoneal cavity until gastrointestinal continuity has been restored.

We prefer the Billroth II over the Billroth I reconstruction in the setting of malignancy since gastrectomy with adequate resection margins may preclude tension-free gastroduodenostomy.

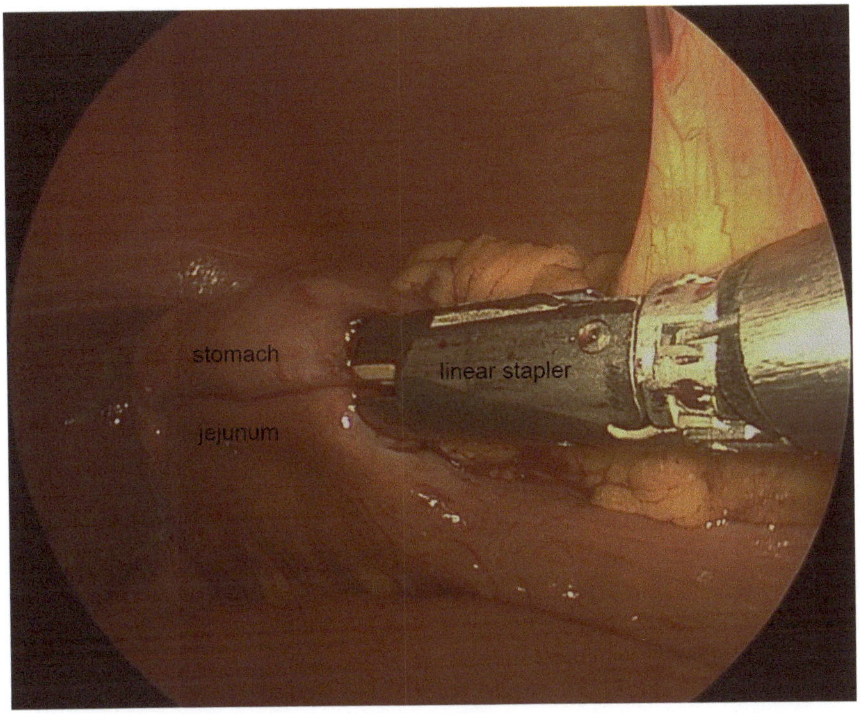


**Fig. 7.7** Creation of the Billroth II gastrojejunostomy using a 60-mm linear stapler with a tan cartridge

To create the anastomosis, we first identify the ligament of Trietz. A loop of jejunum approximately 15–20 cm distal to the ligament of Trietz is brought up ante-colic to the gastric remnant in a tension-free manner. The gastric remnant is then placed in alignment with the antimesenteric border of the jejunum. To avoid parallel staple lines and the potential for ischemia, we align the small bowel at an approximate 30-degree angle away from the gastric staple line. A small enterotomy is made on the antimesenteric border of the jejunum and a small gastrotomy on the gastric remnant. The anastomosis is created with a single firing of the linear stapler with a thin tissue cartridge (Fig. 7.7). The common channel is closed intracorporeally in two layers with an Endostitch device using 2-0 absorbable sutures. A nasogastric tube is always placed and advanced across the anastomosis. The left paramedian trocar site is minimally enlarged (<5 cm) to extract the specimen, which is sent to pathology for frozen section evaluation of the margins. Typically, a 19-French Blake drain is placed adjacent to the anastomosis and brought out through the lateral 5-mm trocar and secured to the skin with a nylon suture. The fascia at the specimen extraction site is re-approximated with standard open techniques. The fascia at the 10/12-mm trocar sites is closed with 0-sutures using the Karter-Thomason device. The skin is closed with absorbable 4-0 sutures and skin glue is applied.

## Postoperative Care and Complications

Postoperative management after laparoscopic distal gastrectomy is the same as after open surgery. Patients are managed on the surgical floor without the need for ICU care. It is our routine to remove the nasogastric tube on postoperative day #3. We do not perform an upper GI study prior to removal of the tube. After the nasogastric tube has been removed, a liquid diet is started and advanced as tolerated. Pain control is initiated with demand-only patient-controlled analgesia (PCA) and transitioned to oral narcotics once the patient has started a diet. Patients are typically discharged home on postoperative day #5 or #6.

Patients are at risk for the same early and late complications observed with open gastric resections. This includes postoperative bleeding that may necessitate reoperation or patients may suffer from prolonged ileus. Anastomotic leak is another potential complication and may require operative repair or revision of the gastrojejunostomy. We have not observed an anastomotic leak in our series. The most feared complication after gastric resection with Billroth II reconstruction is a duodenal stump leak, which historically has had a mortality rate of 50 % [12, 13]. We have not observed this complication is our series. After the immediate postoperative period, there may be late complications that must be appropriately managed. Delayed gastric emptying can occur as can dumping syndrome. Bile reflux gastritis can also occur at any time. These complications can typically be managed with dietary changes and remedial surgery is seldom necessary. On the rare occasion that conservative management is not successful, surgery with conversion from a Billroth II to a Roux-en-Y gastrojejunostomy may be warranted.

## Conclusions

The KLASS group recently reported long-term outcomes after laparoscopic gastrectomy for cancer [14]. They calculated an overall 5-year survival rate after laparoscopic gastrectomy of 78 %. The KLASS 01 trial is an ongoing randomized controlled trial comparing laparoscopic vs. open distal gastrectomy for adenocarcinoma [15]. Initial results from this trial are pending, but another study from Lee et al. [16] compared oncologic outcomes of laparoscopic and open gastrectomy for cancer. This study included over 1,800 patients and found no difference in recurrence-free survival rates. Furthermore, the technique of gastrectomy (open vs. laparoscopic) did not influence outcomes in early or advanced gastric cancer. These studies show that laparoscopic distal gastrectomy with extended lymphadenectomy for gastric adenocarcinoma is a safe and effective procedure when performed by an experienced surgeon with advanced laparoscopic skills. The procedure can typically be performed in a reasonable time with morbidity and mortality comparable to open gastrectomy.

## References

1. Guggenheim DE, Shah MA. Gastric cancer epidemiology and risk factors. J Surg Oncol. 2013;107(3):230–6. doi:10.1002/jso.23262.
2. Jemal A, Bray F, Center MM, Ferlay J, Ward E, Forman D. Global cancer statistics. CA Cancer J Clin. 2011;61(2):69–90. doi:10.3322/caac.20107.
3. Ferlay J, Shin HR, Bray F, Forman D, Mathers C, Parkin DM. Estimates of worldwide burden of cancer in 2008: GLOBOCAN 2008. Int J Cancer. 2010;127(12):2893–917. doi:10.1002/ijc.25516.
4. Ajani JA, Bentrem DJ, Besh S, D'Amico TA, Das P, Denlinger C, et al. Gastric cancer, version 2.2013: featured updates to the NCCN Guidelines. J Natl Compr Canc Netw. 2013;11(5):531–46.
5. Goh P, Tekant Y, Kum CK, Isaac J, Shang NS. Totally intra-abdominal laparoscopic Billroth II gastrectomy. Surg Endosc. 1992;6(3):160.
6. Goh P, Kum CK. Laparoscopic Billroth II gastrectomy: a review. Surg Oncol. 1993;2 Suppl 1:13–8.
7. Azagra JS, Goergen M, De Simone P, Ibanez-Aguirre J. Minimally invasive surgery for gastric cancer. Surg Endosc. 1999;13(4):351–7.
8. Azagra JS, Ibanez-Aguirre JF, Goergen M, Ceuterick M, Bordas-Rivas JM, Almendral-Lopez ML, et al. Long-term results of laparoscopic extended surgery in advanced gastric cancer: a series of 101 patients. Hepatogastroenterology. 2006;53(68):304–8.
9. Uyama I, Sugioka A, Fujita J, Komori Y, Matsui H, Soga R, et al. Purely laparoscopic pylorus-preserving gastrectomy with extraperigastric lymphadenectomy for early gastric cancer: a case and technical report. Surg Laparosc Endosc Percutan Tech. 1999;9(6):418–22.
10. Isobe Y, Nashimoto A, Akazawa K, Oda I, Hayashi K, Miyashiro I, et al. Gastric cancer treatment in Japan: 2008 annual report of the JGCA nationwide registry.

Gastric Cancer. 2011;14(4):301–16. doi:10.1007/s10120-011-0085-6.
11. Japanese Gastric Cancer Association. Japanese classification of gastric carcinoma: 3rd English edition. Gastric Cancer. 2011;14(2):101–12. doi:10.1007/s10120-011-0041-5.
12. Avola FA, Ellis DS. Leakage of the duodenal or antral stump complicating gastric resection. Surg Gynecol Obstet. 1954;99(3):359–67.
13. Larsen BB, Foreman RC. Syndrome of the leaking duodenal stump. AMA Arch Surg. 1951;63(4):480–5.
14. Park do J, Han SU, Hyung WJ, Kim MC, Kim W, Ryu SY, et al. Long-term outcomes after laparoscopy-assisted gastrectomy for advanced gastric cancer: a large-scale multicenter retrospective study. Surg Endosc. 2012;26(6):1548–53. doi:10.1007/s00464-011-2065-7.
15. Kim HH, Han SU, Kim MC, Hyung WJ, Kim W, Lee HJ, et al. Prospective randomized controlled trial (phase III) to comparing laparoscopic distal gastrectomy with open distal gastrectomy for gastric adenocarcinoma (KLASS 01). J Korean Surg Soc. 2013;84(2):123–30. doi:10.4174/jkss.2013.84.2.123.
16. Lee JH, Lee CM, Son SY, Ahn SH, Park do J, Kim HH. Laparoscopic versus open gastrectomy for gastric cancer: long-term oncologic results. Surgery. 2014;155(1):154–64. doi:10.1016/j.surg.2013.06.015.

## Key Operative Steps

1. Gastrectomy and lymphadenectomy are performed in a clockwise set of maneuvers.
2. Divide the gastrocolic ligament in the avascular plane, enter the lesser sac, and expose the anterior surface of the pancreas.
3. Perform intraoperative EGD to confirm the location of the tumor and mark the line of gastric transection.
4. Ligate the right gastroepiploic vessels and harvest nodal tissues (station 6).
5. Divide the duodenum and identify the gastroduodenal artery.
6. Identify and ligate the right gastric artery (station 5).
7. Harvest nodal tissues at station 1.
8. Harvest lymphatic tissues along the proximal proper hepatic artery (station 12) and common hepatic artery (station 8). Along the superior border of the pancreas, expose the celiac axis (station 9), the splenic artery (station 11), and then the left gastric artery (station 7).
9. Ligate the coronary vein to the right of the left gastric artery.
10. Ligate the left gastric artery.
11. Transect the stomach with a linear stapler with thick tissue cartridges.
12. Reconstruct with Billroth II gastrojejunostomy.

# 8 Minimally Invasive Total Gastrectomy

Kaitlyn J. Kelly and Vivian E. Strong

## Introduction

Utilization of minimally invasive approaches for resection of gastric cancer has been increasing rapidly in recent years. Laparoscopic distal gastrectomy for early-stage, distal gastric cancers is well-established and routinely performed in Eastern countries where gastric cancer screening is practiced. Several randomized, prospective trials have confirmed improvements in postoperative outcomes for laparoscopic compared to open distal gastrectomy for patients with early gastric cancer [1–6].

Minimally invasive total gastrectomy (MIS-TG), however, is not as well-established or widely performed. This is primarily due to concerns about the status of the proximal resection margin and technical limitations in the construction of the esophagojejunal anastomosis. Many surgeons feel that this critical step of the operation cannot be performed safely with minimally invasive techniques. To date, no prospective, randomized trial comparing MIS-TG and open total gastrectomy (OTG) has been completed to address this concern.

Multiple small series of MIS-TG have been published, but include a variety of gastroesophageal anastomotic techniques, including intracorporeal and extracorporeal methods [7–9]. These include circular and linear stapling methods and hand-sewn methods with or without construction of a jejunal pouch. Furthermore, these series vary on whether the procedures were performed laparoscopically, with hand-assistance, or with the robotic surgery platform. Given this degree of heterogeneity, the conclusions that can be drawn from these reports are limited, and no single, standardized technique for MIS-TG has been widely embraced. This chapter will describe the technical aspects of MIS-TG for gastric cancer and discuss considerations regarding the learning curve and patient selection. Additionally, the chapter will summarize current literature on MIS-TG with a focus on technique, outcomes, and cost.

## Patient Selection

Patient selection is an important part of successful robotic total gastrectomy (RTG). This is particularly relevant during a surgeon's initial experience. Ideal candidates for RTG are patients

Electronic supplementary material: Supplementary material is available in the online version of this chapter at 10.1007/978-1-4939-1893-5_8. Videos can also be accessed at http://www.springerimages.com/videos/978-1-4939-1892-8.

K.J. Kelly, M.D.
Division of Surgical Oncology, Thornton Hospital and Moores Cancer Center, University of California, San Diego, 3855 Health Sciences Drive, Mail Code 0987, La Jolla, CA 92093, USA
e-mail: k6kelly@ucsd.edu

V.E. Strong, M.D., F.A.C.S. (✉)
Memorial Sloan-Kettering Cancer Center, 1275 York Avenue, New York, NY 10065, USA

Weill Medical College of Cornell University, 525 East 68th Street, New York, NY 10065, USA
e-mail: strongv@mskcc.org

J. Kim and J. Garcia-Aguilar (eds.), *Surgery for Cancers of the Gastrointestinal Tract: A Step-by-Step Approach*, DOI 10.1007/978-1-4939-1893-5_8, © Springer Science+Business Media New York 2015

without significant medical comorbidities; and patients with early-stage disease, small tumors, normal body mass index (BMI), and intestinal-type histology. Patients also ideal for MIS-TG are those undergoing prophylactic TG for hereditary gastric cancer syndrome. These patients nearly always have foci of high-grade dysplasia or intramucosal carcinoma within the stomach, but they do not require more than D1 lymphadenectomy. The critical part of the operation for these patients is that all gastric mucosa is removed with the specimen. Both the proximal and distal margins should be sent for frozen section analysis for these patients to confirm the presence of esophageal and duodenal mucosa, respectively.

As a surgeon's experience with the procedure increases, the incorporation of patients with more advanced disease, neoadjuvant treatment, and higher BMI is reasonable with a low threshold for conversion based on extensive time of operation or difficulty. Consideration should also be given to initiate a prospective clinical trial for these patients as data on safety and efficacy of MIS-TG in this setting is limited. Furthermore, careful prospective recording of clinical and operative data may facilitate collaboration and pooling of data across different institutions. Given the relative rarity of gastric cancer in Western countries, collaboration among different centers is important to gain sufficient numbers of Western gastric cancer patients.

## Technical Aspects of Minimally Invasive Total Gastrectomy

### Patient Positioning and Port Placement

We have previously described patient positioning and technique for MIS gastrectomy [10]. The following description is a modification of the previous text focusing on RTG. MIS-TG is performed with the patient positioned supine on a split-leg table (Fig. 8.1). A beanbag device is helpful for stabilization of the patient during the procedure. The patient's arms can be tucked or placed on arm boards with appropriate padding of elbows and hands and other pressure points. The patient is secured to the table at the shoulders, hips, and knees with tape and/or safety straps. Footboards may also be applied at the feet as a further means to avoid sliding during reverse Trendelenburg positioning. Once patient positioning is completed, it is important to place the patient in steep reverse Trendelenburg as a test to assure stability. For robotic-assisted procedures, it is important that the bed be in reverse Trendelenburg position at approximately 45° prior to docking the robot. Once the robot arms are docked to the port sites, the bed position can no longer be changed without undocking the robot arms.

Port placement for MIS-TG follows the same principles as for any laparoscopic or robotic procedure, which includes placement of the camera port at a distance of 15–20 cm from the target anatomy, and placement of ports at least 5 cm apart for laparoscopic TG (LTG) and at least 8 cm apart for RTG. While multiple variations of port placement have been described, the placement illustrated in Fig. 8.2 is recommended.

Pneumoperitoneum is established via a Veress needle placed off the left costal margin or via an optical viewing trocar. A 10/12-mm trocar is then placed in the midline above or below the umbilicus depending on the patient's body habitus, but with port placement positioned about 15–20 cm from the target anatomy. In the majority of cases, the infraumbilical position is the best trocar position for total gastrectomy, since it is far enough in the caudal direction for omentectomy and the jejunojejunostomy anastomosis, while still providing sufficient reach to and visualization of the hiatus and distal esophagus. For RTG, two additional 8-mm robotic ports are then placed on the left side, at least 8 cm from each other and slightly offset from the plane of the camera port. An additional 12-mm port is placed in the right midclavicular line. This is the port that will be used for stapling and specimen extraction. For RTG, an 8-mm robotic port is placed within this 12-mm port. A 5-mm assistant port is placed further laterally on the right side, approximately at the anterior axillary line. Placement of a

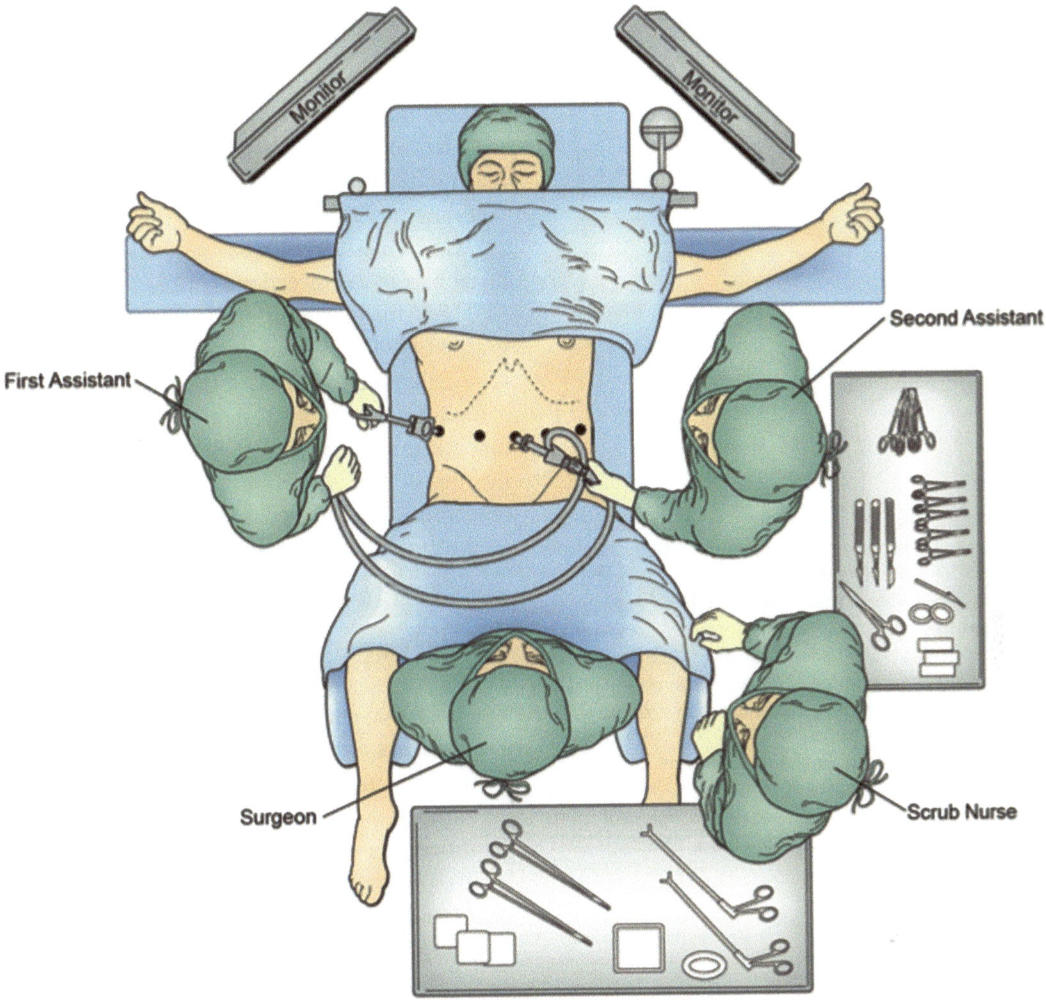


**Fig. 8.1** Illustration of optimal patient position for MIS-TG. The pt is positioned on a split-leg table allowing the primary surgeon to stand between the patient's legs and two assistants to stand on either side of the patient

Nathanson liver retractor, via a small subxiphoid stab-wound incision, facilitates secure retraction of the left lateral lobe of the liver and excellent exposure of the esophageal hiatus.

The abdomen is explored for adhesions and for any evidence of peritoneal or metastatic disease. If the lesion is not appreciable on the extraluminal surface, an endoscope is passed to verify location of the lesion. For gastroesophageal junction tumors, the distal esophagus and Z-line should be carefully examined to localize the proximal extent of the lesion. It is critical to ensure that an adequate esophageal resection margin (2–4 cm from the lesion) can be obtained from the transabdominal approach. Once this is confirmed, the patient is placed in reverse Trendelenburg to approximately 45°. For RTG, the robot is docked from directly over the patient's head. Arms 1 and 3 are docked to the left-sided ports and arm 2 is docked to the right-sided port within the larger 12-mm port (Fig. 8.3). A fenestrated bipolar grasper is placed in arm 2 and an energy sealant device or monopolar scissors is placed in arm 1. Grasping forceps, preferably Cadiere or Prograsp (Intuitive Surgical), are placed in arm 3.

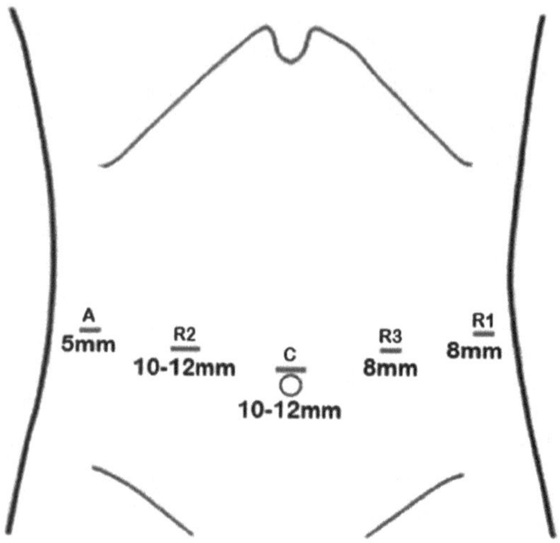


**Fig. 8.2** Illustration of preferred port placement for MIS-TG. A 12 mm port is placed in the midline near the umbilicus. This port is usually above the umbilicus but the final position should be determined by measuring 15–20 cm from the target anatomy. Two additional ports are placed on the patient's left side. These are 8 mm ports for RTG or 5 mm ports for LTG. A 12 mm port is placed on the patient's right mid-clavicular line. For RTG, an 8 mm robotic port is placed within this 12 mm port and can be temporarily removed / reinserted as needed. Finally, a 5 mm assistant port is placed on the right side approximately at the anterior axillary line. All ports should be 5–8 mm apart from each other

## Omentectomy

The procedure commences by retracting the greater omentum cephalad and locating the transverse colon. The omentum is carefully taken off the colon in the avascular plane, proceeding towards the splenic flexure. With careful dissection, the plane between the omentum and the transverse mesocolon is identified and the lesser sac is entered. Visualization of the posterior wall of the stomach confirms entry into the lesser sac. The posterior wall of the stomach is then grasped by the bedside assistant on the patient's right side and is retracted anteriorly and to the right (Fig. 8.4). The omentectomy is carried up towards the spleen allowing visualization of the short gastric vessels, which are ligated with an energy sealant device under direct visualization. This maneuver provides exposure up to the left crus of the diaphragm. The peritoneum overlying the left crus is incised with the energy sealant device, which should allow the crural muscle fibers to be visible. Gentle blunt dissection along the crus exposes the posterolateral aspect of the esophagus. If the port placement does not allow for reach to the esophageal hiatus, the bedside assistant may push the ports further into the abdominal wall, which can then be retracted again for the distal part of the resection.

Then, the posterior wall of the stomach is grasped by an assistant on the patient's left side or utilizing the third arm of the robot in RTG and is retracted toward the patient's left shoulder. The omentectomy then proceeds toward the hepatic flexure of the colon and is completed. The omentum can be placed in the left upper quadrant on the anterior wall of the stomach at this point.

## Greater Curvature Dissection

The posterior attachments between the stomach and pancreas are then divided sharply or with an energy sealant device in the direction of the pylorus. The right gastroepiploic vessels are identified and dissected circumferentially at the level of the superior border of the pancreas at their point of origin from the gastroduodenal vessels (Fig. 8.5). If the linear stapler is to be used, arm 2 of the robot and its 8-mm port is removed from the larger 12-mm port and the linear stapler is used.

## Division of Proximal Duodenum

Attention is then turned towards the suprapyloric region. The gastrohepatic attachments are incised with an energy sealant device in robot arm 1. The right gastric artery is identified and is ligated at its base. The lymphatic tissues along the proper hepatic and common hepatic artery are swept medially toward the specimen and a window is created at the level of the pylorus. The posterior aspect of the pylorus and proximal duodenum is gently elevated off the retroperitoneum with a combination of blunt dissection and use of the energy sealant device. An endovascular linear

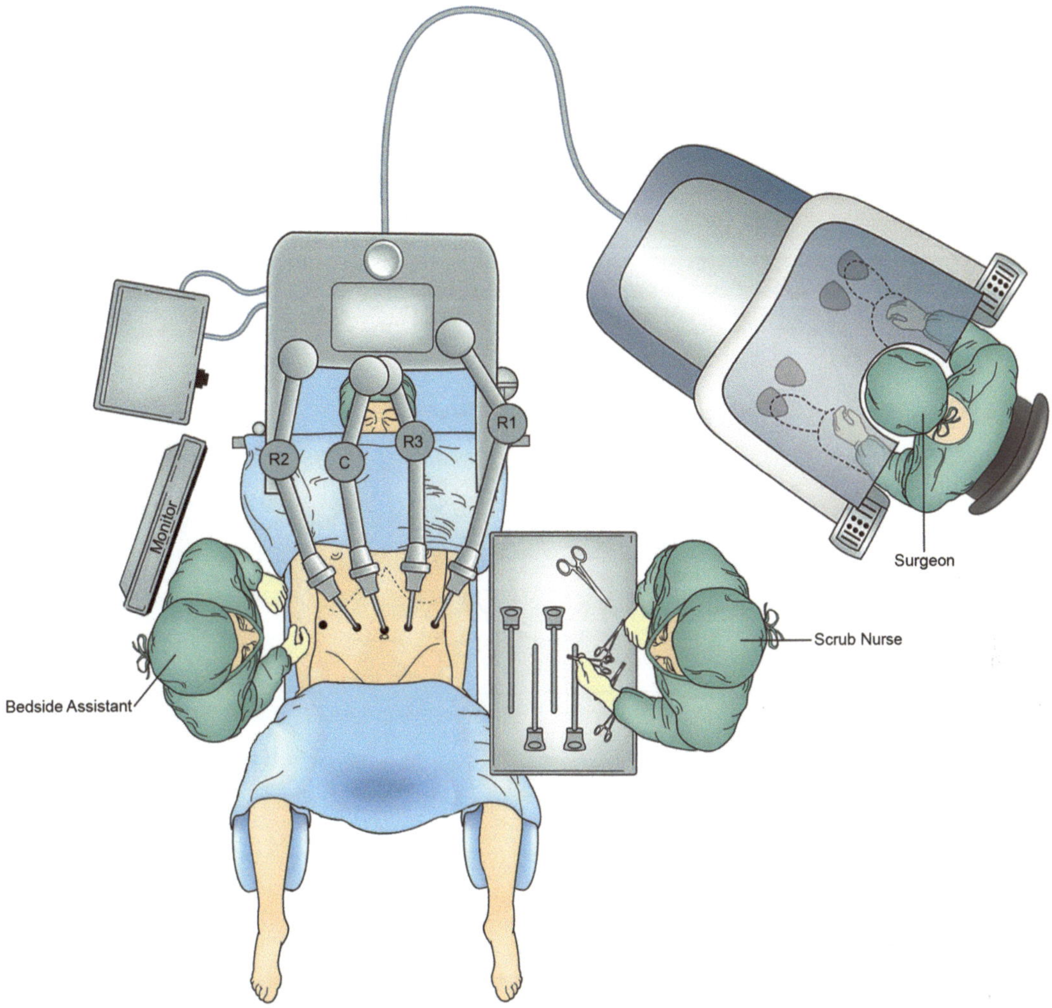


**Fig. 8.3** Illustration of robot position for RTG. The robot is docked from directly over the patient's head

stapler with a blue or green load is then introduced and the proximal duodenum is stapled and divided just distal to the pylorus. We prefer to use bioabsorbable staple line reinforcement on the duodenum (Fig. 8.6).

## Modified D2 Lymphadenectomy (D1 + β)

Next, the stomach can be placed in the left upper quadrant to facilitate exposure of the D2 lymph nodes (Fig. 8.7). The dissection that was started previously along the proper hepatic artery is continued along the common hepatic artery toward the celiac axis and proximal splenic artery. The left gastric vein and artery are identified at the celiac axis and all surrounding lymph nodes carefully swept up en bloc with the specimen. The vessels are then divided at their origin at the celiac axis with the endovascular linear stapler or with clips.

## Division of the Distal Esophagus

The gastrohepatic attachments are then further incised up to the level of the esophageal hiatus

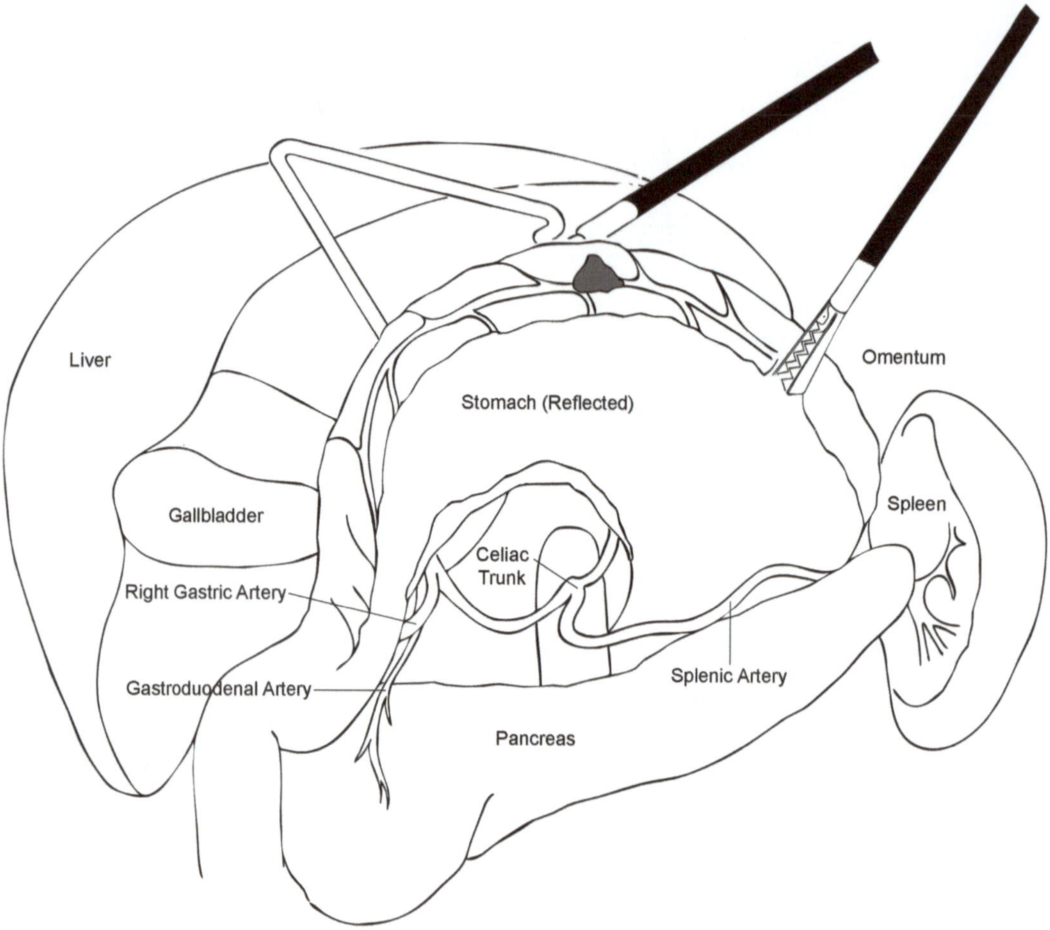


**Fig. 8.4** Illustration of the view provided when the posterior wall of the stomach is grasped and elevated. This is a key maneuver in MIS-TG

**Fig. 8.5** Photo of the origin of the right gastroepiploic vessels. The right gastroepiploic vein often shares a common trunk with the right colic vein (Henle's trunk)

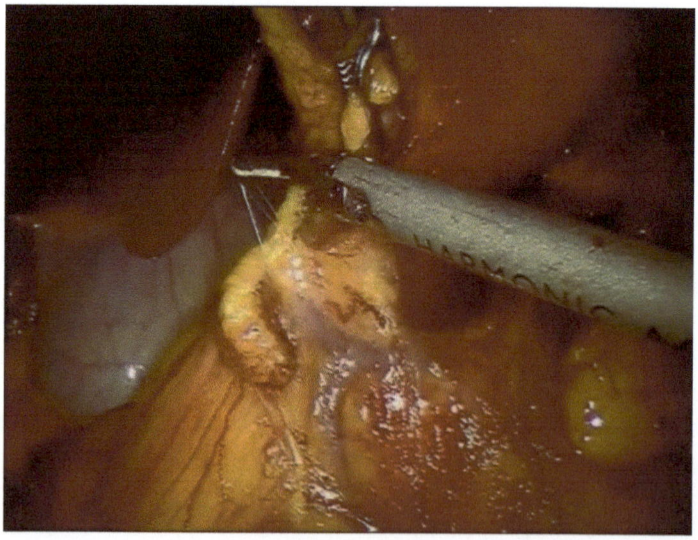

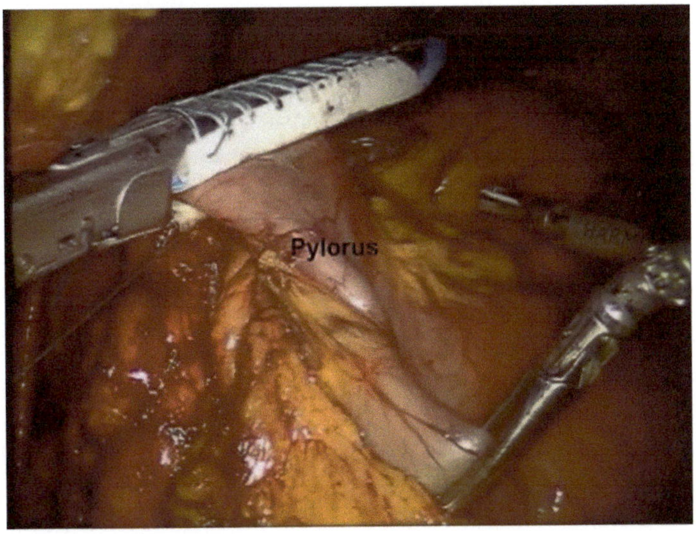


**Fig. 8.6** Photo of the proximal duodenum being divided just distal to the pylorus. A linear stapler with bioabsorbable reinforcement is preferred

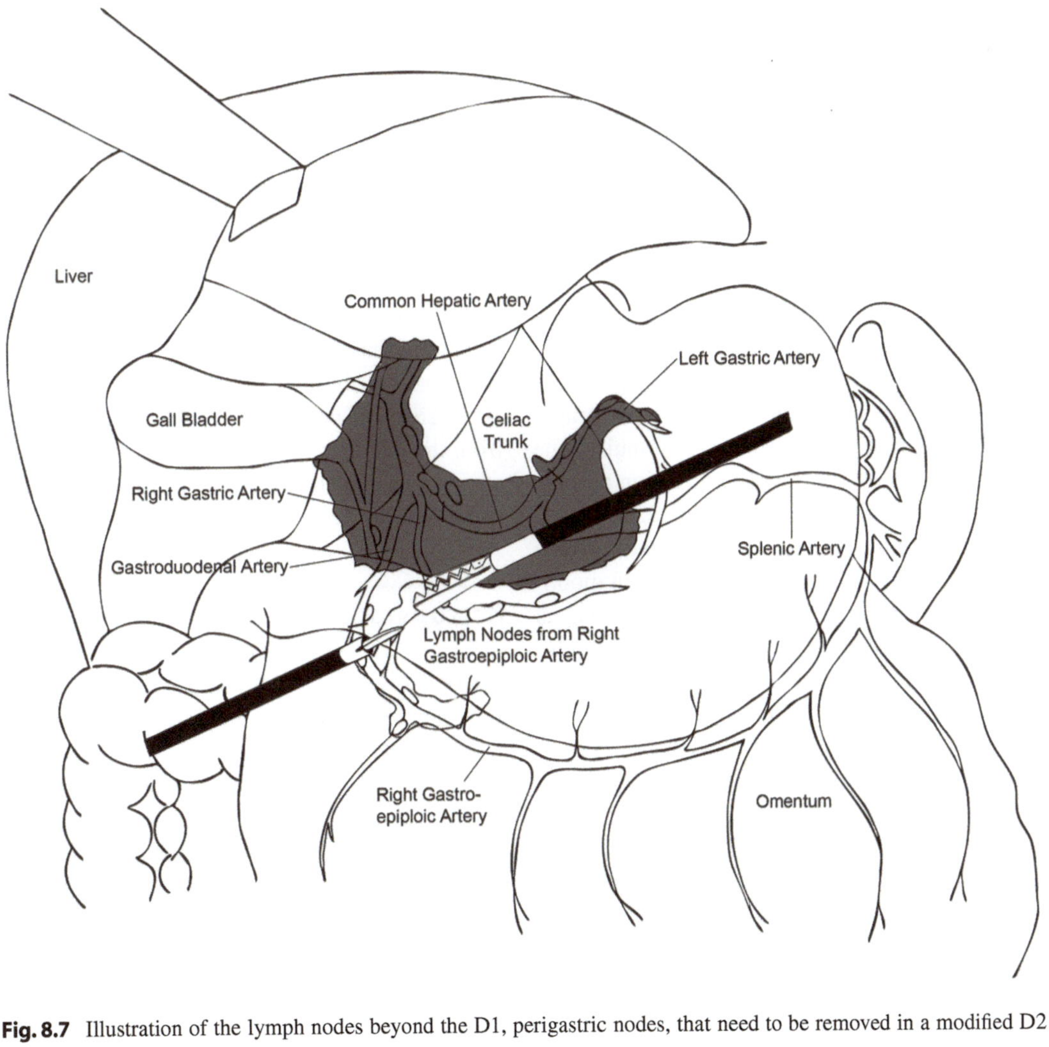


**Fig. 8.7** Illustration of the lymph nodes beyond the D1, perigastric nodes, that need to be removed in a modified D2 lymphadenectomy

with the energy sealant device. The level 1 and 3 lymph nodes are dissected with the proximal stomach up to the right crus of the diaphragm and esophagus. The peritoneal fat and fat pad overlying the esophagus are opened with the energy sealant device and the distal esophagus is circumferentially dissected. The distal esophagus is then divided with a reticulating linear stapler (blue load).

## Specimen Retrieval

At this point, the specimen is placed in a specimen retrieval bag and is removed via the umbilical port site which is enlarged about 1.5 cm after changing the camera position to the right-sided 12-mm port site. The camera port is then replaced and the 8-mm robotic port attached to arm 2 is placed within the 12-mm right-sided port site after returning the camera to its initial position at the umbilical port. The proximal margin is marked with a stitch and is sent for frozen section analysis to confirm microscopic clearance of disease. Attention is then turned to the reconstruction.

## Reconstruction

Roux-en-Y esophagojejunostomy is performed for restoration of gastrointestinal continuity. The colon is elevated in a cephalad direction and the ligament of Treitz (LOT) is identified. A mobile piece of jejunum approximately 30–40 cm downstream from the LOT is selected based on mobility and tension-free reach to the esophageal hiatus and is used for reconstruction. The jejunum is then transected with a linear stapler with a blue load and the Roux limb is measured out to about 60–70 cm at which point the jejunojejunostomy is created with another firing of the linear stapler with a blue load. The resultant enterotomy is closed with a 2-0 silk running suture. The Roux limb is then prepared for esophagojejunostomy, which is an end-to-side anastomosis created with a 25-French circular stapler. To facilitate this, we prefer to use a transoral anvil (OrVil, Covidien) (Fig. 8.8). This device is an anvil connected to a nasogastric tube. The device is passed transorally usually by the anesthesiologist. Once the tip of the tubing is visible against the stapled end of the distal esophagus, a small esophagotomy is made with electrocautery to facilitate passage of the tubing through the wall of the esophagus. Care is taken to prevent contact between the contaminated tubing and the abdominal viscera. The tubing is grasped and pulled out of the abdomen via the 12-mm port. Robot arm 2 is undocked to facilitate removal of the tube in RTG. The tubing is then gently detached from the end of the anvil and is removed through the 12-mm port. The stapler is inserted into the Roux limb after removing the staple line with the energy sealant device. The anvil and spike are then connected and the stapler is fired. The open end of the Roux limb is then closed with a linear stapler.

Other options for the esophagojejunal anastomosis include using a linear stapler in the prepared Roux limb. The limb is positioned posterior to the esophageal stump and after creating the esophagotomy and enterotomy, a linear stapler is fired with closure of the remaining enterotomy with a running 2-0 silk suture. One other option is to hand sew the anastomosis in a single or double layer reconstruction. No single technique has been definitively shown to be superior, so the choice is based on surgeon experience and comfort level. Mesenteric defects from the jejunojejunostomy and Petersen's space are sutured closed in a running fashion with 3-0 vicryl suture.

## Postoperative Care

Postoperatively, nasoesophageal/nasojejunal decompression is not necessary and is not recommended. In the absence of abdominal distention or evidence of ileus, patients are started on sips of clear liquids on postoperative day #2. This consists of ice chips and small-volume clear liquids ($\leq$60 ml per 8 h nursing shift). If this is well tolerated, the diet is advanced to clear liquid tray the following day, then full liquids, and finally a soft bariatric diet (six small meals per day). Patients are discharged home on the soft

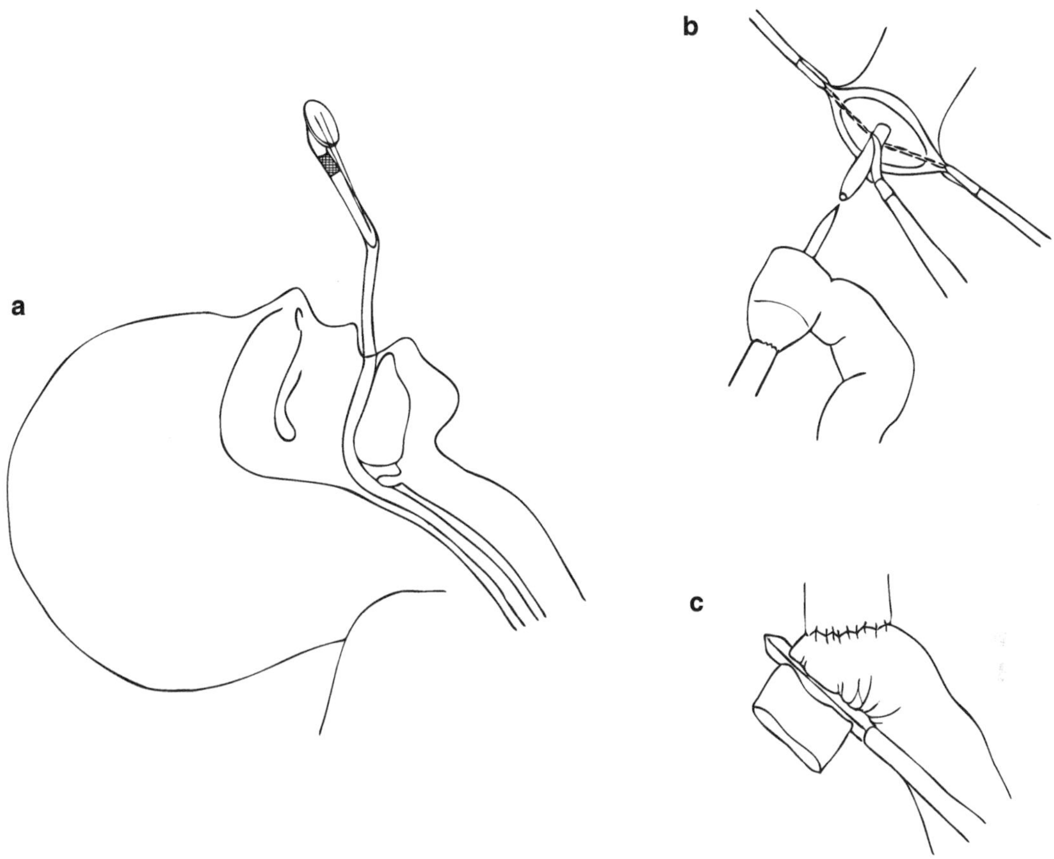


**Fig. 8.8** Illustration of esophagojejunal anastomosis using the OrVil™ device (Covidien, USA). (**a**) The anvil is passed trans-orally by the anesthesiologist or a surgical assistant. (**b**) An end-to-side anastomosis is created by passing a 25 mm EEA stapler into the Roux limb. (**c**) The remaining open end of the Roux limb is closed with a linear stapler

diet for 2–3 weeks before advancing to solid food. We do not perform routine radiographic studies to evaluate for subclinical anastomotic leaks. If patients develop tachycardia, fever, or other evidence of leak, contrast-enhanced computed tomography (CT) or an esophogram with water-soluble oral contrast is performed.

## Postoperative Outcomes

While the preponderance of data on minimally invasive gastric resection for cancer focuses on distal or subtotal gastrectomy, there are several retrospective series and meta-analyses that focus on MIS-TG [7, 8, 11, 12]. A recent meta-analysis comparing 2,313 patients undergoing LTG ($n=955$) versus OTG ($n=1,358$) found that LTG was associated with improved short-term outcomes including decreased blood loss, less postoperative pain, quicker return of bowel function, shorter hospital stay, and decreased postoperative morbidity [12]. The decrease in perioperative morbidity was primarily a reflection of decreased wound infections and there was no significant difference in anastomotic leak or stricture rates. Operative time was longer for the LTG group and long-term oncologic outcomes were not reported.

Comparisons of the robotic platform to both conventional laparoscopy and open surgery have also been performed. A meta-analysis by Marano et al. included 7 studies and 1,967 patients and robotic gastrectomy ($n=404$) was compared to both laparoscopic ($n=845$) and open gastrectomy ($n=718$) [13]. The robotic platform was associated with shorter length of stay compared to open surgery. Moreover, the robotic platform demonstrated a significant reduction in blood loss compared to the laparoscopic approach. On the other hand, robotic gastrectomy was associated with significantly longer operative time compared to both laparoscopic and open gastrectomy. Importantly, surgical morbidity and lymph node retrieval were not significantly different between the robotic gastrectomy and laparoscopic or open gastrectomy groups.

## Cost of Robotic Gastrectomy

The cost of the robotic surgery platform is limiting in the current economy. In Eastern countries, patients pay out-of-pocket for the extra costs of robotic-assisted procedures. In the United States, hospitals charge significantly more for robotic-assisted procedures than for open or laparoscopic surgeries to offset the costs of the robots, instruments, and technical support. It is estimated that RTG costs approximately $4,400 more per case than LTG [14]. While most surgeons agree that the technical advantages of the robot definitely allow for more precise dissection and lymphadenectomy in some procedures, particularly gastrectomy, prostatectomy, and proctectomy, it is unknown whether the increased cost will continue to be justified in the absence of measurable clinical benefits over laparoscopy.

## Summary

Current data suggest that utilization of minimally invasive approaches in total gastrectomy for cancer is associated with improved short-term postoperative outcomes compared to OTG. While data on MIS-TG with robotic-assistance are limited, use of the robot may allow for more precise dissection and D2 lymphadenectomy than with standard laparoscopy. This advantage comes with significantly increased cost, and it is unclear whether it will translate into clinical benefits for patients. It is reasonable to hypothesize that decreased postoperative morbidity, decreased blood loss and need for transfusion, and more precise lymphadenectomy may eventually translate into improved long-term oncologic outcomes. More prospective studies of MIS-TG are needed to clarify the role of laparoscopic and robotic approaches to total gastrectomy for gastric cancer.

## References


1. Hayashi H, Ochiai T, Shimada H, Gunji Y. Prospective randomized study of open versus laparoscopy-assisted distal gastrectomy with extraperigastric lymph node dissection for early gastric cancer. Surg Endosc. 2005;19(9):1172–6. doi:10.1007/s00464-004-8207-4.
2. Huscher CG, Mingoli A, Sgarzini G, Sansonetti A, Di Paola M, Recher A, et al. Laparoscopic versus open subtotal gastrectomy for distal gastric cancer: five-year results of a randomized prospective trial. Ann Surg. 2005;241(2):232–7.
3. Kim HH, Hyung WJ, Cho GS, Kim MC, Han SU, Kim W, et al. Morbidity and mortality of laparoscopic gastrectomy versus open gastrectomy for gastric cancer: an interim report–a phase III multicenter, prospective, randomized Trial (KLASS Trial). Ann Surg. 2010;251(3):417–20. doi:10.1097/SLA.0b013e3181cc8f6b.
4. Kim YW, Baik YH, Yun YH, Nam BH, Kim DH, Choi IJ, et al. Improved quality of life outcomes after laparoscopy-assisted distal gastrectomy for early gastric cancer: results of a prospective randomized clinical trial. Ann Surg. 2008;248(5):721–7. doi:10.1097/SLA.0b013e318185e62e.
5. Lee JH, Han HS, Lee JH. A prospective randomized study comparing open vs laparoscopy-assisted distal gastrectomy in early gastric cancer: early results. Surg Endosc. 2005;19(2):168–73. doi:10.1007/s00464-004-8808-y.
6. Kitano S, Shiraishi N, Fujii K, Yasuda K, Inomata M, Adachi Y. A randomized controlled trial comparing open vs laparoscopy-assisted distal gastrectomy for the treatment of early gastric cancer: an interim report. Surgery. 2002;131(1 Suppl):S306–11.
7. Shim JH, Yoo HM, Oh SI, Nam MJ, Jeon HM, Park CH, et al. Various types of intracorporeal esophagojejunostomy after laparoscopic total gastrectomy for gastric cancer. Gastric cancer. 2013;16(3):420–7. doi:10.1007/s10120-012-0207-9.
8. Corcione F, Pirozzi F, Cuccurullo D, Angelini P, Cimmino V, Settembre A. Laparoscopic total gastrectomy in gastric cancer: our experience in 92 cases.

Minim Invasive Ther Allied Technol. 2013;22(5): 271–8. doi:10.3109/13645706.2012.743919.
9. Liu XX, Jiang ZW, Chen P, Zhao Y, Pan HF, Li JS. Full robot-assisted gastrectomy with intracorporeal robot-sewn anastomosis produces satisfying outcomes. World J Gastroenterol. 2013;19(38):6427–37. doi:10.3748/wjg.v19.i38.6427.
10. Kelly KJ, Vivian ES. Robotic utilization in gastric cancer surgery. In: Hochwald S, editor. Minimally Invasive Foregut Surgery for Malignancy: Principles and Practice. New York: Springer; 2014.
11. Nagai E, Ohuchida K, Nakata K, Miyasaka Y, Maeyama R, Toma H, et al. Feasibility and safety of intracorporeal esophagojejunostomy after laparoscopic total gastrectomy: inverted T-shaped anastomosis using linear staplers. Surgery. 2013;153(5): 732–8. doi:10.1016/j.surg.2012.10.012.
12. Wang W, Zhang X, Shen C, Zhi X, Wang B, Xu Z. Laparoscopic versus open total gastrectomy for gastric cancer: an updated meta-analysis. PLoS One. 2014;9(2):e88753. doi:10.1371/journal.pone.0088753.
13. Marano A, Choi YY, Hyung WJ, Kim YM, Kim J, Noh SH. Robotic versus laparoscopic versus open gastrectomy: a meta-analysis. J Gastric cancer. 2013;13(3):136–48. doi:10.5230/jgc.2013.13.3.136.
14. Park JY, Jo MJ, Nam BH, Kim Y, Eom BW, Yoon HM, et al. Surgical stress after robot-assisted distal gastrectomy and its economic implications. Br J Surg. 2012;99(11):1554–61. doi:10.1002/bjs.8887.

## Key Operative Steps

1. Explore abdomen for adhesions and peritoneal carcinomatosis. Ensure that 2–4 cm of adequate proximal margin can be obtained.
2. If the lesion cannot be appreciated on the extraluminal surface, perform intraoperative endoscopy.
3. Dock the robot.
4. Dissect the omentum from the colon in the avascular plane proceeding towards the splenic flexure and enter the lesser sac.
5. Grasp the posterior wall of the stomach and retract anteriorly and to the right. Ligate the short gastric vessels with energy sealant device up to the left crus.
6. Incise the peritoneum over the left crus and expose the posterolateral aspect of the esophagus.
7. Retract the stomach to the left side and proceed with omentectomy towards the hepatic flexure. Place fully mobilized omentum in the left upper quadrant.
8. Divide the posterior attachments between the stomach and the pancreas sharply or with an energy sealant device.
9. Dissect the right gastroepiploic vessels at the level of the superior border of the pancreas near the point of origin from the gastroduodenal vessels. The linear stapler can be used for this maneuver.
10. Incise the gastrohepatic attachments near the suprapyloric region. Identify and ligate the right gastric artery.
11. Dissect the lymphatic tissues along the proper hepatic and common hepatic artery towards the specimen creating a window at the level of the pylorus.
12. Mobilize the posterior aspect of the pylorus and proximal duodenum and divide the duodenum with a linear stapler. Use a bioabsorbable staple line reinforcement.
13. Continue dissecting lymphatic tissues toward the celiac axis and proximal splenic artery.
14. Identify and ligate the left gastric vein and artery. Dissect all lymphatic tissues with the specimen.
15. Further incise gastrohepatic attachments to the level of the esophageal hiatus. Level 1 and 3 lymph nodes are dissected with the proximal stomach up to the right crus and esophagus.
16. Mobilize distal esophagus and divide it with a linear stapler.
17. Place specimen in a specimen bag and remove via the umbilical port site.
18. A Roux limb is prepared 30–40 cm downstream from the ligament of Treitz. Transect jejunum with a linear stapler.
19. Create jejunojejunostomy 60–70 cm downstream from the transected jejunum.
20. Perform esophagojejunostomy with a transoral anvil device and a circular stapler.

# 9 Open Total Gastrectomy and Splenectomy

Han-Kwang Yang and Seung-Young Oh

## Incision

Upper midline incision from the xiphoid to approximately 2–3 cm above the umbilicus is required for total gastrectomy (Fig. 9.1). If necessary, the incision can be extended to below the umbilicus, e.g. for an obese patient. For the initial diagnostic exploration, a relatively small incision should be considered.

## Peritoneal Cavity Exploration

To evaluate peritoneal seeding or distant metastasis, careful exploration of the peritoneal cavity should be performed. If there is a suspicious lesion for peritoneal seeding or other distant metastasis, intraoperative frozen biopsy is required. For suspected malignant ascites, cytologic washings may be helpful. Evaluation for resectability is also essential during peritoneal cavity exploration. Invasion of the aorta, diaphragm, pancreas, or other adjacent organs should be checked. If there is no evidence of distant metastasis and primary gastric cancer is resectable, abdominal incision can be extended for the radical operation.

To obtain an optimal operative field and avoid unexpected injury to the spleen, it is helpful to place a surgical pad behind the spleen. Sometimes, dividing the triangular ligament and flipping over the left lateral section of the liver is necessary to widely expose the gastroesophageal junction and distal esophagus. Traction in four diagonal directions and pushing the diaphragm upward with a self-retraining retractor is useful to obtain an adequate operative field for total gastrectomy (Fig. 9.2).

## Total Gastrectomy With D2 Lymph Node Dissection

### Total Omentectomy

Omentectomy starts from the middle of the transverse colon and is usually performed to the left side first. To develop an adequate dissection plane for total omentectomy, it is necessary for the assistant to spread the transverse mesocolon downward with appropriate tension. During omentectomy, it is important not to injure the transverse colon or vasa recta around the colonic wall. The necessity of omental bursectomy is controversial. A randomized controlled trial to evaluate the clinical benefit of bursectomy for cT3-4a gastric cancer is ongoing in Japan.

Electronic supplementary material: Supplementary material is available in the online version of this chapter at 10.1007/978-1-4939-1893-5_9. Videos can also be accessed at http://www.springerimages.com/videos/978-1-4939-1892-8.

H.-K. Yang, M.D., Ph.D., F.A.C.S. (✉)
S.-Y. Oh, M.D.
Department of Surgery, Seoul National University College of Medicine, 28 Yongon-Dong, Chongno-Gu, Seoul 110-744, South Korea
e-mail: hkyang@snu.ac.kr

J. Kim and J. Garcia-Aguilar (eds.), *Surgery for Cancers of the Gastrointestinal Tract: A Step-by-Step Approach*, DOI 10.1007/978-1-4939-1893-5_9, © Springer Science+Business Media New York 2015

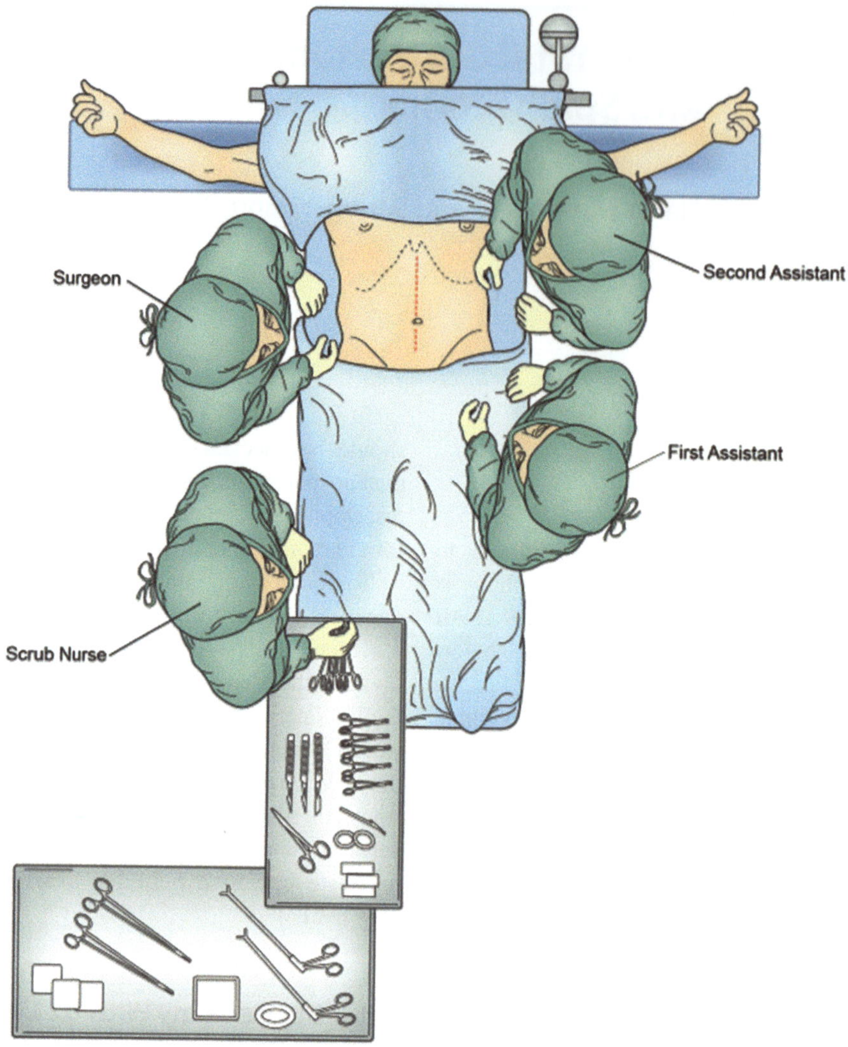


**Fig. 9.1** Operative positioning for open total gastrectomy

## Left Side Omentectomy With Dissection of Lymph Node Station 4sb

To complete dissection of lymph node (LN) station 4sb, it is mandatory to ligate the root of the left gastroepiploic artery (LGEA). Division of the splenocolic ligament is useful to expose the root of the LGEA and lower pole of the spleen. During dissection, it is easy to injure the inferior polar artery towards the lower pole of the spleen or pancreatic tail, which may cause partial infarction of the spleen or lead to pancreatic fistula.

## Right Side Omentectomy With Dissection of Lymph Node Station 6

Right side omentectomy continues toward the hepatic flexure of the colon and the second portion of the duodenum. Wrapping and lifting up the stomach using surgical gauze by the assistant is useful to help develop the appropriate surgical field. Dissection along the middle colic vein as well as accessory right colic vein is helpful to find an avascular plane for safe approach to the area of lymph node station 6. Following the avascular plane, the dissection

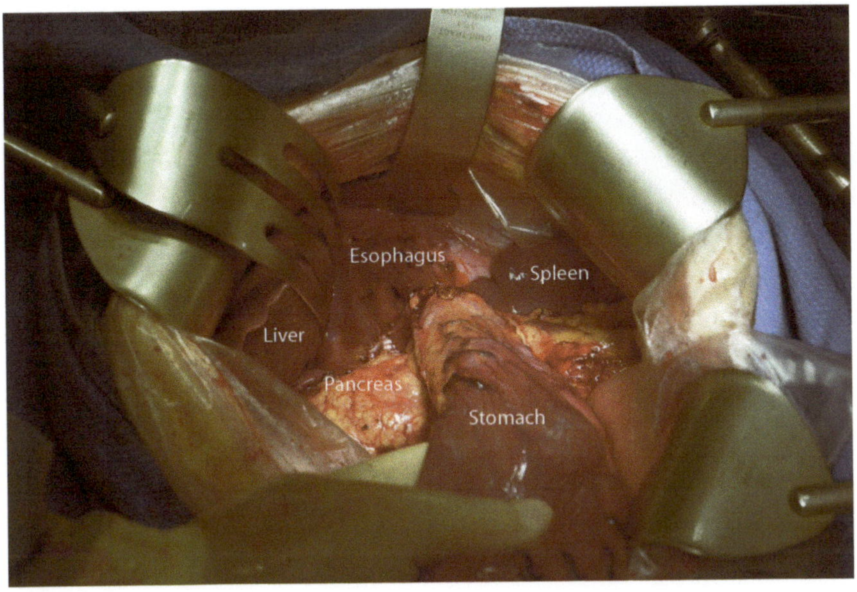


**Fig. 9.2** A self-retaining retractor is used to provide optimal exposure of the operative field

eventually leads to the gastrocolic trunk and superior mesenteric vein (SMV). Careful dissection is mandatory not to injure these named vessels. Using the avascular plane, omental bursectomy may be easier for right-sided omentectomy than for left-sided omentectomy. Meticulous dissection of the gastrocolic trunk and anterior surface of the pancreatic head can expose the root of the right gastroepiploic vein (RGEV). After identification of the anterior superior pancreaticoduodenal vein (ASPDV) and gastrocolic trunk, the RGEV can be ligated just distal to the ASPDV. According to the Japanese classification of gastric carcinoma guideline third edition [1], it is optional to dissect LNs around the SMV (i.e., LN number 14v) for D2 LN dissection.

Complete dissection around the pancreatic head and gastroduodenal artery (GDA) can expose the root of the right gastroepiploic artery (RGEA). After ligation of the RGEA at its root, careful dissection and ligation of the infrapyloric artery is also required. Energy device (ultrasonic or bipolar) is helpful to dissect not only the infrapyloric artery but also the small branches to the posterior wall of the duodenum from the GDA.

## Dissection of Lymph Node Stations 5 and 12

Division between LN stations 5 and 8 can effectively expose the medial side of the proper hepatic artery as well as the root of the right gastric artery (RGA). To develop a good surgical field, it is useful for the assistant to roll down the first portion of duodenum to the caudal side to make appropriate tension. During dissection of LN station 12 (i.e., hepatoduodenal ligament LNs along the proper hepatic artery in the caudal half between the confluence of the right and left hepatic ducts and the upper border of the pancreas), it is important not to injure the hepatic artery, bile duct, and portal vein.

After careful dissection of the hepatoduodenal ligament, the root of the RGA can be identified and ligated. For sufficient mobilization of the duodenum, one or two supraduodenal vessels can also be ligated.

## Duodenal Transection

A linear stapler can be used for duodenal transection (Fig. 9.3). After transection, the

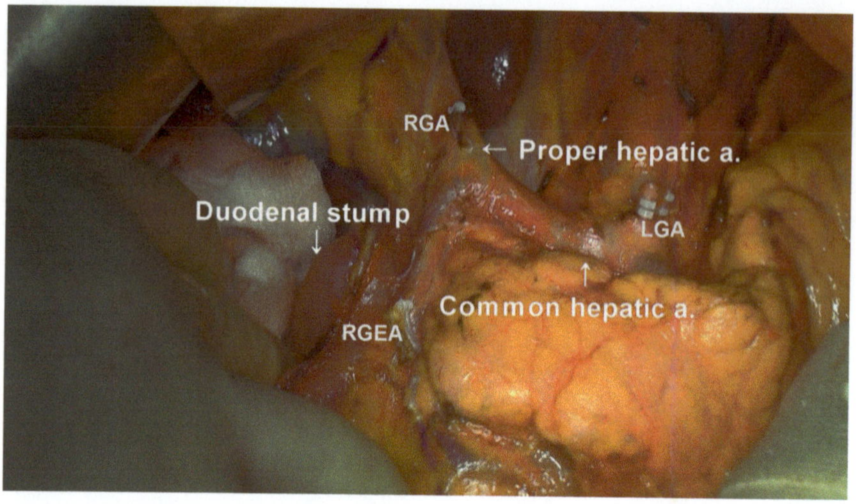


**Fig. 9.3** Intraoperative photo showing the duodenal stump and clips on the divided right gastroepiploic artery (RGEA), right gastric artery (RGA), and left gastric artery (LGA)

operator should be careful to obtain hemostasis of the staple line. Attempts to obtain hemostasis with electrocautery may cause postoperative duodenal stump leakage. Reinforcement of the staple line with Lambert sutures, even though it may not always be necessary, can be useful to prevent duodenal stump leakage.

## Splenectomy for Dissection of Lymph Node Station 10

For early gastric cancer (EGC) in the upper third of the stomach or the gastroesophageal junction, dissection of LN station 10 or splenectomy is not essential. During total gastrectomy for advanced gastric cancer (AGC), splenectomy can be considered in tumors (1) located on the greater curvature or (2) with lymph node enlargement near the splenic artery or vein to facilitate complete D2 LN dissection including the splenic hilar LNs (i.e., LN station 10).

Mobilization of the distal pancreas and spleen is helpful to make a better surgical field. After division of the splenocolic ligament, dissection of the lienorenal ligament and line of Toldt, which are usually avascular planes, is required to mobilize the spleen and the distal pancreas. After mobilization, lifting up on the spleen is useful for safe dissection around the splenic vessels and splenic hilum (Fig. 9.4). During these procedures, careful approach is necessary because it is easy to injure not only the vessels but also the parenchyma of the pancreas. After splenic hilar dissection, the splenic artery and vein can be identified and ligated. To avoid unwanted congestion of the spleen, ligation of the splenic artery first is recommended. The necessity of splenectomy is controversial. A randomized controlled trial to evaluate splenectomy in total gastrectomy for proximal gastric carcinoma is ongoing (ClinicalTrials.gov, NCT00112099).

## Dissection of Lymph Node Station 4sa

For total gastrectomy without splenectomy, meticulous LN dissection of station 4sa should be considered. After ligation of the LGEA, dissection of the gastrosplenic ligament toward the upper pole of the spleen is performed to dissect LN station 4sa. During this procedure, careful dissection and ligation of the short gastric arteries is required not to injure the main splenic vessels or splenic parenchyma. The surgeon should note that the superior polar artery of the spleen is sometimes located close to the upper pole of spleen as well as the gastric fundus.

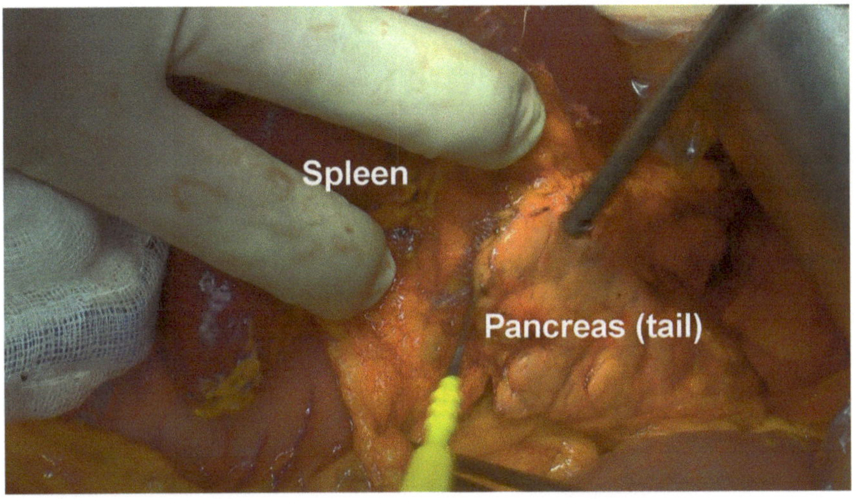


**Fig. 9.4** Intraoperative photo showing the mobilization of the distal spleen and pancreas to allow safe dissection around the splenic hilum

## Suprapancreatic Lymph Node Dissection

To expose the suprapancreatic LNs effectively, it is important for the assistant to expose the superior border of the pancreas. Finding the plane between LNs and the splenic artery can be helpful. Dissection of the suprapancreatic LNs can usually be performed from the right (LN station 8) to the left (LN station 11p) side. However direction of the dissection can be changed according to the convenience of procedures. From the medial side of the hepatoduodenal ligament and common hepatic artery, meticulous en bloc LN dissection is necessary not to disrupt metastatic LNs. Simple sharp dissection of LNs can cause spillage of lymphatic contents intraoperatively which may contain metastatic cancer cells. Therefore, ligation with clips or energy device can be helpful to seal the lymphatics. However, the activated blade of energy devices (e.g., ultrasonic dissector) can damage the walls of major vessels, which may cause serious intraoperative bleeding or postoperative pseudoaneurysmal change. Therefore, the active blade of the energy-based device should be always placed away from the patient side.

The splenic artery often has an unpredictable tortuous pathway. Therefore, it is easy to injure splenic vessels during the dissection of LN stations 11p and 11d, even though exposure of the splenic vein is sometimes required for complete D2 LN dissection. It is also common to injure small branches from the splenic artery towards the upper pole of the spleen or pancreas, which may cause infarction of splenic upper pole or pancreatic fistula. Preoperative review of the pathway of the splenic artery using abdominal computed tomography (CT) scan is helpful to prevent unwanted intraoperative injury to the splenic vessels. During dissection of suprapancreatic LNs and its related retroperitoneal space, careful attention is also required to differentiate the left adrenal gland, especially for advanced gastric cancer in the posterior wall of the upper third of the stomach.

After dissection of the celiac trunk and ventral side of the abdominal aorta, the root of the left gastric artery (LGA) can be exposed (Fig. 9.5). Because the left gastric vessels are the only vessels for the stomach at this point, ligation of the LGA first before the coronary vein is recommended to avoid unwanted congestion of the stomach. Suture ligation is not essential for the LGA; double clips or simple double ligation is usually sufficient.

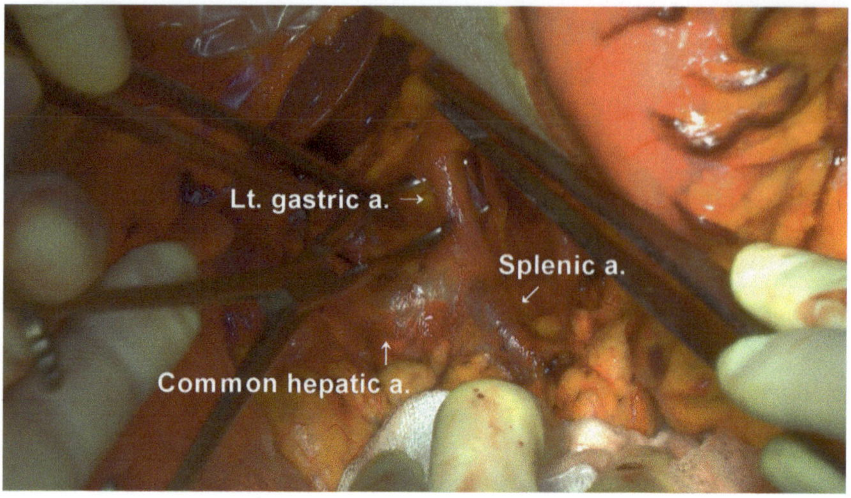


**Fig. 9.5** Intraoperative photo demonstrating exposure of the root of the left gastric artery

## Dissection of LN Stations 1 and 2

Dissection of LN stations 1 and 2 around the esophagus is performed along the diaphragmatic crus and esophageal hiatus. The anterior and posterior vagus nerves are also transected after complete isolation. During the dissection of the diaphragmatic crus, the inferior phrenic artery is also identified and ligated. In case of esophageal invasion of gastric cancer or adenocarcinoma of the gastroesophageal junction, dissection of infradiaphragmatic LNs, paraesophageal LNs in the diaphragmatic esophageal hiatus, and supradiaphragmatic LNs might be necessary, even though evidence demonstrating benefit of these procedures has not yet been confirmed. To enhance exposure of the esophagus, division of the diaphragmatic arch can be added.

## Esophageal Transection

Once dissection around the esophagus is complete, a purse-string clamp is applied with sufficient proximal resection margin. Careful attention should be paid to the esophageal resection and intraoperative frozen section confirmation of a negative proximal resection margin is mandatory.

During preparation of the esophageal stump, spillage of intraluminal contents into the peritoneal cavity should be avoided because of potential tumor cell spillage as well as microbial contamination. Since we use a circular stapler for our reconstruction, we insert the anvil and clamp a full layer of the esophageal wall with 3 Allis clamps toward the 1, 5, and 9 o'clock positions. If there is a relatively wide gap in between the purse-string, reinforcing sutures can be considered. Safe and secure esophageal stump including full layers of the esophageal wall is fundamental for successful esophagojejunostomy.

## Reconstruction

Roux-en-Y esophagojejunostomy using a circular stapler is the most common reconstruction method after total gastrectomy. The size of the circular stapler depends on the diameter of the jejunal Roux limb as well as that of esophagus. Usually, a 25-mm stapler is recommended.

Careful preparation of the Roux limb for esophagojejunostomy is important for successful anastomosis. Enough arterial supply and adequate venous drainage is critical to the Roux limb preparation. In addition, adequate length of the Roux limb toward the esophageal stump is also

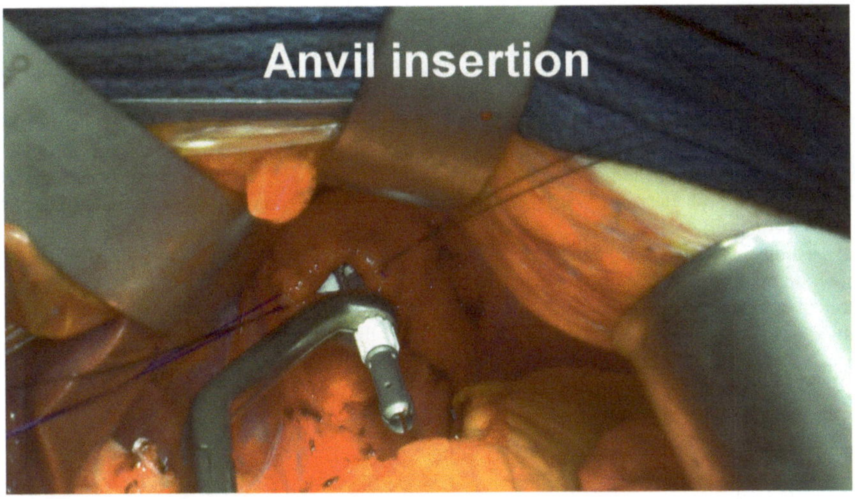


**Fig. 9.6** Intraoperative photo demonstrating insertion of the anvil into the end of the esophagus in preparation for esophagojejunostomy with the circular stapler

required to avoid unnecessary tension of the esophagojejunostomy. To prepare the Roux limb, the proximal jejunum is transected about 20 cm from the ligament of Treitz. The circular stapler is inserted through the distal end of the transected jejunum and then connected to the anvil, which was already placed in the esophageal stump (Fig. 9.6). End-to-side esophagojejunostomy is performed. For AGC, antecolic anastomosis is usually recommended whereas retrocolic anastomosis can be an alternative for EGC. During circular stapling, unexpected kinking of the jejunum at the anastomosis site should be avoided. To avoid kinking or slippage of the jejunal loop, tightening of the jejunal loop to the circular stapler using a vessel loop can be an option. After esophagojejunostomy, the jejunal stump is closed with the linear stapler.

Jejunojejunostomy is performed around 40 cm distal to the esophagojejunostomy by either hand-sewn method (end-to-side) or linear stapling method (side-to-side). To avoid internal herniation, the intermesenteric space between the afferent and efferent jejunal loop is closed. To prevent Petersen's hernia, the space between the transverse mesocolon and jejunal Roux limb can also be closed.

After completion of the anastomosis, a Levin tube may be introduced to the afferent loop through the jejunojejunostomy to identify postoperative delayed bleeding at the anastomosis site. Two closed suction drains are put into the left upper quadrant and the right upper quadrant. A right-sided drain runs through the foramen of Winslow and the LN dissection site of the suprapancreatic area towards the pancreas tail. The left-sided drain runs through the subphrenic space towards the posterior side of the esophagojejunostomy.

## Reference

1. Japanese Gastric Cancer Association. Japanese classification of gastric carcinoma: 3rd English edition. Gastric Cancer. 2011;14(2):101–12. doi:10.1007/s10120-011-0041-5.

## Key Operative Steps

1. Begin with omentectomy from the middle of the transverse colon and towards the left.
2. For proper dissection of lymph node station 4sb, the root of the left gastroepiploic artery must be ligated. Division of the splenocolic ligament is useful to expose this artery.
3. Continue omentectomy towards the hepatic flexure. Follow transverse mesocolic veins to find the avascular plane leading to the gastrocolic trunk and superior mesenteric vein. Expose and divide the root of the right gastroepiploic vessels. Dissect lymph node station 6.

4. Expose the proximal proper hepatic artery and root of the right gastric artery and dissect lymph node stations 12 and 5, respectively.
5. Divide the duodenum with a linear stapler. Reinforcement of the staple line is optional.
6. Consider splenectomy for advanced gastric cancer with serosal invasion located along the greater curvature or for bulky lymphadenopathy in the splenic hilum for dissection of lymph node station 10.
7. For total gastrectomy without splenectomy, meticulous dissection of the gastrosplenic ligament near the upper pole of spleen should be considered for lymph node station 4sa.
8. Expose the superior border of the pancreas to dissect from right to left, lymph node stations 8, 11p, and 11d.
9. Expose the celiac axis and left gastric artery and dissect lymph node stations 9 and 7, respectively. Ligate the left gastric artery before ligating the coronary vein.
10. Dissect lymph node stations 1 and 2 along the diaphragmatic crus and esophageal hiatus.
11. Identify and ligate the inferior phrenic artery.
12. Once the esophagus is fully mobilized, place a purse-string clamp on the esophagus.
13. Prepare Roux limb approximately 20 cm downstream from ligament of Treitz.
14. Perform end-to-side esophagojejunostomy with circular stapler.
15. Create jejunojejunostomy 40 cm downstream from the esophagojejunostomy.
16. Close intermesenteric space to prevent internal hernia.
17. Place two closed suction drains.

# Open Pancreaticoduodenectomy for Peri-Ampullary Cancers

**10**

Kaitlyn J. Kelly and Andrew M. Lowy

## Introduction

Pancreaticoduodenectomy is indicated for neoplasms of the head of the pancreas, the distal bile duct, the ampulla, and the peri-ampullary duodenum. While procedure-related mortality has been reduced significantly over the past two to three decades, the morbidity associated with this procedure remains high. Well-characterized complications of this procedure include, but are not limited to pancreatic fistula, delayed gastric emptying, and post-pancreatectomy hemorrhage. Multiple variations in the technique of pancreaticoduodenectomy have been investigated and described as means to reduce complications, including pylorus preservation, pancreatic duct stenting, Braun entero-enterostomy, and pancreaticogastrostomy [1–5]. Despite this, no specific technique has been convincingly shown to improve outcomes, and thus no specific variation has been widely adopted.

Regardless of variations in technique, it is clear that surgeon experience is an important predictor of outcome. Meticulous attention to detail is required for each individual step of the procedure to minimize the incidence of complications. This chapter breaks down the procedure of open pancreaticoduodenectomy into individual steps and discusses management of complex intraoperative situations that may be encountered.

K.J. Kelly, M.D. • A.M. Lowy, M.D. (✉)
Division of Surgical Oncology, Moores Cancer Center, University of California, San Diego, 3855 Health Sciences Drive, Mail Code 0987, La Jolla, CA 92093, USA
e-mail: k6kelly@ucsd.edu; alowy@ucsd.edu

## Patient Selection

Pancreaticoduodenectomy is indicated for premalignant and malignant lesions involving the head of the pancreas, the peri-ampullary duodenum, and the distal bile duct. It is also appropriate for symptomatic benign lesions and for conditions when malignancy cannot be definitively excluded without resection. For patients with known or presumed malignancy, high-quality, contrast-enhanced cross-sectional imaging with computed tomography (CT) or magnetic resonance imaging (MRI) should be performed. Most institutions have pancreas-specific imaging protocols with arterial and portal venous phase imaging for characterization of lesions and their associations with the mesenteric vasculature. Imaging should be recent, ideally within 30 days of surgery, to ensure that no significant disease progression has occurred in the interval between imaging and surgery. Unexpected intraoperative findings of locally advanced disease or vascular invasion should therefore be relatively rare.

J. Kim and J. Garcia-Aguilar (eds.), *Surgery for Cancers of the Gastrointestinal Tract: A Step-by-Step Approach*, DOI 10.1007/978-1-4939-1893-5_10, © Springer Science+Business Media New York 2015

## Patient Positioning

In the operating room the patient is placed in the supine position. The patients' arms are placed on arm boards or can be tucked depending on the size of the patient and surgeon preference. If the arms are left out, the arm boards should be placed cephalad so that a fixed retractor can still be comfortably placed caudal to the arm board. The surgeon generally stands on the patient's left side and the assistant on the patient's right side (Fig. 10.1).

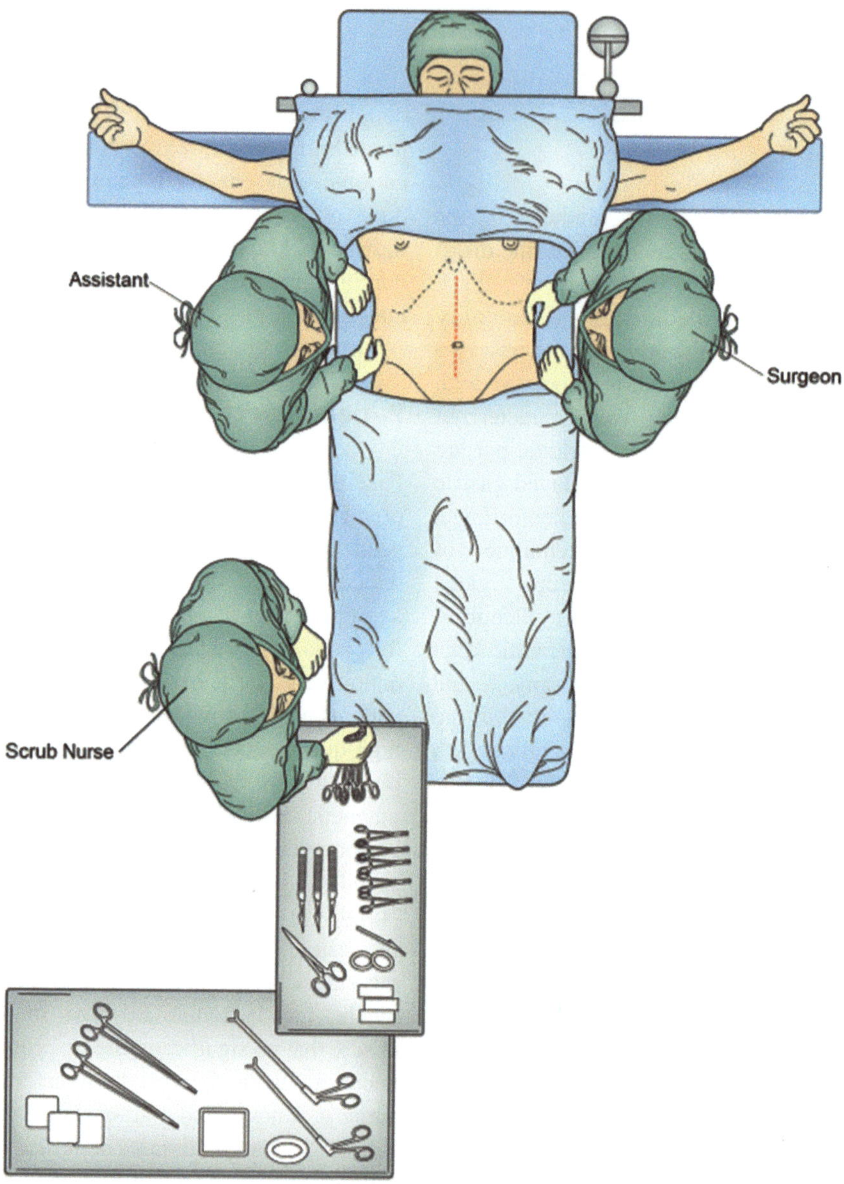


**Fig. 10.1** Patient positioning with both arms tucked to the side. The surgeon stands to the left and the assistant to the right of the patient

## Surgical Technique

### Exploration and Exposure

We recommend diagnostic laparoscopy to evaluate for clinically occult metastatic disease. This may be performed via open technique Hasson port placed in-line with the planned incision. The peritoneal cavity is then systematically inspected for ascites, peritoneal or liver nodules, or other evidence of metastatic disease. If any suspicious lesions are identified, an additional 5-mm port is placed to facilitate laparoscopic biopsy. Any suspicious lesions are sent for frozen section examination before proceeding.

Once absence of metastatic disease is confirmed, a laparotomy incision is made. We prefer a midline vertical incision from the xiphoid process to just above or just below the umbilicus, depending on the length of the patient's torso. A horizontal Chevron-type incision is also feasible. The two have been shown to be equivalent in terms of postoperative pain and postoperative hernia formation. The midline incision preserves the integrity of the rectus muscles and has been shown to result in decreased wound infections [6]. The pre-peritoneal fatty tissue is excised to facilitate exposure and the falciform ligament is divided between clamps and ties or with an energy-sealing device. The liver and the celiac trunk are palpated for liver masses or abnormal celiac lymph nodes, respectively. A fixed retractor is then assembled. We prefer the Thompson retractor (Thompson Surgical Instruments, Traverse City, MI).

### Dissection of the Inferior Border of Pancreas

The stomach is grasped and elevated by the assistant, whereas the transverse colon is grasped and placed inferiorly by the surgeon. The lesser sac is entered by dividing the greater omentum between the gastroepiploic vessels and the transverse colon. Entry into the lesser sac is confirmed by visualization of the posterior wall of the stomach. This opening should be extended along the greater curvature of the stomach, following the gastroepiploic vessels, but should be stopped prior to reaching the short gastric vessels. The opening is then similarly extended toward the distal stomach and the origin of the gastroepiploic vessels. It is important for the assistant to continue holding the stomach straight up in the air to expose this area. The avascular attachments between the posterior wall of the stomach and the pancreas are divided with electrocautery. The right gastroepiploic vein is identified and is carefully followed down to the superior mesenteric vein (SMV). The right gastroepiploic vein often shares a common trunk with the right colic vein, known as the gastrocolic trunk or Henle's trunk (Fig. 10.2). The trunk may include the middle colic vein as a trifurcation. Careful dissection should be performed along the left side of the venous trunk until the SMV is reached. The right gastroepiploic vein can be ligated and divided at this point to prevent tearing or this step can be performed later once final determination of resectability has been made.

Once the SMV is identified, it is critical to determine that there is an adequate length of vein uninvolved by tumor to proceed safely with resection. This typically requires a minimum of 2–3 cm of infra-pancreatic SMV to allow for placement of a vascular clamp to permit vascular reconstruction. It is acceptable to begin a tunnel between the anterior surface of the SMV and the neck of the pancreas, however significant dissection at this stage is strongly discouraged as vascular control of inflow and outflow has not been obtained and exposure is severely limited at this stage of the operation. Furthermore, in most cases, high quality preoperative imaging should clearly define the status of the plane behind the pancreatic neck. If an attempt to dissect this plane is made at this stage, any resistance during dissection should lead to this maneuver being immediately aborted. If small-volume bleeding is encountered, it is best controlled by applying pressure for some time, as there is no exposure to control it directly. If there is high-volume bleeding that will not stop with pressure, vascular control of the portal vein above and SMV below must be obtained while holding direct pressure. If necessary, the neck of the pancreas should be divided to expose the underlying source of

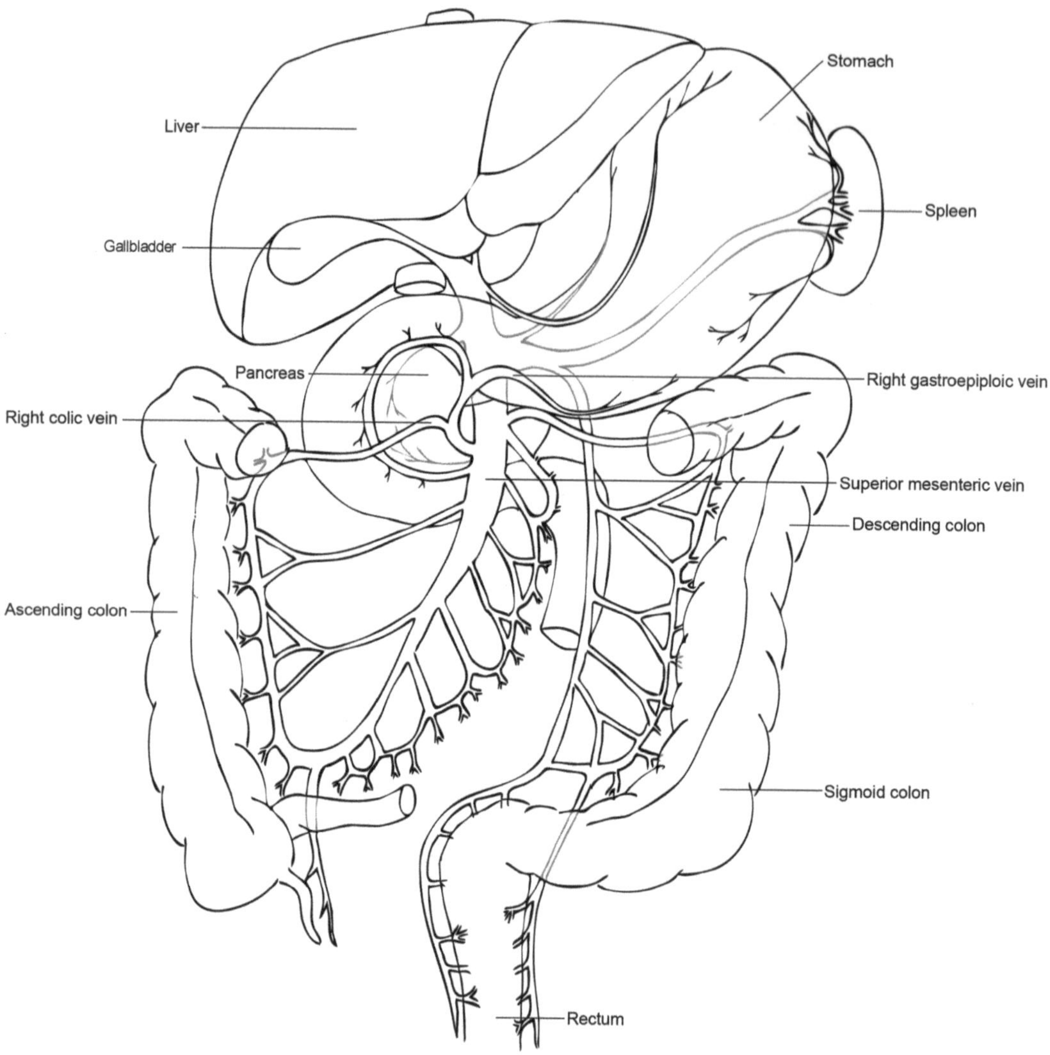


**Fig. 10.2** Illustration of the venous confluence of the right gastroepiploic and right colic veins. These veins drain into the superior mesenteric vein as a common trunk, which may also include the middle colic vein. These veins are easily torn with excessive traction and are a common site of bleeding in pancreaticoduodenectomy

bleeding. Next, we typically prefer to identify the superior mesenteric artery (SMA) just posteromedial to the SMV. This will help define the right lateral border of the SMA and later facilitate the uncinate dissection.

## Mobilization of the Hepatic Flexure

The transverse colon is grasped and elevated. Any attachments to the gallbladder are divided. The hepatic flexure attachments are divided with an energy sealant device exposing Gerota's fascia of the right kidney and the proximal duodenum. There is a discrete, avascular tissue plane between the colon mesentery and Gerota's fascia. This plane should be widely opened so that the colon can be packed caudally, maximizing exposure of the duodenum.

## Kocher Maneuver

The duodenum is gently rolled to the patient's left side by the surgeon, placing the underlying retroperitoneal attachments on tension. These attachments within an avascular plane are then divided with electrocautery, staying close to the edge of the duodenum. Care should be taken to avoid injury to the retroperitoneal structures in this region, including the right gonadal vessels, the right renal vein, and the inferior vena cava. This dissection should be continued under the head of the pancreas until the left renal vein and ligament of Treitz are reached. Tumor adherence to the inferior vena cava or aorta or abnormal lymphadenopathy in this region signifies advanced unredectable disease.

## Dissection of the Porta Hepatis

### Hepatic Artery

Attention is then turned to the supra-pyloric region. The gastrohepatic ligament is opened and the stomach is again grasped and elevated. This maneuver tents up the right gastric artery making the location of this typically small vessel apparent. The artery and surrounding tissue is divided at the left lateral aspect of the porta hepatis with an energy sealant device.

Next, the hepatic artery and associated hepatic artery lymph node are identified along the superior border of the pancreas. The node may be difficult to appreciate in obese patients, when it is covered by adipose tissue that must be opened to identify the plane between the node and the pancreatic parenchyma. This fatty tissue should be opened carefully, layer-by-layer until the anatomy is apparent. The lymph node is then removed and should be sent for frozen section analysis, since the finding of metastatic disease will impact the decision to proceed.

Removal of the hepatic artery lymph node provides exposure of the gastroduodenal artery (GDA) and common hepatic artery (CHA). The CHA should be dissected circumferentially to fully visualize its course and the GDA takeoff. The GDA is dissected circumferentially, ideally for a distance of 1–2 cm. The GDA should be gently occluded with a vessel loop or small vascular clamp and the proper hepatic artery should then be palpated to ensure that it still has a strong pulse. If occlusion of the GDA diminishes the pulse in the proper hepatic artery, this indicates narrowing of the celiac axis or variant hepatic arterial anatomy.

Once proper hepatic artery flow is confirmed, the GDA is ligated and divided. We prefer to divide the vessel sharply between two right-angle clamps leaving an approximately 1-cm stump of GDA coming off the CHA to allow for embolization of the stump should post-pancreatectomy hemorrhage develop. The proximal end is secured by 3-0 or 4-0 Prolene sutures followed by 3-0 silk ties. This vessel may also be divided with a vascular stapler if preferred.

### Portal Vein

Division of the GDA allows for exposure of the portal vein (PV), which lies posterior to the GDA (Fig. 10.3). The GDA stump is gently retracted upward and the anterior surface of the portal vein is exposed. The space between the anterior surface of the PV and the neck of the pancreas is bluntly dissected with the goal of communicating with the space inferior to the neck of the pancreas. This should be performed very carefully and should again be aborted if any resistance is met. A vessel loop may then be passed around the neck of the pancreas to facilitate relocation of the tunnel later in the procedure.

### Common Bile Duct

Attention is then turned back to the porta hepatis and the gallbladder should be removed if the patient has not had prior cholecystectomy. It is not necessary to keep the gallbladder attached to the remainder of the specimen. The cystic duct is ligated and the gallbladder is passed off as a separate specimen to facilitate exposure. The common bile duct (CBD) is identified and is dissected circumferentially. This should be done by identifying the right lateral aspect of the PV and dissecting from left to right around the CBD. Performing this dissection from right to left can result in injury to the portal vein. There is often nodal and fatty tissue posterior to the bile duct and this area should be carefully palpated for the presence of a replaced or accessory right hepatic artery before it is inadvertently divided. Once the absence of a vessel is confirmed, this tissue can be divided with an energy sealant device, taking care to keep these lymph nodes with the specimen.

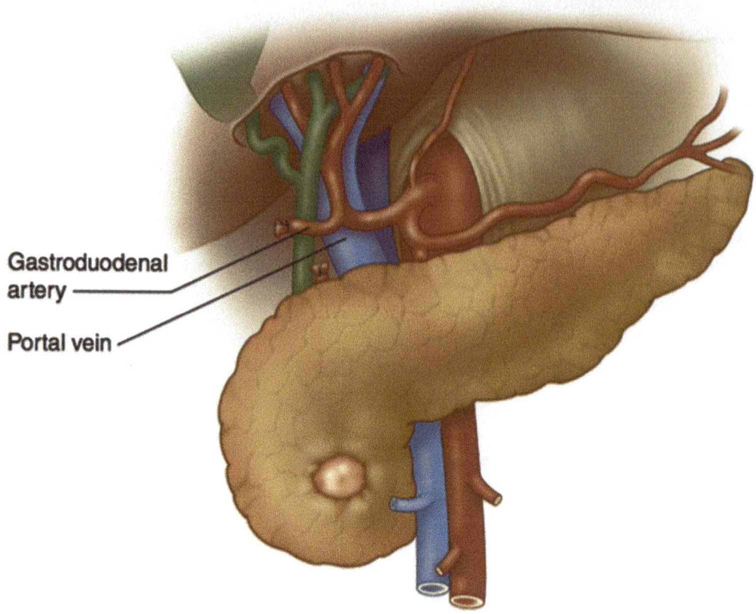


**Fig. 10.3** Illustration of the anatomic position of the portal vein behind the gastroduodenal artery. Division of the gastroduodenal artery and elevation of the trunk provide exposure of the anterior surface of the portal vein above the pancreas

The CBD is then sharply divided. We recommend angling the scissors or knife so that the posterior wall of the CBD is left slightly longer than the anterior wall to facilitate creation of the hepaticojejunostomy during the reconstruction. There is often bleeding from the lateral longitudinal arteries of the bile duct. This can be controlled with electrocautery or with placement of a bulldog clamp on the CBD. The latter method also prevents spillage of bile during the remainder of the procedure. If a biliary stent was placed preoperatively, it is removed at this point and should be sent for culture. The culture results may be useful should the patient develop a surgical site infection postoperatively. At this point, a portion of the bile duct may be sent for frozen section analysis. The distal bile duct is typically oversewn with a silk suture to facilitate hemostasis.

## Division of the Stomach

Attention is next turned to the stomach. We often perform a standard pancreaticoduodenectomy including a small portion of the antrum and pylorus with the specimen. Multiple randomized, controlled trials have confirmed no difference in outcomes with standard versus pylorus-preserving techniques. Any remaining gastrohepatic ligament attachments are cleared for about 3–4 cm proximal to the pylorus. A target area on the greater curvature side of the stomach is selected and is similarly cleared of any remaining omental attachments. The stomach is then divided with a linear stapler. After assuring hemostasis on the staple line, the proximal stomach can then be packed into the left upper quadrant.

## Division of the Proximal Jejunum

Attention is next turned to the jejunum. The ligament of Treitz is identified from the left side and the jejunum is divided with a linear stapler at a site where the mesentery is long enough to comfortably reach the right side of the mesenteric vessels. The mesentery to the proximal jejunum is then divided immediately adjacent to the bowel wall with an energy sealant device. Straying away from the peripheral-most aspect of the mesentery at the junction with the bowel wall could result in catastrophic injury to the SMA. The mesentery can usually be divided as

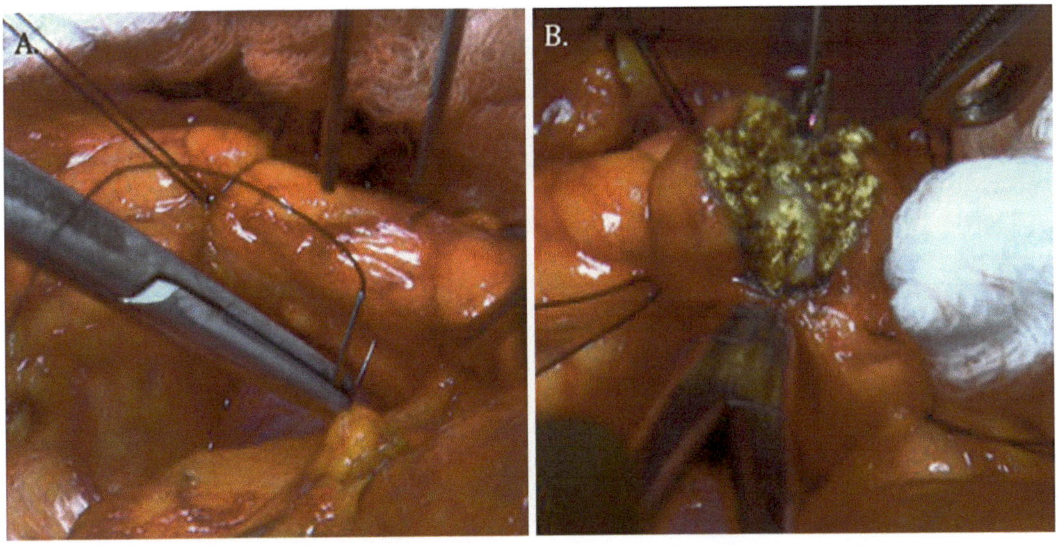


**Fig. 10.4** Division of the pancreas. (**a**) Intraoperative image depicting placement of stay sutures on either side of the neck of the pancreas prior to transection. (**b**) Image demonstrating transection of the pancreatic neck with electrocautery. A Kelly clamp is positioned to protect the underlying portal vein

one layer initially, but as the ligament of Treitz is approached, it becomes thicker and may need to be taken in two layers. Care should be taken to identify the inferior mesenteric vein in this region to avoid injury to this vessel.

The ligament of Treitz itself may be divided with electrocautery. The goal is to enter into the space that was created on the right side of the mesenteric vessels during the Kocher maneuver. Once this is achieved, the divided edge of the mesentery should be carefully inspected for hemostasis. Bleeding from this area is common. The proximal jejunum is then gently passed beneath the SMA to the right side of the abdomen. There are often remaining attachments at the ligament of Treitz that are easier divided after passing the jejunum to the right side.

## Division of the Pancreas

Attention is next turned back to the neck of the pancreas. The transection line is marked on the anterior capsule with electrocautery. Stay sutures are then placed on both sides of this transection line at both the inferior and superior edges of the gland (four total) (Fig. 10.4a). They are tied down gently against the pancreatic capsule and are left long with hemostat clamps placed on the ends to facilitate retraction of the gland. The purpose of these sutures is to prevent bleeding from the intra-pancreatic vessels when the gland is divided.

A Kelly clamp or other curved, blunt instrument is placed under the neck of the pancreas to protect the SMV-PV. The pancreas is first divided with electrocautery in the anterior and inferior aspect of the gland (Fig. 10.4b). Once the duct is identified, any bleeding from the adjacent cut parenchyma on the remnant side can be controlled with electrocautery. The remnant side is then mobilized off the retroperitoneum and splenic vein for a distance of 1–2 cm.

## Dissection of the Head and Uncinate Process

At this point, attachments remain between the uncinate process and the retroperitoneum and the lateral aspect of the PV. We generally approach the dissection anteriorly first, gently freeing the head and uncinate process off the SMV-PV. The specimen is retracted toward the right and is dissected off the right lateral aspect of the PV. There is consistently a large venous branch at the cephalad aspect of the retropancreatic PV that should be ligated and divided with clips or ties. The remaining branches are generally small enough to be controlled with cautery or clips. The first jejunal branch of the SMV generally takes off at the right lateral aspect but abruptly turns posteriorly and courses behind the PV. This branch may or may not need to be ligated and divided.

Once the specimen is freed from the SMV-PV, the PV is rolled to the left and the SMA is identified. The plane between the pancreatic parenchyma and retroperitoneal fat is identified and the retroperitoneal fat is divided along the SMA in a caudal to cephalad direction. Retraction of the specimen laterally and cephalad is key to facilitate exposure. The medial extent of the dissection is the right lateral border of the SMA. Most of the attachments, aside from the inferior pancreaticoduodenal artery can be divided with an energy sealant device, but occasionally other small arterial branches may need to be ligated with clips or ties. During this portion of the dissection, a replaced right hepatic artery will be encountered and if not involved by tumor, should be preserved. Once the SMA dissection is complete, the specimen is oriented and sent to pathology and the surgical bed is irrigated and thoroughly inspected for hemostasis.

## Reconstruction

### Pancreaticojejunostomy

Next an avascular area on the transverse colon mesentery is identified and opened with electrocautery. The proximal jejunum is then passed through this defect and is comfortably approximated to the remnant pancreas and bile duct. The pancreaticojejunal anastomosis is performed first. The side of the jejunum is approximated to the cut edge of the pancreas in an end-to-side fashion, approximately 2–3 cm from the stapled end. We prefer to perform the anastomosis in two layers. A row of interrupted 3-0 silk sutures is placed from the posterior edge of the pancreas through the seromuscular layer of the jejunum starting at the superior end of the cut surface of the pancreas. These sutures are not immediately tied but are kept separate and organized with hemostat clamps. Once all sutures are placed, they are tied. After this, ideally the cut edge of the pancreas should be facing anteriorly, or nearly parallel to the floor to provide excellent exposure of the pancreatic duct.

Once the posterior row is complete encompassing the entire cephalocaudad width of the pancreas, the duct-to-mucosa anastomosis is performed. A small enterotomy is made on the jejunum adjacent to the pancreatic duct. A duct-to-mucosa anastomosis is then performed with interrupted, 4-0 absorbable sutures. Approximately 4–8 stitches are placed depending on the size of the duct, starting with the central posterior suture. In cases of a small pancreatic duct, it is helpful to place the anterior central stitch through the pancreatic duct only first, leaving the needle on, as a means of tenting the duct open. The three posterior sutures are placed in an in-to-out fashion so that the knots are on the inside, and the anterior sutures are placed out-to-in with the knots on the outside. It is critical to place these sutures carefully avoiding excess needle sticks to the pancreas and obtaining solid, full-thickness bites of the pancreatic duct wall with each suture. Once all of the sutures are placed, they are gently tied down sequentially, starting first with the posterior row. For small pancreatic ducts, use of a 5-French pediatric feeding tube is useful as a stent to avoid narrowing the duct (Fig. 10.5). We do not suture the tube in place, since it will then pass naturally into the gastrointestinal tract. Once the duct-to-mucosa anastomosis is complete, an anterior row of 3-0 silk sutures is placed from the pancreatic capsule to the seromuscular layer of the jejunum, covering the duct-to-mucosa suture line.

### Hepaticojejunostomy

A site on the jejunal limb lying in proximity to the cut end of the bile duct is selected for creation of the hepaticojejunostomy. We prefer to perform this anastomosis with running sutures when the duct is dilated, and interrupted sutures

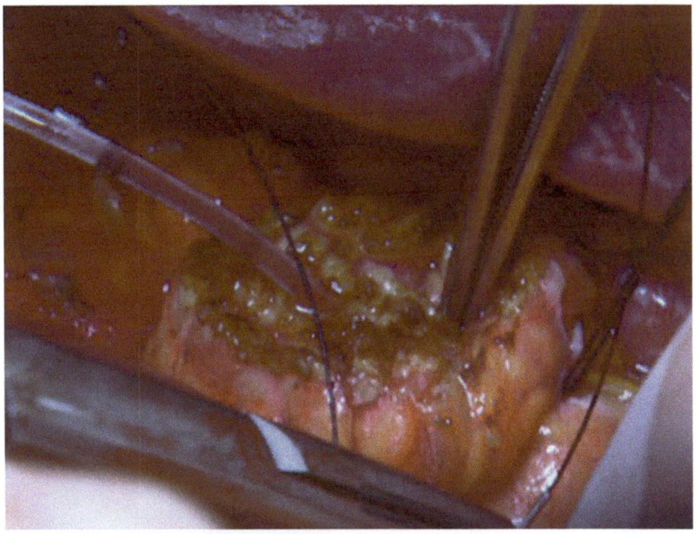

**Fig. 10.5** Image of a 5-French pediatric feeding tube placed within a small pancreatic duct as a stent

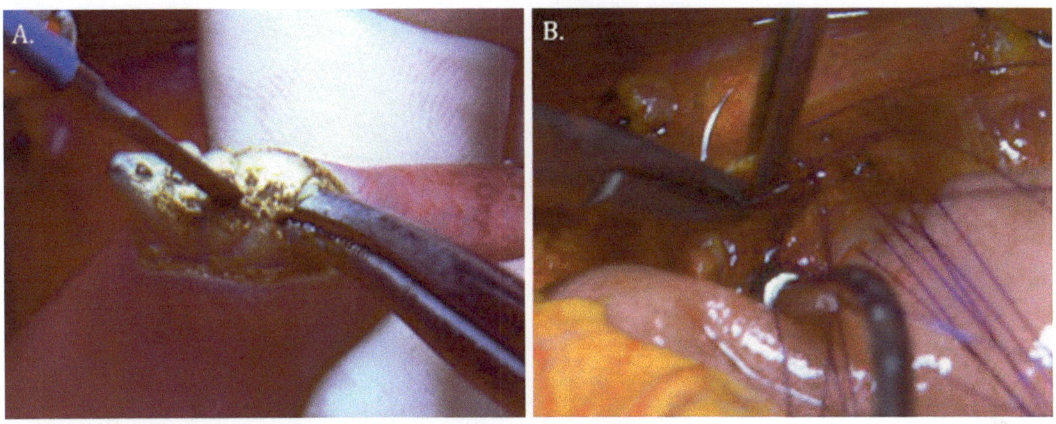


**Fig. 10.6** Hepaticojejunostomy. (**a**) Image of jejunal enterotomy making sure to adequately open the mucosa as well as the serosa. (**b**) Creation of interrupted, single-layer hepaticojejunal anastomosis

when it is small. In either case, the anastomosis is started by placing two corner stay sutures aligning the cut end of the duct and the side of the jejunum. An enterotomy is made in the jejunum with electrocautery (Fig. 10.6a) and the posterior layer of the anastomosis is performed taking full-thickness bites of the bowel wall and the duct (Fig. 10.6b). This can be done as one running suture or as several interrupted sutures positioned with the knots on the inside. The anterior row is then performed in the same fashion with single layer full-thickness running or interrupted sutures now with the knots positioned on the outside. The corner stay sutures are then tied down. This anastomosis is performed with 3-0 or 4-0 absorbable sutures depending on the size of the duct. We often place a clean laparotomy pad behind this anastomosis once it is complete and leave it in place while the gastrojejunostomy is performed to demonstrate whether there is any leakage of bile. Once these anastomoses are complete, the transverse mesocolon defect is inspected and is approximated with interrupted 3-0 sutures if necessary. We also routinely suture the edge of this defect to the serosa of the jejunal limb.

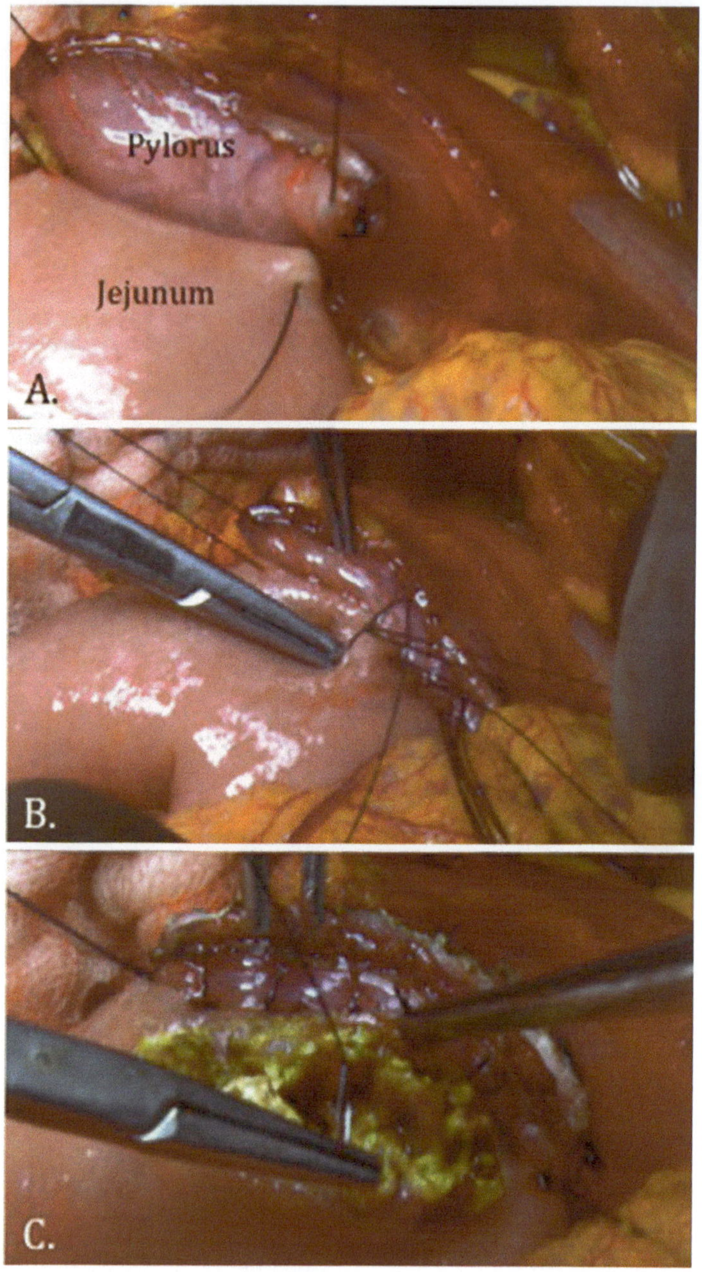


**Fig. 10.7** Duodenojejunostomy in a pylorus-preserving pancreaticoduodenectomy. (**a**) The stapled pylorus and jejunum are aligned with stay sutures. (**b**) A posterior row of Lembert 3-0 silk sutures is placed. (**c**) The staple line is removed and the jejunum is opened for placement of a running inner layer of full-thickness sutures

## Gastrojejunostomy

For the final anastomosis, a segment of jejunum approximately 30–40 cm downstream from the hepaticojejunostomy is selected and is brought into proximity of the gastric remnant in a retro- or antecolic position for creation of a double-layered, end-to-side gastrojejunostomy. Stay sutures of 3-0 silk or absorbable sutures are placed to align the gastric staple line with the anti-mesenteric border of the jejunum (Fig. 10.7a). A line demarcating the position of the planned jejunal enterotomy is marked on the bowel with electrocautery to serve as a guide in placing the posterior layer of stitches. The staple line serves as the guide on the stomach side.

The outer serosal layer is placed with running or interrupted sutures, taking care to maintain a straight, horizontal line and not migrate along the radial aspect of the jejunum (Fig. 10.7b). The gastric staple line is then removed with electrocautery and the jejunum is opened. An inner posterior layer of running 3-0 absorbable sutures is then placed (Fig. 10.7c). We use single double-armed sutures in the center of the posterior row and run each needle around their respective corners to meet on the anterior wall. An anterior outer serosal layer is then performed in the same fashion as the posterior layer. In creating this anastomosis, the jejunum can be oriented so that the efferent aspect is on the left or right sides. Care should be taken to avoid rolling excessive tissue into the efferent limb to prevent mechanical problems with gastric emptying. We prefer to place a nasogastric tube for decompression of the gastric remnant for the first 24-h postoperatively.

### Final Inspection

Once the reconstruction is complete, all anastomoses are inspected. The laparotomy pad behind the hepaticojejunostomy is inspected for bile leakage. The abdomen is irrigated with sterile saline and the operative bed is inspected for hemostasis, focusing on the divided edge of the proximal jejunal mesentery and GDA stump. We do not routinely utilize drains but prefer to place them only for high-risk pancreatic anastomoses, particularly those with small pancreatic ducts and soft gland consistency.

## Complex Situations

### Vascular Involvement

In cases of tumor involvement of the SMV-PV and/or the CHA, vascular resection and reconstruction is required to achieve margin-negative resection. For venous involvement, the uncinate process must be completely freed from the SMA and retroperitoneum prior to approaching the SMV-PV. The dissection should be carried out so that the only remaining attachment to the specimen is the involved segment of vein. Proximal and distal vascular control is achieved and the involved segment is then excised with tenotomy scissors. In most cases, primary repair is possible. This may require division of the splenic vein to allow for approximation of the defect. If there is concern that primary repair may not be possible, maneuvers such as mobilizing the liver to bring the PV down and incising the peritoneum on the small bowel mesentery to allow the SMV to move cephalad can provide extra length. If these maneuvers are not adequate, a graft is required. Autologous vein is preferred. The left renal vein makes an ideal graft because of its size and because it does not require external areas to be prepared and draped. The internal jugular vein is also an excellent conduit. Smaller defects can be repaired using saphenous vein patches.

In cases of hepatic arterial involvement, the specimen should similarly be dissected free of all attachments except the involved arterial segment so that vascular control can be achieved. The involved segment is then excised and reconstruction is performed with primary repair or with an interposition graft if primary repair is not possible.

### Inability to Locate the Pancreatic Duct

In rare cases, the pancreatic duct may not be identifiable after division of the pancreatic parenchyma. In this situation, it is helpful to assess the specimen for the location of the duct in the head of the pancreas, where it is larger in caliber. This may help to localize the duct in the remnant. If this is not successful, an invaginated pancreaticojejunostomy or pancreaticogastrostomy must be performed as a duct-to-mucosa anastomosis is not possible. For a pancreaticojejunostomy, a posterior anastomosis is created between the posterior capsule of the pancreas and the serosa of the jejunum. The jejunal staple line is removed and the entire cut end of the pancreatic remnant is invaginated into the jejunum. An anterior row of capsule to serosa sutures is then performed. A recent randomized, controlled trial comparing invaginated pancreaticojejunostomy to pancreaticogastrostomy reported decreased incidence of pancreatic fistula with pancreaticogastrostomy [4].

Pancreaticogastrostomy is created by invaginating the cut end of the pancreas through the posterior wall of the stomach. An anterior gastrotomy must be made first to expose the posterior wall of the stomach from inside the lumen. Stay sutures are placed through and through the pancreas. A posterior gastrotomy is then made and the pancreas is gently pulled up into the stomach using the stay sutures. An anastomosis is then created between the gastric serosa and the pancreas capsule on the outside of the stomach.

## Conclusions

Pancreaticoduodenectomy is a technically challenging procedure with high perioperative morbidity. Surgeon experience is a strong predictor of outcome [7]. Early in their practice, surgeons should initially select uncomplicated cases without evidence of vascular involvement and should have a more experienced partner available for assistance. Meticulous attention to detail for each step of the procedure is key to performing a successful resection and minimizing perioperative complications.

## References

1. Hochwald SN, Grobmyer SR, Hemming AW, Curran E, Bloom DA, Delano M, et al. Braun enteroenterostomy is associated with reduced delayed gastric emptying and early resumption of oral feeding following pancreaticoduodenectomy. J Surg Oncol. 2010;101(5):351–5. doi:10.1002/jso.21490.
2. Kawai M, Tani M, Hirono S, Miyazawa M, Shimizu A, Uchiyama K, et al. Pylorus ring resection reduces delayed gastric emptying in patients undergoing pancreatoduodenectomy: a prospective, randomized, controlled trial of pylorus-resecting versus pylorus-preserving pancreatoduodenectomy. Ann Surg. 2011;253(3):495–501. doi:10.1097/SLA.0b013e31820d98f1.
3. Pessaux P, Sauvanet A, Mariette C, Paye F, Muscari F, Cunha AS, et al. External pancreatic duct stent decreases pancreatic fistula rate after pancreaticoduodenectomy: prospective multicenter randomized trial. Ann Surg. 2011;253(5):879–85. doi:10.1097/SLA.0b013e31821219af.
4. Topal B, Fieuws S, Aerts R, Weerts J, Feryn T, Roeyen G, et al. Pancreaticojejunostomy versus pancreaticogastrostomy reconstruction after pancreaticoduodenectomy for pancreatic or periampullary tumours: a multicentre randomised trial. Lancet Oncol. 2013;14(7):655–62. doi:10.1016/S1470-2045(13)70126-8.
5. Tran KT, Smeenk HG, van Eijck CH, Kazemier G, Hop WC, Greve JW, et al. Pylorus preserving pancreaticoduodenectomy versus standard Whipple procedure: a prospective, randomized, multicenter analysis of 170 patients with pancreatic and periampullary tumors. Ann Surg. 2004;240(5):738–45.
6. Seiler CM, Deckert A, Diener MK, Knaebel HP, Weigand MA, Victor N, et al. Midline versus transverse incision in major abdominal surgery: a randomized, double-blind equivalence trial (POVATI: ISRCTN60734227). Ann Surg. 2009;249(6):913–20. doi:10.1097/SLA.0b013e3181a77c92.
7. Schmidt CM, Turrini O, Parikh P, House MG, Zyromski NJ, Nakeeb A, et al. Effect of hospital volume, surgeon experience, and surgeon volume on patient outcomes after pancreaticoduodenectomy: a single-institution experience. Arch Surg. 2010;145(7):634–40. doi:10.1001/archsurg.2010.118.

## Key Operative Steps

1. Explore to evaluate for occult metastatic disease.
2. Enter the lesser sac and expose the inferior border of the pancreas.
3. Mobilize the hepatic flexure to expose Gerota's fascia and the duodenum.
4. Perform a wide Kocher maneuver to the left renal vein and ligament of Treitz.
5. Dissect the porta hepatis: open the gastrohepatic ligament, divide the right gastric artery, resect the common hepatic artery lymph node, divide the gastroduodenal artery, perform cholecystectomy, and divide the common bile duct.
6. Transect the antrum of the stomach or proximal duodenum.
7. Divide the proximal jejunum and the mesentery to it up to the ligament of Treitz.
8. Transect the neck of pancreas.
9. Pass the distal duodenum and proximal jejunum underneath the superior mesenteric vessels to the right side of the abdomen and dissect the head and uncinate process of the pancreas from the superior mesenteric vein-portal vein and from the right lateral aspect of the superior mesenteric artery.
10. Perform reconstruction: pancreaticojejunostomy, hepaticojejunostomy, and gastrojejunostomy/duodenojejunostomy.

# Laparoscopic Pancreaticoduodenectomy

# 11

Palanisamy Senthilnathan and Chinnusamy Palanivelu

## Introduction

Laparoscopic pancreatic surgery represents one of the most sophisticated and advanced applications of laparoscopy in the current surgical practice. But the adoption of laparoscopic pancreaticoduodenectomy (LPD) has been relatively slow due to the proximity of the pancreas to major vessels, its retroperitoneal location, and the need for prolonged and meticulous intracorporeal suturing. With enormous development in technology coupled with improved anatomical knowledge and refined skills, LPD has grown out of its infancy and is an established procedure today. Although safety and outcomes are well-documented, patient selection remains the key, especially during the period of initial experience. In recent years, an increasing number of LPDs have been performed and reported from centers around the world. However, LPD is associated with a long learning curve, technically difficult reconstruction, and prolonged operative time. As experience with LPD has increased, data demonstrating technical feasibility, comparable perioperative results, and acceptable oncologic outcomes are forthcoming.

## Historical Perspectives

Bernheim reported the use of diagnostic laparoscopy in a patient with a pancreatic mass in 1911 [1]. Later, Cuschieri in 1978 and Warshaw in 1986 performed laparoscopic staging for the detection of metastases and tumor ingrowth [2, 3]. A wide variety of pancreatic laparoscopic resections, ranging from enucleation to distal pancreatic resection, have since been performed with successful outcomes. It was not until 1992 that the first minimally invasive pancreaticoduodenectomy (MIPD) was performed; Gagner and Pomp successfully accomplished the procedure with the intent to treat chronic pancreatitis [4]. This technique took approximately 600 min to complete and had a 30-day hospital stay. Since this first description more than 20 years ago, a large number of single-institution series of minimally invasive (laparoscopic-assisted, totally laparoscopic, and more recently robotic) pancreaticoduodenectomy performed for a variety of indications have been reported. Several recent articles with larger sample sizes have been published over the last few years. Our group has two decades long experience in managing various

Electronic supplementary material: Supplementary material is available in the online version of this chapter at 10.1007/978-1-4939-1893-5_11. Videos can also be accessed at http://www.springerimages.com/videos/978-1-4939-1892-8.

P. Senthilnathan, M.S., DNB GI Surgery, F.A.C.S. (✉)
C. Palanivelu, M.S., MCh GI Surgery,
F.A.C.S., F.R.C.S.
Division of Minimally Invasive & HPB Surgery, GEM Centre for Liver and Pancreas, GEM Hospital & Research Centre, 45, Pankaja Mill Road, Ramanathapuram, Coimbatore 641028, Tamilnadu, India
e-mail: senthilnathan94@yahoo.com

J. Kim and J. Garcia-Aguilar (eds.), *Surgery for Cancers of the Gastrointestinal Tract: A Step-by-Step Approach*,
DOI 10.1007/978-1-4939-1893-5_11, © Springer Science+Business Media New York 2015

pancreatic diseases by the minimal access method. Regarding LPD, we have one of the largest series of cases, with our last publication of a series of 75 cases demonstrating excellent outcomes in relation to blood loss and length of hospital stay with comparable morbidity and mortality to the open approach [5].

## Indications for Operation

Selection of the patient is extremely important for the success of the procedure. The stress must be on judiciously selecting early and small periampullary lesions during the initial period of the learning curve. With growing experience, LPD may be attempted for most periampullary tumors and tumors in the pancreatic head, with exceptions for patients with poor performance status, hostile abdomen due to multiple previous surgeries, extensive comorbidities, borderline resectability, and vascular invasion. The preferred indications include ampullary tumors, distal common bile duct tumors, early pancreatic head carcinoma (<3 cm), and duodenal carcinoma.

## Preoperative Investigations

The routine preoperative workup for LPD is no different from the open approach albeit with a few modifications. It includes full blood counts, liver function tests, and radiological investigations. Side viewing endoscope is done for all the periampullary lesions.The main imaging modality to assess the pancreatic and periampullary pathology is triphasic computed tomography (CT) with pancreatic protocol. It provides fairly good information about the tumor and its relation to the vascular structures. It is better to find the anomalous arterial anatomy preoperatively so that intraoperative accidental injury to these vessels can be avoided. Alternatively, magnetic resonance imaging (MRI) is employed especially in renal compromised patients. Endoscopic ultrasound (EUS) not only refines the information obtained by CT scan but also allows tissues to be sampled [6]. It is the authors practice to selectively perform EUS for patients with suspected vascular involvement, uncharacteristic imaging on CT scan, and associated chronic pancreatitis. Positron emission tomography (PET) is selectively employed for patients with high degree of suspicion of metastatic disease, such as lymphadenopathy extending beyond the peripancreatic nodal group and poorly differentiated histologic grades. The tumor markers carbohydrate antigen (CA) 19-9 and carcino-embryonic antigen (CEA) are included in the routine workup.

## Preoperative Preparation

Preoperative preparation for LPD is similar to any other major surgery. However, there are a few points worth mentioning. Patients with significant comorbidities like ischemic heart disease and higher American Society of Anesthesiology (ASA) grades are generally avoided in the initial stages of one's learning curve. Patients should also be nutritionally adept to withstand the stress of major surgery. Incentive spirometry should ideally be started 5 days prior to surgery to optimize the respiratory function in all patients, irrespective of the existing lung function. The role of preoperative biliary drainage in patients with obstructive jaundice is questionable but cholangitis is an absolute indication for biliary decompression prior to surgery. Patients are then stabilized and taken for surgery after a minimum of 4 weeks. The other indication for preoperative biliary decompression is a very high bilirubin level even without cholangitis. Different centers have different cut-off values and we drain the biliary system if the serum bilirubin level is >20 mg%. The role of preoperative bowel preparation for major surgeries like LPD is controversial, however it facilitates good laparoscopic exposure in the peripancreatic region with a collapsed transverse colon. Central venous access prior to the procedure in all patients is preferable and preoperative antibiotics are routinely given at the time of induction of anesthesia.

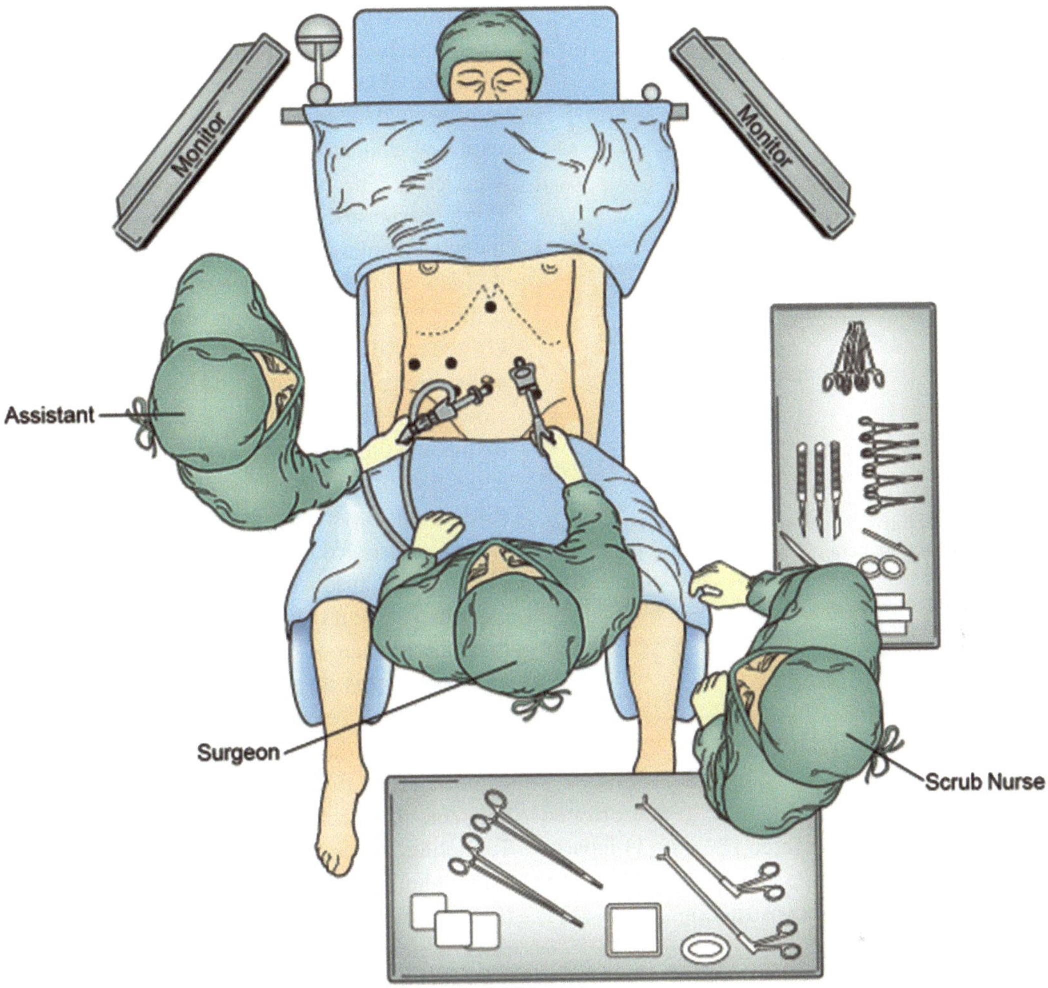


**Fig. 11.1** Operative positioning of the patient. The surgeon stands between the legs for most part of the operation

## Operative Details

### Team Setup and Port Placement

The procedure is undertaken under general anesthesia with endotracheal intubation and standard intraoperative monitoring. The patient is placed in reverse Trendelenburg position with the legs split. The monitor is placed at the head end of the patient. The surgeon stands between the legs of the patient for most part of the procedure (Fig. 11.1). At select steps of the operation, like hepatic flexure mobilization or the performance of hepaticojejunostomy, the operating surgeon stands on the left side. Pneumoperitoneum is created at the umbilical/supra-umbilical area and the remaining ports are then placed. Generally, seven ports are required to complete the entire procedure laparoscopically (Fig. 11.2).

### Instrumentation

High quality imaging systems are preferable. Routine hand instruments including bowel graspers and needle holders are also used. The special instruments, which are very useful for resection include ultrasonic shears (Ethicon), specialized bipolar coagulation probes, endoscopic gastrointestinal (GIA) linear staplers, and laparoscopic ultrasound probes (LUS) with 7–10 MHz frequency.

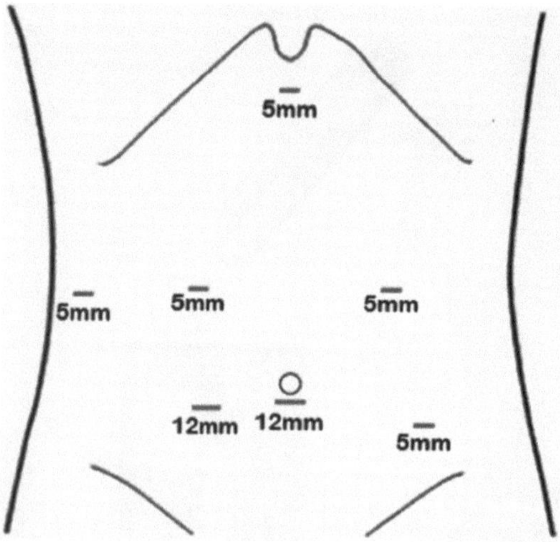


**Fig. 11.2** Operative placement of ports. Seven ports are utilized and the camera alternates between the midline and right abdominal port. The left subcostal port is utilized for retraction of the gallbladder and the subxiphoid port is utilized for liver retraction

## Technical Description

The technique of LPD is similar to that of open surgery. It involves the three phases: (1) laparoscopic staging and assessment of resectability, (2) resection, and (3) reconstruction.

### Phase I

Laparoscopic staging of periampullary and pancreatic lesions is entirely different from the conventional method. The tactile sensation of the open method is replaced by LUS and Doppler examination. It is important to get adequate exposure and various measures for exposure include cranial traction of the gallbladder, right-sided table tilt, tacking the falciform ligament to the anterior abdominal wall, and mobilization of the right colon and hepatic flexure. Initially, any free fluid in the peritoneal cavity is aspirated and sent for cytology. Then a systematic examination of the peritoneum is performed and suspicious deposits are biopsied. Specific areas that should be examined include the sub-diaphragmatic regions, the falciform ligament, and the pelvis. Then, a systematic inspection of the liver is performed on all surfaces, which is facilitated by reverse Trendelenburg and left lateral tilt of the table. The gastrohepatic omentum overlying the caudate lobe of the liver is opened thereby exposing caudate lobe, celiac axis, and inferior vena cava. The hepatic artery is also visualized. Portal, perigastric, and celiac axis lymph nodes are biopsied if enlarged.

LUS is performed to evaluate small hepatic lesions (<1 cm) that are not usually identified by CT scan. All segments of the liver are examined sequentially by moving and rotating the probe slowly. The hepatoduodenal ligament is evaluated by placing the probe transversely. The portal vein and superior mesenteric vein (SMV) and artery (SMA) are examined and their relation to the tumor is assessed. The pancreas is examined by placing the transducer through the window in the gastrohepatic and gastrocolic omentum directly onto the surface of the gland. Gentle rotation of the probe at this stage allows for evaluation of the celiac axis and proximal hepatic artery.

Division of the gastrocolic trunk opens up the anterior aspect of the SMV to approach the plane between the neck of the pancreas and SMV. Tunneling behind the neck is safely performed using blunt irrigation and a suction instrument (Fig. 11.3). Resectability can be easily assessed in early periampullary lesions but may be difficult with pancreatic head carcinoma, particularly in association with chronic pancreatitis when LUS cannot accurately assess and stage the disease.

### Phase II

#### Mobilization of the Pancreatic Head

To start, Cattell-Braasch maneuver is performed followed by an extended Kocher maneuver. The Cattell-Braasch maneuver is best performed by standing on the left side of the patient; and surgeon moves to right side of the patient for kocherization. The colo-hepatic peritoneum is incised and the hepatic flexure is mobilized down. This exposes the entire second and third part of the duodenum up to the neck of the pancreas. Kocherizing the duodenum is facilitated by retracting it anteriorly and medially by an atraumatic bowel grasper

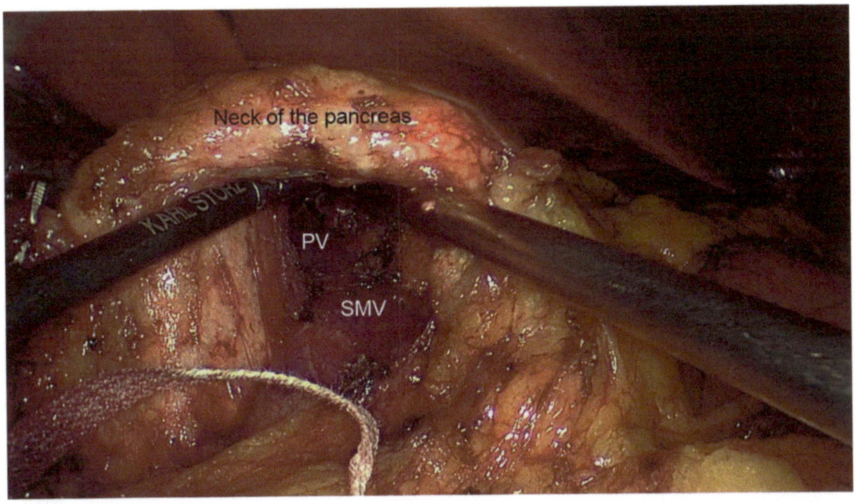


**Fig. 11.3** Dissection of the neck of the pancreas away from the superior mesenteric vein (SMV) and portal vein (PV). The pancreas is lifted in the air and an umbilical tape will be placed around the neck

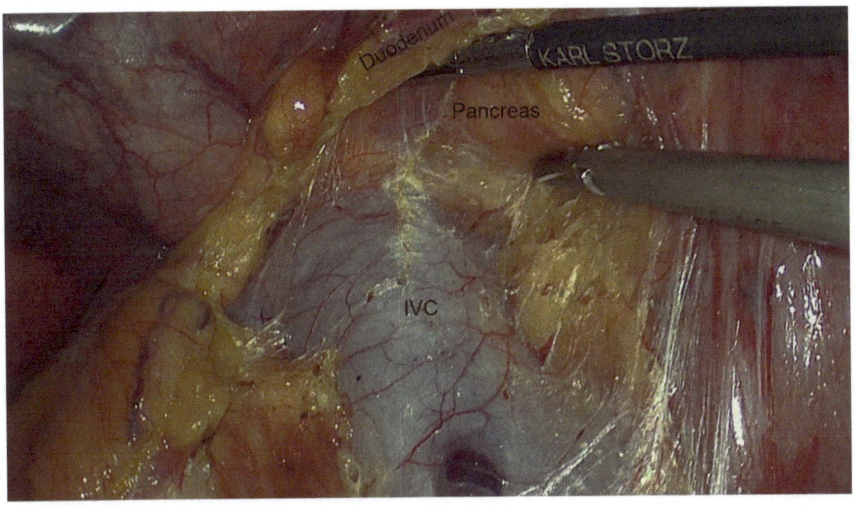


**Fig. 11.4** Kocherization of the duodenum. The inferior vena cava (IVC) is clearly seen along with the posterior aspect of the head of the pancreas

through the subxiphoid port. The duodenum and pancreas are dissected free to the left border of the aorta (Fig. 11.4). The right gastroepiploic vein and artery are clipped and divided and the first portion of the duodenum is skeletonized. On the suprapyloric side, the right gastric artery is divided thus freeing the pylorus and the first portion of the duodenum. Depending on the nature of the tumor and oncological requirement, either the pylorus or first portion of the duodenum is divided using an endo-GIA stapler.

The dissection of portal structures begins with decompression of the gallbladder as it provides better visualization of the structures in the porta hepatis. Calot's triangle is dissected and the cystic artery and duct are clipped and divided. The gallbladder is left attached to the liver until the reconstruction is over as it provides good retraction of the liver. The common hepatic duct is transected above the level of the cystic duct junction and all fibro-fatty and lymphatic tissues along the hepatoduodenal ligament are cleared

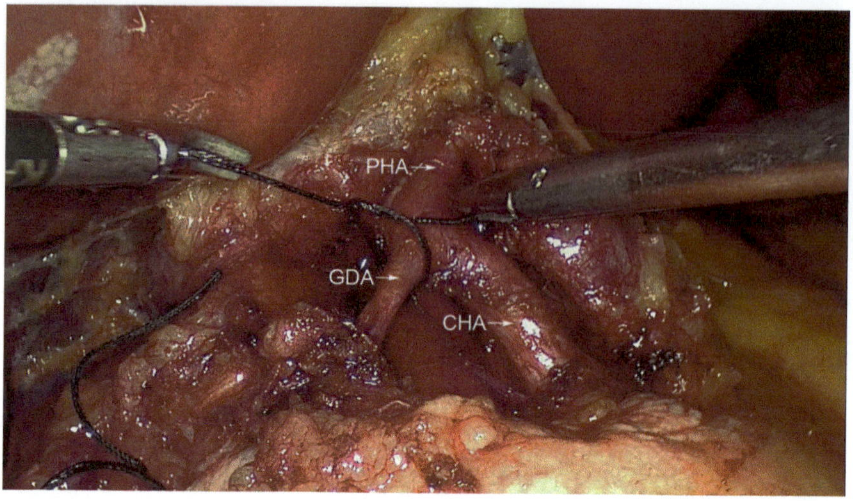


**Fig. 11.5** Ligation of the gastroduodenal artery close to its origin from the common hepatic artery (CHA). The proper hepatic artery (PHA) is also identified

exposing the proper hepatic artery and portal vein. Bile spillage from the cut end of the hepatic duct is avoided by applying an endo-bulldog clamp. The hepatic artery is then traced along the superior border of the pancreas in the gastrohepatic omentum where the gastroduodenal artery may be identified and ligated near its origin from the common hepatic artery (Fig. 11.5). Dissection is continued towards the celiac axis along the superior border of pancreas taking lymphatic tissues with the specimen.

### Infra-Colic Dissection

The peritoneum lateral to the duodenojejunal flexure is incised. The inferior mesenteric vein is carefully retracted to the left and the ligament of Treitz is divided. The jejunum about 10 cm distal to the ligament of Treitz is divided using an endoscopic GIA stapler. Jejunal vessels of the proximal jejunum and duodenum are divided using ultrasonic shears (Ethicon). Care should be taken while dividing the proximal jejunal tributaries that drain to the SMV posterior to the superior mesenteric artery (SMA). These jejunal branches also receive small tributaries from the uncinate process of the pancreas. Hence, extreme care should be taken in delineating these branches to avoid bleeding. The free end of the jejunum is delivered into the supracolic compartment.

### Resection of Pancreas

The patient is tilted to the left in reverse Trendelenburg position, which facilitates exposure of the pancreas. The camera is placed in the right lateral port instead of the supra-umbilical port. Pancreatic transection at the neck begins after placing stay sutures at the superior and inferior borders on either side of the transection line to help in retraction and hemostasis. Pancreatic transection is performed using ultrasonic shears (Ethicon) while the area of the suspected pancreatic duct is divided with scissors to avoid injury to the ductal mucosa.

### Resection of Uncinate Process

A hook retractor or an umbilical tape is applied across the root of the small bowel mesentery to give traction anteriorly and to the left. This maneuver clearly exposes the uncinate process to facilitate its resection and lymph node clearance along the right border of the SMA. The inferior pancreaticoduodenal artery is controlled and clipped by retracting the SMV medially. All other venous tributaries and small vessels of the uncinate process are identified separately, clipped, and divided. Great care is taken not to injure any of the major vessels (Fig. 11.6). Similarly, the pancreatic neck vein that drains posteriorly into the portal vein can be controlled between the

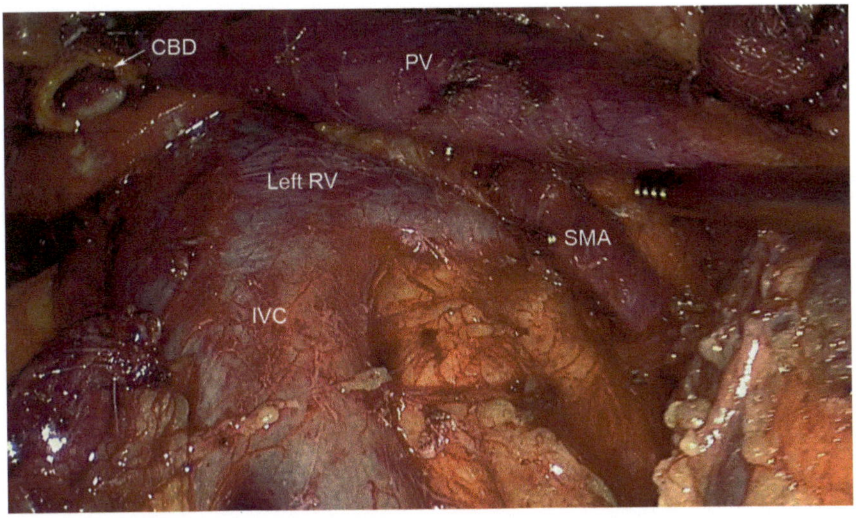


**Fig. 11.6** At the completion of resection, the major vessels should be visible. The inferior vena cava (IVC), left renal vein (RV), portal vein (PV), and superior mesenteric artery (SMA) are clearly identified. The open common bile duct (CBD) is also visible

common bile duct and portal vein. Following complete mobilization, the specimen is placed in an endoscopic specimen bag introduced through a 10-mm port and is left in the upper quadrant.

## Phase III

### Pancreaticojejunal Anastomosis

The divided end of the jejunum is brought up to the supracolic compartment in a retrocolic fashion. The pancreatic stump is mobilized for a length of 2–3 cm to facilitate the pancreatic anastomosis. Pancreaticojejunal reconstruction is done by end-to-side duct-to-mucosa technique using 4-0 polydioxanone sutures (Ethicon). The technique begins by placement of seromuscular sutures from the jejunum to the posterior pancreatic capsule using interrupted 3-0 polypropylene sutures. This places the jejunal loop in alignment with the pancreatic stump, which facilitates the subsequent pancreatic duct-to-mucosa anastomosis to be tension free. Six to eight interrupted duct-to-mucosa sutures are placed starting at the 6'o clock position and continued on either side (Fig. 11.7). The knots are placed preferably outside the lumen to prevent obstruction to the flow of pancreatic juice. The anterior seromuscular sutures are then placed to complete the anastomosis. Stenting the anastomosis is optional and may be preferred in cases of a non-dilated pancreatic duct. If the pancreas is soft and the duct is small, a dunking or invagination technique may be performed.

### Hepaticojejunostomy

Approximately 7–8 cm distal to the pancreaticojejunal anastomosis, the hepaticojejunostomy is performed by creating a small enterotomy in the jejunum and anastomosing it to the cut end of hepatic duct. It is a single-layer anastomosis with 4-0 polydioxanone sutures (Ethicon) placed in interrupted manner starting on posterior border (Fig. 11.8). It is easier to perform the anastomosis from right to left for the posterior layer with the knots placed inside the lumen. Anteriorly, the sutures are placed sequentially from the corners to the center. If the duct is dilated, the anterior layer can be completed using a continuous suture. The anastomosis is better performed with the surgeon standing on the left side of the patient.

### Duodenojejunal Anastomosis

The final reconstruction involves restoration of gastrointestinal continuity by performing a duodenojejunal or gastrojejunal anastomosis.

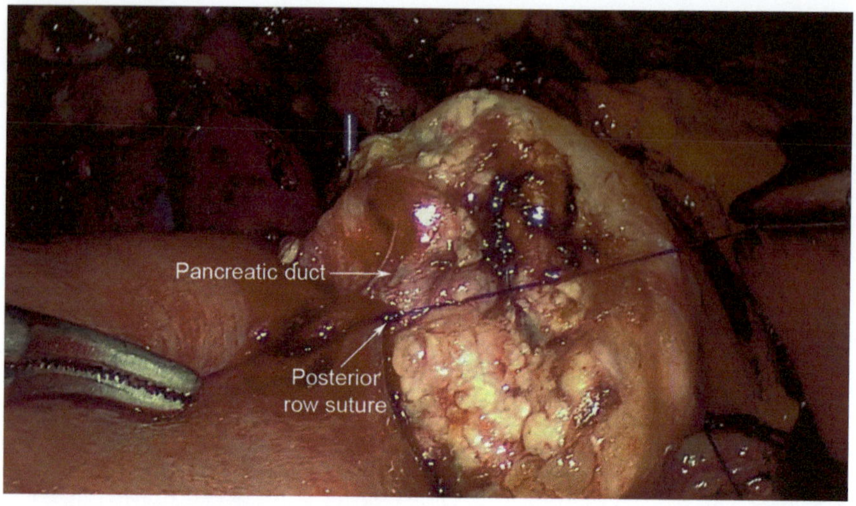


**Fig. 11.7** Duct-to-mucosa anastomosis of the pancreaticojejunostomy. The posterior row suture has been placed

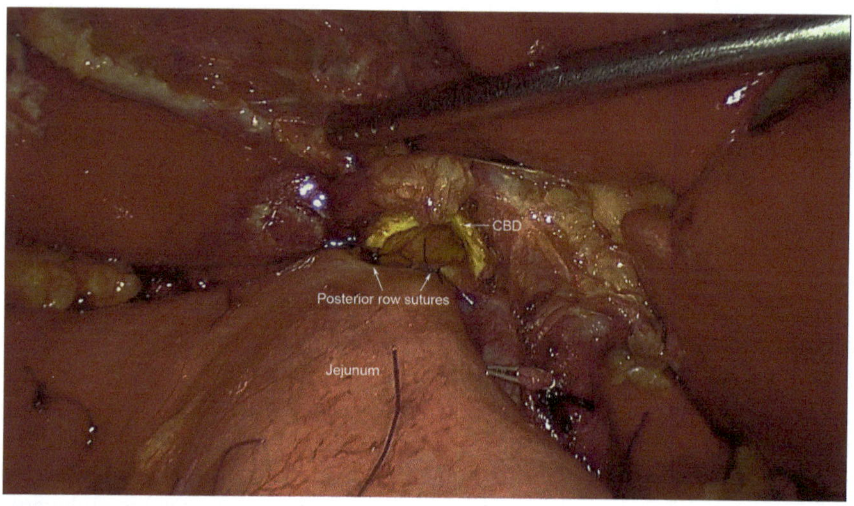


**Fig. 11.8** Single layer hepaticojejunostomy. The posterior row of interrupted sutures has been completed

About 40 cm distal to the hepaticojejunostomy, a duodenojejunostomy is performed in an antecolic fashion using 2-0 polydioxanone sutures (Ethicon) placed in a continuous, extra-mucosal fashion (Fig. 11.9). For classical resection a gastrojejunostomy is performed using an endoscopic gastrointestinal (GIA) linear stapler on the dependent posterior aspect of the stomach. Nasojejunal and nasogastric tubes are used for feeding and decompression, respectively. Though the placement of drains following pancreaticoduodenectomy is a contentious issue, it is preferable to place at least one drain near the pancreatic anastomotic site through one of the lateral port sites. The specimen in the specimen bag is removed through a Pfannenstiel incision.

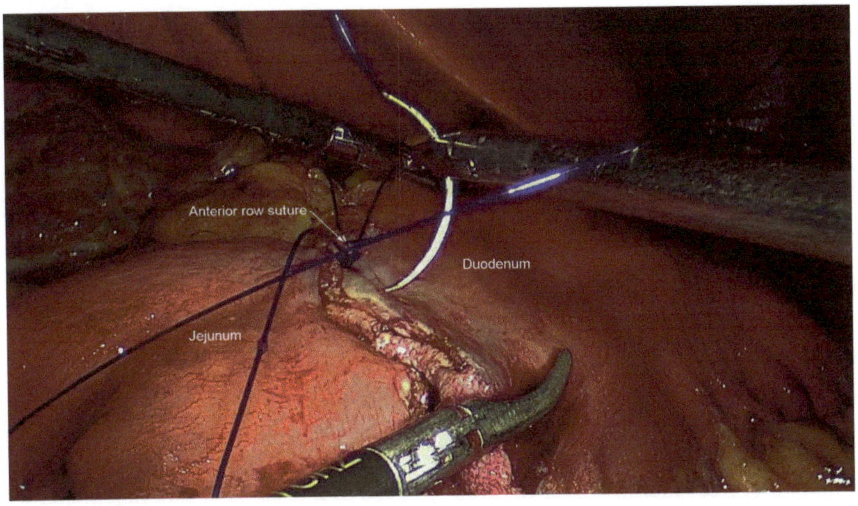


**Fig. 11.9** The final anastomosis of the reconstruction is the duodenojejunostomy. The anterior row of sutures is being completed

## Evolution and Technical Variations

LPD continues to evolve in its own right. In the two decades of its performance it has undergone various modifications in technical details. This section highlights the important changes that have taken place in the evolution of a standardized technique for LPD. We also comment on some of the variations in technique that are described in the literature.

- With experience, indications for LPD can be extended to include larger tumors and obese patients. In fact, for obese patients LPD is now a preferred indication as it avoids wound-related complications.
- The midline camera port can be changed to the right lateral port. Interchanging the camera between the midline and lateral port gives different views suited for different stages of the procedure. The lateral camera port provides better vision during kocherization, pancreatic transection, and uncinate dissection.
- Laparoscopic adaptation of an artery first technique is possible and the best available route is via a mesenteric approach. This provides the opportunity to assess arterial involvement with minimal mobilization. The inferior border of the pancreas must be well defined to undertake this approach.
- In the early learning period, it may be better to attempt resection alone by laparoscopy and slowly graduate to total LPD. The hepaticojejunostomy may be attempted by the laparoscopic method while the remaining anastomoses can be performed through a small incision. Later, complete reconstruction can be performed laparoscopically.
- In the event of a high-risk pancreatic anastomosis (i.e., soft pancreas, undilated duct, or increased intraoperative blood loss), a Roux-en-Y reconstruction is an option to reduce the morbidity of a postoperative anastomotic leak.
- Portal vein involvement necessitating portal vein resection was considered a contraindication to LPD. But as experience grows, even portal vein reconstruction is now being performed in limited centers [7].
- Generally, the specimen is removed by enlarging one of the port site incisions. This has been replaced by a small Pfannenstiel incision, which not only gives better cosmesis but also reduces postoperative pain.

## Complications

### Intraoperative

LPD is a formidable surgical procedure that requires adequate experience and expertise. Bleeding is the most common reason for conversion to an open procedure. The vessels generally injured during the resection phase are the gastrocolic trunk, branches of the SMV, and the hepatic artery. Most bleeding can be controlled laparoscopically, however it is better to avoid injury to these vessels altogether by proper traction, clear visualization, and correct identification of structures. For major injuries, especially to the portal vein and hepatic artery, proximal control is essential and can be controlled by an endoscopic bulldog clamp. In our own reported series, one patient had minor injury to the portal vein that was managed by intracorporeal suturing. Another patient had left gastric vein injury that was controlled with a clip. Finally, a patient had gastrocolic vein avulsion from the SMV due to excess retraction. Bleeding was controlled by intracorporeal suturing after applying a bulldog clamp. Other factors associated with conversion to an open procedure include chronic pancreatitis and bulky and borderline resectable tumors.

### Postoperative

Since LPD involves multiple resections and reconstructions, complications are expected and are to be managed the same way as in open surgery. The general postoperative morbidity ranges from 26 to 42 %, which is comparable to the open approach [5, 8]. The main morbidity after LPD is pancreatic fistula. It is the underlying cause of complications like intraabdominal collection, delayed gastric emptying, and delayed hemorrhage. Undrained collections in symptomatic patients should be managed using radiological guidance. Postoperative hemorrhage can be secondary or delayed due to pancreatic fistula. If bleeding is suspected by drop in hemoglobin levels, patient is treated conservatively with blood products and radiologic intervention. If bleeding is sudden and massive with an unstable patient, urgent surgical intervention is needed. The role of laparoscopy is very limited in these conditions. Finally, bile leaks are relatively innocuous and tend to resolve with conservative management; and port site and wound infections are not a major problem with LPD.

## Present Status of LPD

Over the past 20 years LPD has grown to acceptance as a feasible option in patients with pancreatic and periampullary malignancies. From the earliest report [4], a large number of patients have successfully undergone LPD [9, 8]. In our own institution, LPD was started after sufficient experience in other major laparoscopic procedures like colectomy, gastrectomy, and choledochal cyst excision. The authors reported an early experience of 42 patients in 2007, which showed excellent perioperative outcomes [10]. At that time, few other studies confirmed the feasibility of the procedure [11]. Over the years numerous technical modifications have been made leading to our follow-up report on 75 patients [5]. We reported a mean operative time of 357 min and blood loss of 74 mL with no conversions and an overall postoperative morbidity rate of 26.7 %. Pancreatic fistula developed in 5 patients reflecting an improvement in our learning curve as with other series [12]. Oncologically, the margin status and lymph node yield in LPD are comparable to the open approach. Asbun and colleagues discovered better perioperative outcomes for laparoscopy in terms of blood loss and hospital stay when reviewing their own series [13]. Other reports have observed similar findings [14–16].

## Summary

LPD has crossed the feasibility stage and has come to be an acceptable alternative to the open approach in select centers across the world.

The available evidence suggests comparable immediate postoperative and short-term outcomes to open surgery. However, issues such as long-term oncologic outcomes and a prolonged learning curve must be addressed to gain widespread acceptance and practice of LPD.

## References


1. Bernheim IV BM. Organoscopy: cystoscopy of the abdominal cavity. Ann Surg. 1911;53(6):764–7.
2. Cuschieri A, Hall AW, Clark J. Value of laparoscopy in the diagnosis and management of pancreatic carcinoma. Gut. 1978;19(7):672–7.
3. Warshaw AL, Tepper JE, Shipley WU. Laparoscopy in the staging and planning of therapy for pancreatic cancer. Am J Surg. 1986;151(1):76–80.
4. Gagner M, Pomp A. Laparoscopic pylorus-preserving pancreatoduodenectomy. Surg Endosc. 1994;8(5):408–10.
5. Palanivelu C, Rajan PS, Rangarajan M, Vaithiswaran V, Senthilnathan P, Parthasarathi R, et al. Evolution in techniques of laparoscopic pancreaticoduodenectomy: a decade long experience from a tertiary center. J Hepatobiliary Pancreat Surg. 2009;16(6):731–40. doi:10.1007/s00534-009-0157-8.
6. Castillo C. Endoscopic ultrasound in the papilla and the periampullary region. World J Gastrointest Endosc. 2010;2(8):278–87. doi:10.4253/wjge.v2.i8.278.
7. Kendrick ML, Sclabas GM. Major venous resection during total laparoscopic pancreaticoduodenectomy. HPB (Oxford). 2011;13(7):454–8. doi:10.1111/j.1477-2574.2011.00323.x.
8. Zureikat AH, Breaux JA, Steel JL, Hughes SJ. Can laparoscopic pancreaticoduodenectomy be safely implemented? J Gastrointest Surg. 2011;15(7):1151–7. doi:10.1007/s11605-011-1530-x.
9. Kendrick ML, Cusati D. Total laparoscopic pancreaticoduodenectomy: feasibility and outcome in an early experience. Arch Surg. 2010;145(1):19–23. doi:10.1001/archsurg.2009.243.
10. Palanivelu C, Jani K, Senthilnathan P, Parthasarathi R, Rajapandian S, Madhankumar MV. Laparoscopic pancreaticoduodenectomy: technique and outcomes. J Am Coll Surg. 2007;205(2):222–30. doi:10.1016/j.jamcollsurg.2007.04.004.
11. Dulucq JL, Wintringer P, Mahajna A. Laparoscopic pancreaticoduodenectomy for benign and malignant diseases. Surg Endosc. 2006;20(7):1045–50. doi:10.1007/s00464-005-0474-1.
12. Kim SC, Song KB, Jung YS, Kim YH, Park do H, Lee SS, et al. Short-term clinical outcomes for 100 consecutive cases of laparoscopic pylorus-preserving pancreatoduodenectomy: improvement with surgical experience. Surg Endosc. 2013;27(1):95–103.
13. Asbun HJ, Stauffer JA. Laparoscopic vs open pancreaticoduodenectomy: overall outcomes and severity of complications using the Accordion Severity Grading System. J Am Coll Surg. 2012;215(6):810–9. doi:10.1016/j.jamcollsurg.2012.08.006.
14. Gumbs AA, Rodriguez Rivera AM, Milone L, Hoffman JP. Laparoscopic pancreatoduodenectomy: a review of 285 published cases. Ann Surg Oncol. 2011; 18(5):1335–41. doi:10.1245/s10434-010-1503-4.
15. Lei P, Wei B, Guo W, Wei H. Minimally invasive surgical approach compared with open pancreaticoduodenectomy: a systematic review and meta-analysis on the feasibility and safety. Surg Laparosc Endosc Percutan Tech. 2014;24(4):296–305. doi:10.1097/sle.0000000000000054.
16. Langan RC, Graham JA, Chin AB, Rubinstein AJ, Oza K, Nusbaum JA, et al. Laparoscopic-assisted versus open pancreaticoduodenectomy: early favorable physical quality-of-life measures. Surgery. 2014; 156(2):379–84. doi:10.1016/j.surg. 2014.03.018.


## Key Operative Steps

1. Place the patient in supine position on a split leg table.
2. Seven trocars/ports are generally needed to complete LPD.
3. Perform laparoscopic staging using LUS. May require division of the gastrocolic trunk and opening the plane posterior to the neck of the pancreas.
4. Perform Cattell-Braasch maneuver followed by wide kocherization of the duodenum.
5. Skeletonize the duodenum and divide the right gastric artery.
6. Divide the pylorus/duodenum with a laparoscopic GIA stapler.
7. Start the portal dissection with decompression of the gallbladder. Clip and divide the cystic artery and duct but do not remove the gallbladder. It will be used for retraction.
8. Transect the common hepatic duct above the level of the cystic duct. Place a bulldog clamp.
9. Clear all lymphatic tissues to fully visualize the proper hepatic artery and portal vein.
10. Identify and divide the gastroduodenal artery.
11. Take down the ligament of Treitz and divide the proximal jejunum.
12. Divide the pancreas at the neck.
13. Retract the small bowel mesentery to the left and expose the uncinate process. Retract the SMV to the left and resect the uncinate process close to the SMA.
14. Place the specimen into an endoscopic retrieval bag.
15. Bring the divided end of the jejunum up to the pancreas and perform a duct-to-mucosa anastomosis.
16. Perform single-layer hepaticojejunostomy.
17. Perform antecolic single-layer duodeno jejunostomy.

# Robotic Technique for Pancreaticoduodenectomy

**12**

Bhavin C. Shah, Amer H. Zureikat, Herbert J. Zeh III, and Melissa E. Hogg

## Historical Perspective

In 1935, Allen Oldfather Whipple reported the first successful complete duodenectomy with pancreatic head resection performed as a two-stage procedure [1]. The first recorded one-stage procedure for complete excision of the head of the pancreas and the entire duodenum (OPD) by Whipple was reported in 1941 [2]. In the minimally invasive era, the first laparoscopic pancreaticoduodenectomy (LPD) was reported in 1994 by Michel Gagner [3], but the minimally invasive approach to this procedure has not been adopted universally except at specialized centers [4–7]. This is primarily due to limitations such as difficulty in complex reconstruction, two-dimensional imaging, limited surgical training, and lack of range in laparoscopic instrumentation. Hand assistance with laparoscopic resection and partial open reconstruction has been used in some centers but has failed to gain popular traction [3, 7–9].

Using the robotic platform overcomes many of the shortcomings of laparoscopy with improved three-dimensional imaging, 540° movement of surgical instruments, improved dexterity, and precision in complex tasks like dissection and intracorporeal suturing [10–12]. In 2010, Giulianotti and colleagues reported the first large series of robotic pancreatic resections where 134 patients underwent various pancreatic procedures of which 60 patients underwent robotic pancreaticoduodenectomy (RPD) [7].

At the University of Pittsburgh, we have adapted a combined robotic and laparoscopic approach for RPD with encouraging early experience in periampullary lesions [13]. We have continued to modify our technique over the past 5 years to improve style and efficiency. Recently Zureikat et al., reported 250 consecutive robotic procedures which included 132 RPD with low mortality and morbidity rates [14]. The mean operative time for RPD was 529 ± 103 min and conversion to an open procedure was required in 11 patients (9 %) [14]. One hundred and six (80.3 %) RPD were performed for pancreatic cancer and an R0 resection was achieved in 87.7 % ($n$ = 93 of 106) with a median lymph node harvest of 19 [14]. We have clearly shown that the procedure can be safe and feasible with good outcomes [13, 14].

Electronic supplementary material: Supplementary material is available in the online version of this chapter at 10.1007/978-1-4939-1893-5_12. Videos can also be accessed at http://www.springerimages.com/videos/978-1-4939-1892-8.

B.C. Shah, M.D. • A.H. Zureikat, M.D.
H.J. Zeh III, M.D. • M.E. Hogg, M.D. (✉)
Division of Surgical Oncology, University of Pittsburgh Medical Center, Pittsburgh, PA, USA
e-mail: hoggme@upmc.edu

J. Kim and J. Garcia-Aguilar (eds.), *Surgery for Cancers of the Gastrointestinal Tract: A Step-by-Step Approach*, 131
DOI 10.1007/978-1-4939-1893-5_12, © Springer Science+Business Media New York 2015

## Indication and Preoperative Evaluation

Indications for RPD are the same as for OPD with the exception when vascular resection and reconstruction are anticipated and when the patient cannot tolerate pneumoperitoneum. The indications include, but are not limited to cholangiocarcinoma, duodenal cancer, ampullary cancer, pancreatic adenocarcinoma, pancreatic acinar cell carcinoma, pancreatic neuroendocrine tumor, intrapapillary mucinous neoplasms (IPMN), mucinous cystic neoplasms (MCN), chronic pancreatitis, and other less common etiologies.

All patients must have a preoperative pancreatic protocol triple-contrast computed tomographic (CT) scan to stage the tumor, identify the configuration of the arterial anatomy, and determine tumor freedom from and abutment or encasement of the portal vein (PV), superior mesenteric vein (SMV), superior mesenteric artery (SMA), and hepatic arteries. Endoscopic ultrasound (US) allows fine needle aspiration (FNA) for cytologic diagnosis, to demonstrate nodal disease, and to further characterize vascular involvement of the tumor. Endoscopic retrograde cholangiopancreatogram (ERCP) allows brushings for cytology, provides a cholangiogram to delineate ductal anatomy, and offers therapeutic decompression of the biliary tree using plastic stents, covered metal stents, and uncovered metal stents. Serum CA19-9 levels are obtained preoperatively for all patients as a prognostic marker for pancreatic cancer and cholangiocarcinoma.

Based on preoperative work-up, patients with pancreatic cancer are classified as resectable, borderline resectable, locally advanced, or as metastatic [15–17]. Resectable patients are either taken to surgery or given neoadjuvant therapy on clinical trial. Borderline resectable patients are all given neoadjuvant chemotherapy ± radiotherapy. Locally advanced patients are given systemic therapies and if they respond, these patients will be reevaluated for surgical consideration. Patients with venous encasement that will need a formal portal vein resection with interposition graft are not approached robotically.

## Anatomic Highlights/Landmarks

- Ligament of Treitz. The identification and division of the ligament of Treitz is performed laparoscopically from the patient's right side following a Kocher maneuver. This dissection is critical for freeing the retroperitoneal attachments to the duodenum and pancreas. It is of critical importance to dissect directly onto the duodenum and not get into the mesentery encasing the SMV and SMA. This dissection is complete when the proximal portion of the jejunum can be pulled into the right upper quadrant (RUQ).
- Hepatic artery lymph node. This lymph node is large even when it is not pathologic and it is easy to identify. Once identified and removed, the common hepatic artery (CHA), the PV, and the gastroduodenal artery (GDA) can be easily identified. This lymph node is highly vascular and friable and removing it whole with the "no touch" technique is recommended to avoid venous oozing.
- Superior pancreaticoduodenal vein or vein of Belcher. This vessel is usually located at the superior aspect of the pancreas and enters into the PV posteriorly. It is easy to avulse and may create significant bleeding from the PV. It is best to locate this vessel after the pancreatic neck dissection, but not to ligate it until the end of pancreatic resection. This allows for ease of stapling or suture ligation to control potential hemorrhage.
- First jejunal branch of the SMV (Fig. 12.1). This branch is usually quite large and may have several branches to the uncinate process. Ligating these branches without injuring the first jejunal is tedious but critical to free the inferior border of the uncinate from the small bowel mesentery allowing for better visualization of the lateral wall of the SMA.

## Preoperative Preparation

All patients undergo a bowel prep the day before surgery and are nil per os (NPO) after midnight. Patients are considered for paravertebral blocks

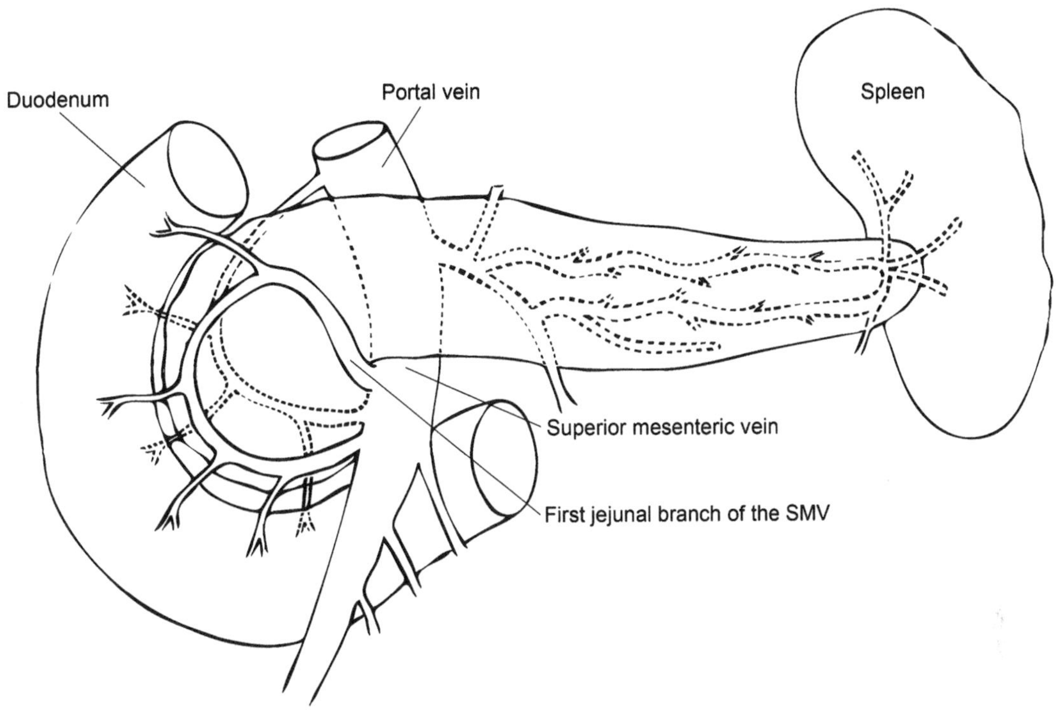


**Fig. 12.1** Important venous anatomy of the pancreas, including the first jejunal vein

for postoperative pain control in the preoperative holding area. Preoperative prophylaxis includes sequential compression stockings, subcutaneous heparin 5,000 units, and intravenous antibiotics that are administered within 1 h of skin incision and re-dosed throughout the operation as indicated. After induction of general anesthesia, all patients undergo arterial line placement and central line placement in addition to a Foley catheter and a nasogastric tube (NGT).

## Operative Positioning

The patient is placed supine on a split-leg table with the right arm tucked and left arm extended 60° on an arm board (Fig. 12.2a). The bed, arm board, and leg components are all padded with Pigazzi pink pad (Xodus Medical, New Kensington, PA) or crate sponges (Table 12.1). All pressure points are protected with sponge rolls and a Velcro chest strap is used to secure the patient to the bed. The legs are abducted to the "B" notch setting, and secured in place with padding under the knee to avoid leg hyperextension. Footboards are used to secure patients on the bed since the patient will be in reverse Trendelenburg for the procedure. The patient is also secured to the table with blankets, sheets, and overlying tape at the shin and feet for additional padding anteriorly. An upper-body warming blanket is used to keep patient warm. The operating table is repositioned at a 90° angle from the anesthesia machine to allow for future robot docking over the head (Fig. 12.2b).

## Port Placement

Port placement is a key component to a successful RPD. Standard laparoscopic ports including a 5-mm optical separator, two 12-mm ports, four 5-mm ports, and a GelPOINT (Applied Medical, Rancho Santa Margarita, CA) are used for initial dissection. The left upper quadrant (LUQ) optical separator and the two RUQ 5-mm trocars are replaced with 8-mm robotic ports prior to docking (Fig. 12.3). In general, all ports should be a hands breadth apart from each other. Also, the camera port should be 2–3 fingers breadth to the patient's right of the umbilicus to allow best visualization of the PV during the uncinate dissection. The ports may need to be shifted higher or lower depending on patient size, which can be best assessed by evaluating the distance from the xiphoid to the umbilicus. The location and size of the gel port should take into account the location of the inferior epigastric vessels. We make sure the location of the port is low so the LUQ robot arm does not conflict with it, but not too low to prevent the stapler, clip-applier, etc. from reaching the porta hepatis. For smaller patients, the GelPOINT Mini (Applied Medical, Rancho Santa Margarita, CA) is better. This can be placed at the beginning of the case with a 12-mm trocar through it or later in the case after the specimen is removed to prevent air leak from the extraction site.

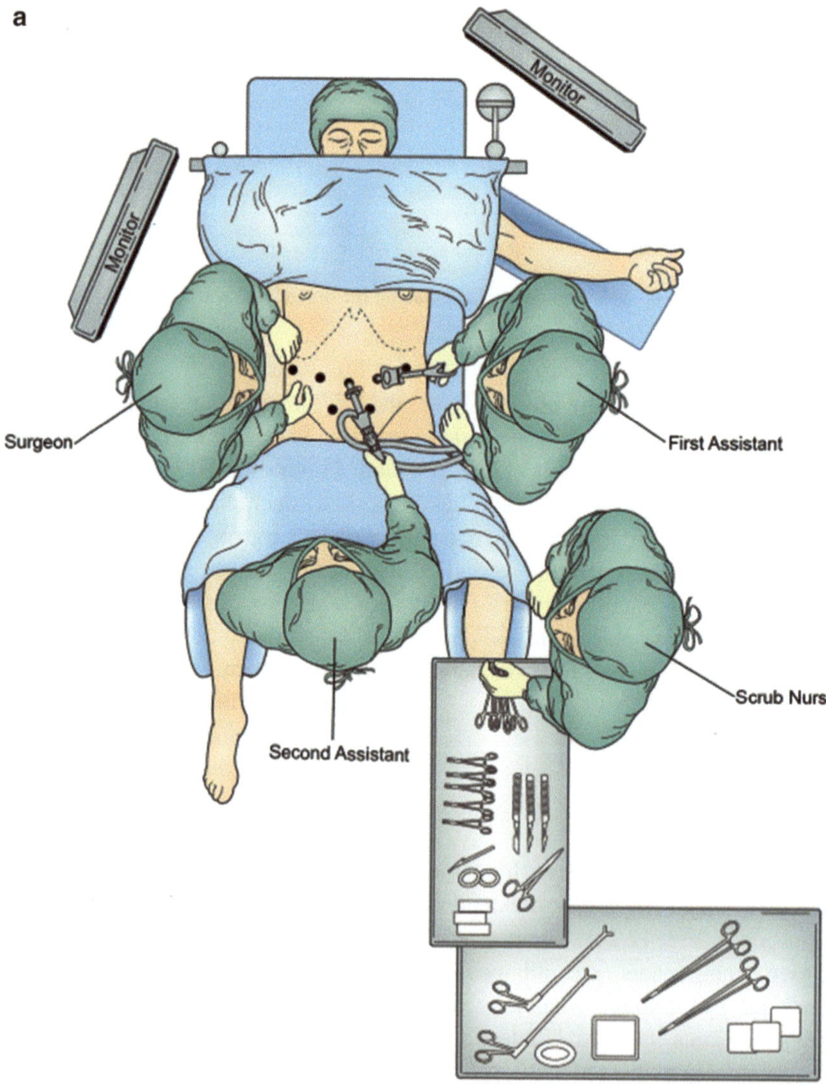


**Fig. 12.2** (**a**) Patient positioning for laparoscopic mobilization and (**b**) patient positioning for robotic pancreatectomy

b

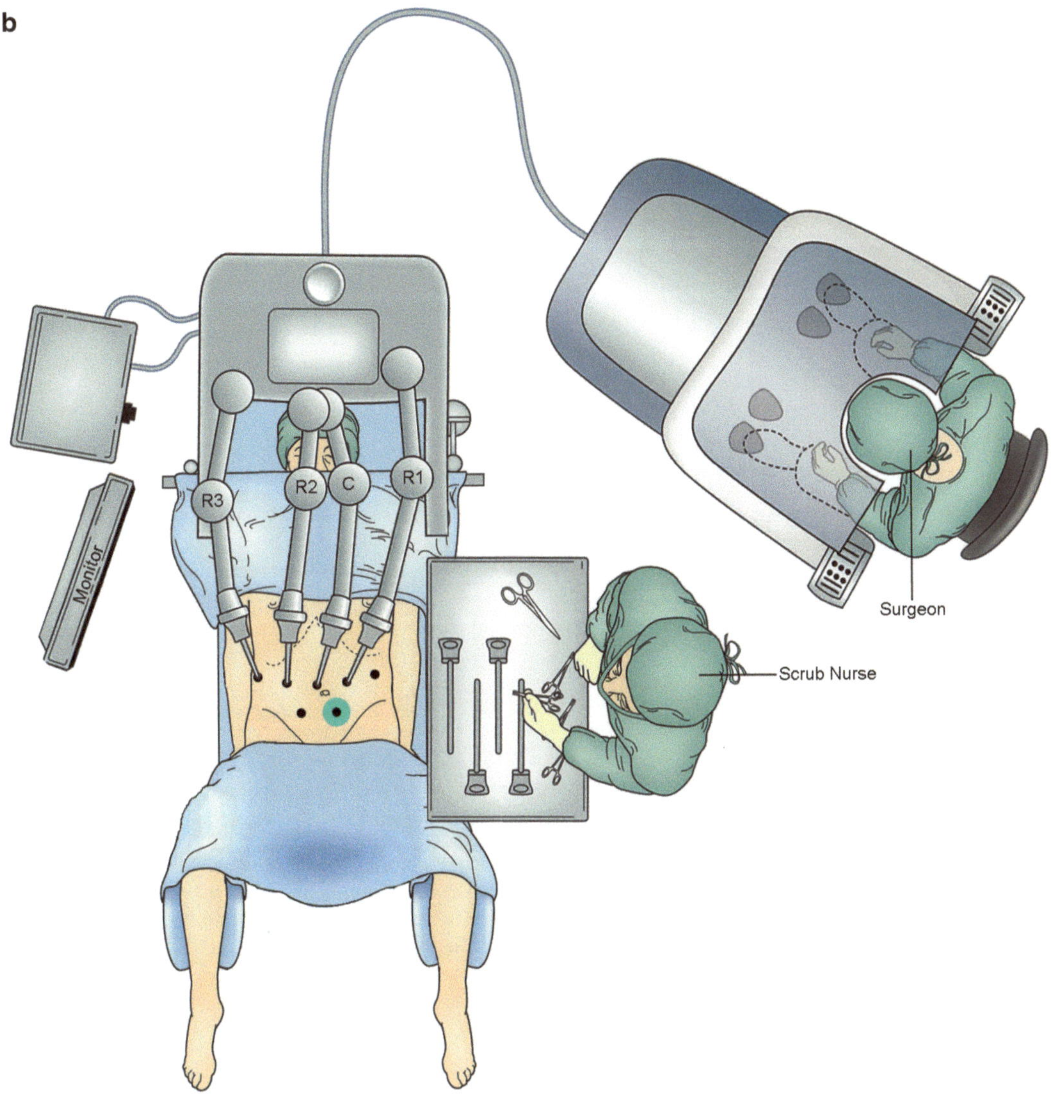


**Fig. 12.2** (continued)

## Operative Procedure

### Laparoscopic Mobilization and Assessment of Resectability

The roles of the surgeon and assistant are summarized in Table 12.1. A 1-cm incision is made through the left rectus muscle one hands breadth to the left and 1 in. above the level of the umbilicus. A 0°, 5-mm camera is placed through an optical separator trocar and inserted under direct visualization in the left upper abdomen. This trocar will be converted to the R1 trocar (Fig. 12.3). After diagnostic laparoscopy we place other ports under direct visualization. A total of seven ports are placed with the camera port placed 2–3 cm to the right and above the level of the umbilicus. Then a 5-mm port is placed a hands breadth to the right of the camera. Another 5-mm port is placed a hands breadth lateral to this port. These will be exchanged later with robot ports R2 and R3, respectively. The first assistant port is placed a hands breadth below the camera port and splits

**Table 12.1** Equipment table

| Positioning | General laparoscopic | Specific laparoscopic | Robotic[i] | Open |
|---|---|---|---|---|
| 3″ silk tape | 0, 30° cameras, 5 mm[d] | 2-0 Ticron Endo Stitch[c] | 4-Arm da Vinci drape kit | 19-Fr Round Blake × 2[l] |
| Blue foam rolls | 0, 30° cameras, 10 mm[d] | Battery powered suction irrigator[g] | 8 mm disposable obturator | Bovie[c] |
| Egg crate | 5, 10 mm Endoclip appliers[c] | Bulldogs[h] | 8 mm ports × 3 | Pancreatic stents (sizes 4, 5, or 7)[n] |
| Foot boards | 5, 12 mm bladeless Versaports[c] | Carter Thomason[m] | Cadiere forceps | Slush drape for sterile cover |
| Left arm board | Alligator × 2 | DHELP[e] | Disposable bipolar cord | Closesure |
| Pigazzi Pink Pad[a] | Camera, light cord[d] | Endo-GIA Stapler[c] | Disposable monopolar cord | Surgicel, Nu-Knit, Gelfoam[l] |
| Pillowcases × 4 | Duckbill × 4 (2 short, 2 long) | Endocatch 10 mm × 2[c] | Fenestrated bipolar | Thompson retractor[j] |
| Velcro chest strap | Insufflators × 2 | Endocatch 15 mm[c] | Hook cautery | Triad[c] |
| Split-leg bed | LigaSure 5 mm blunt tip[c] | Endo Stitch[c] | Large needle driver × 2 | Ultrasound machine[k] |
| Upper body bare hugger[o] | Mediflex retractor[f] | Gelpoint gelport[b] | Prograsp × 2 | Umbilical tapes cut to 6″[c] |
| Warm blankets × 2 | Optical separator[b] | Hemolok appliers[h] | Scissor cautery | Yellow vessel loops cut to 6″ |
| | General laparoscopic instruments | Lapra-Ty (Applier-KA200/ Clips-XC200)[l] | Suture cut needle driver | General open instrument |
| | | Stapler loads angled tip Gold 45 and 60[c] | General robotic instrument | |
| | | Stapler loads purple 45 and 60[c] | | |

Citations: [a]Xodus medical, [b]Applied Medical, [c]Covidien, [d]Storz, [e]New Wave Surgical, [f]Velmed, [g]Stryker, [h]Aesculap, [i]Intuitive, [j]Thompson, [k]Aloka, [l]Ethicon, [m]Cook Surgical, [n]Hobbs Medical, [o]Arizant Healthcare

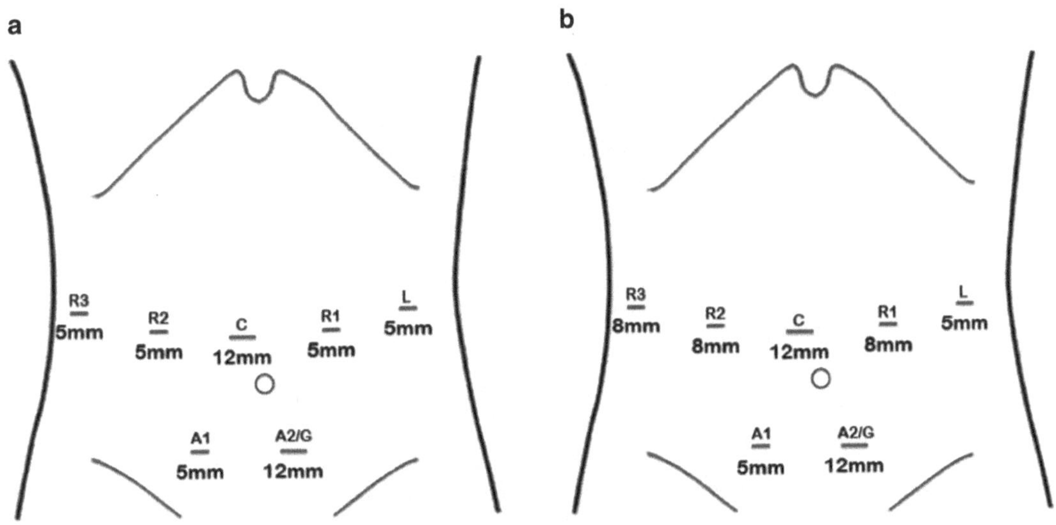


**Fig. 12.3** (**a**) Port placement for laparoscopic mobilization and (**b**) port placement for robotic pancreatectomy indicating the position of the assistant ports (A), robotic ports (R), camera port (C), and gel port (G)

the distance between the camera and R2 port. For the left lower quadrant assistant port, it can be approached in two ways. One method is to make an extraction incision (3–4 cm) medial to the epigastric vessels through the rectus muscle low enough that the gel port does not conflict with arm R1. Once the gel port is placed, the insufflation tubing is connected to it and a 12-mm trocar is placed through it. The second method is to place a 12-mm port and make an extraction incision when the specimen is removed and place the gel port prior to reconstruction.

A stitch is placed laparoscopically to retract the falciform ligament superiorly with the Carter-Thomason CloseSure System (Cooper Surgical, Trumbull, CT) suture-passing device. This aids liver retraction and provides better exposure. If liver retraction is inadequate, a 5-mm port is placed laterally in the LUQ anterior axillary line through which a Mediflex liver retractor (Mediflex® Surgical Products, Islandia, NY) is placed. The Mediflex retractor has several moving parts and requires trial and error to place and use effectively. It may require readjustment throughout the case.

The lesser sac is entered through the gastrocolic omentum using a blunt tip 5-mm LigaSure device (Covidien, Mansfield, MA) below the gastroepiploic vessels and extending halfway up the greater curvature. All posterior adhesions from the stomach to the pancreas are ligated and upon retraction of the stomach cranially, the left gastric pedicle and GDA are identified. Careful dissection is used to separate the transverse mesocolon from the gastroepiploic vein pedicle as the dissection heads toward the hepatic flexure. Care should be taken not to avulse the middle colic or gastroepiploic veins.

Cattell-Braasch maneuver is performed and the entire right colon is mobilized along the white line of Toldt to the appendix, which aids in duodenal exposure especially in obese patients. Once this is done, the duodenum is in full view. Kocherization of the duodenum is completed to expose the foramen of Winslow, the inferior vena cava (IVC), left renal vein, SMA, and the ligament of Treitz. This is the point at which resectability is assessed.

Fibers attaching the posterior duodenum to the retroperitoneum are taken with the LigaSure device. The pancreatic head and uncinate are dissected from the retroperitoneal attachments up to the SMA origin. An extended Kocher maneuver is performed to release the ligament of Treitz from the right side and release the first part of jejunum. Next, the proximal jejunal loop is pulled

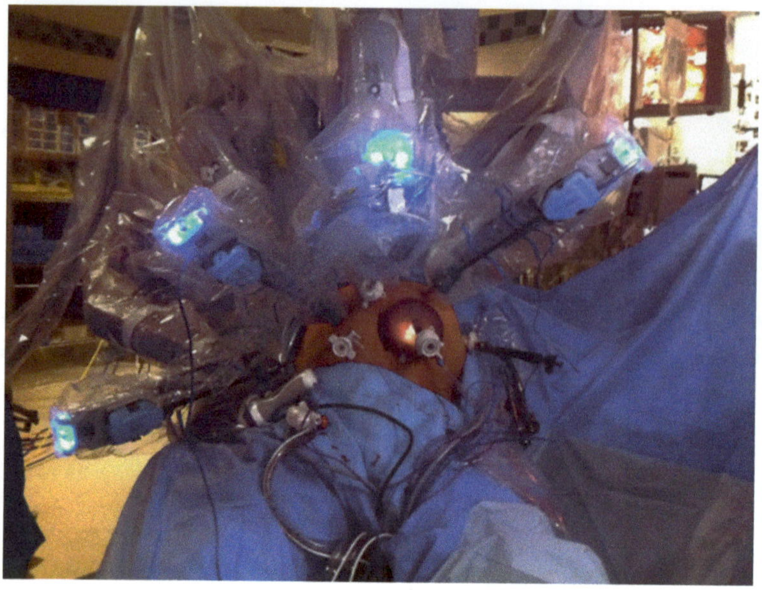

**Fig. 12.4** Intraoperative photo of a docked robot during pancreaticoduodenectomy

into the right supracolic compartment through the ligament of Treitz. A window through the mesentery is created and the proximal jejunum is divided using a laparoscopic linear stapler with a 60-mm gold load (Covidien) with a tip about 10 cm from the duodenojejunal ligament.

The mesentery of the transected jejunum is ligated serially with the LigaSure until the level of the uncinate process. It is critical to complete this step as it sets up the later portions of the venous dissection. The duodenum is rolled to expose the pancreas posteriorly and the soft tissue fibers directly attaching the duodenum to the pancreatic head are ligated, allowing the duodenum to be "rolled off" the pancreas.

The gastrohepatic ligament is inspected for a replaced left hepatic artery and then divided through the *pars flaccida* avascular plane. The right gastric artery (RGA) is ligated flush with the lesser curvature to clear an area on the lesser curvature for the linear stapler. A corresponding area is chosen on the greater curvature where the gastrocolic omentum is further dissected towards the stomach. The area of transection of the stomach or proximal duodenum is defined depending on the type of procedure planned (pylorus-preserving or classic pancreaticoduodenectomy). It is critical to have anesthesia withdraw the NGT back into the esophagus prior to firing the stapler across the stomach. We divide the stomach with a linear stapler with a 60-mm purple load.

Attention then turns to the jejunum in the RUQ. Jejunum (50 cm) is pulled into the RUQ and labeled with proximal and distal seromuscular Endo Stitch 2–0 ticron suture (Covidien) placement. The transverse colon is then retracted cranially to identify the ligament of Treitz from the left infracolic side of the patient. The jejunum is pulled back through the ligament of Treitz to identify the marking stitches. Once identified, the bowel is grasped and pulled antecolic in isoperistaltic fashion with two duckbill graspers. This loop is positioned in left upper abdomen and sutured to the stomach with an Endo Stitch to keep the isoperistaltic orientation. This allows for quick and easy identification for the gastrojejunostomy (GJ) reconstruction. The 12-mm camera port is closed using the Carter Thomason suture-passing device with 0-vicryl sutures. The two RUQ and one LUQ 5-mm ports are exchanged for 8-mm robot ports.

## Robotic Resection

The Da Vinci Robotic system (Intuitive Surgical, Sunnyvale, CA) is docked as shown in Fig. 12.4 with the robot positioned over the head of the patient with two robotic arms on the right side, one arm on the left, and the camera port in the same location as the laparoscopic procedure. The robotic surgeon sits at the console while the laparoscopic assistant stands between the patient's legs and operates using ports A1 and A2. The camera holder is no longer needed. Dissection starts with a monopolar hook in R1, the fenestrated bipolar in R2, and a ProGrasp (Intuitive) in R3. A 30° camera (facing down) is used. The assistant starts with the LigaSure and suction irrigator.

The first step is identification and dissection of the hepatic artery lymph node. This lymph node is dissected using the robotic hook with monopolar cautery and divided with the LigaSure and removed as the first step to expose the porta hepatis. The lymph node is placed into a 10-mm specimen bag and sent off to pathology. Removal of this node creates a window for exposure of the CHA.

The "no touch" technique is used when dissecting vasculature. The vessels are retracted without grabbing the vessel or just by grasping the soft tissue lymphatic network that encases the vessels. R3 is used to grasp the specimen side of the gastric/duodenal staple line, which is pulled to the left. The CHA is lifted by the closed bipolar (R2) and the hook (R1) is used to dissect the artery off the portal vein (PV). Once the PV is identified, the lymphatic soft tissue is dissected off the pancreas neck creating a cranial landing zone on the neck for subsequent pancreatic transection.

The CHA is followed distally to identify the RGA, GDA, and the right and left branches of the hepatic artery (RHA and LHA, respectively). The RGA is always in a plane anterior to the CHA and GDA and can be found near the origin of the GDA or often traced back from the specimen. This is typically clipped proximally with a 5-mm clip and then divided with an energy sealant device. The GDA is circumferentially dissected but not ligated. R1 is switched to a bipolar dissector to pass a vessel loop around the GDA. Of note, bipolar cautery will not work when two bipolar instruments are used simultaneously. The vessel loop is clipped at its end to hold it in place.

R3 is moved off the specimen side of the staple line and used to retract the gallbladder cranially to better expose the porta hepatis. The assistant rolls the specimen medially to the patient's left to aid in exposure of the lateral porta hepatis as well. The lateral aspect of the CBD is mobilized and the peri-portal lymph nodes are dissected with the duct. Careful inspection for a replaced RHA is mandatory here. The CBD is carefully skeletonized off the PV in preparation for ligation of the CBD.

The specimen is rolled back to its native position and R3 retracts the stomach/duodenum staple line for retraction. Prior to ligation of the GDA, and if there is doubt about the presence of a replaced RHA, we use intraoperative laparoscopic/robotic ultrasound with Doppler flow to confirm pulsatile flow in hepatic arteries after clamping the GDA. The GDA is transected with a 45-mm gold stapler load with an angled tip. A 10-mm clip is placed on the GDA stump to mark its location.

Next, the CBD is isolated and dissected off the PV. Again, careful inspection for a replaced RHA is done. Once the CBD is isolated, a vessel loop is passed around it for retraction. The CBD is divided distal to the cystic duct junction (except in distal cholangiocarcinoma) with a 60-mm gold stapler load with an angled tip.

The inferior border of the pancreas is then dissected to look for the SMV under the pancreatic neck. This dissection should proceed slowly and carefully due to the absence of haptic feedback as these vessels are fragile and can easily bleed. The intent is to identify the right gastroepiploic vein, middle colic vein, trunk of Henle (if present), and SMV. Before any structures are divided, it is paramount to visualize the SMV above as it runs under the pancreas and below as it courses through the mesocolon. Once all venous structures have been identified, the right gastroepiploic vein is divided with a vascular stapler load or energy sealant device.

The SMV is dissected off the posterior neck of the pancreas. The tunnel is carefully created by lifting up the pancreatic neck with a closed bipolar in R2 and gingerly pushing down on the SMV with the hook monopolar parallel to the vein in R1. R3 grasps the duodenal/gastric staple line pulling it upwards and to the left. The assistant aids

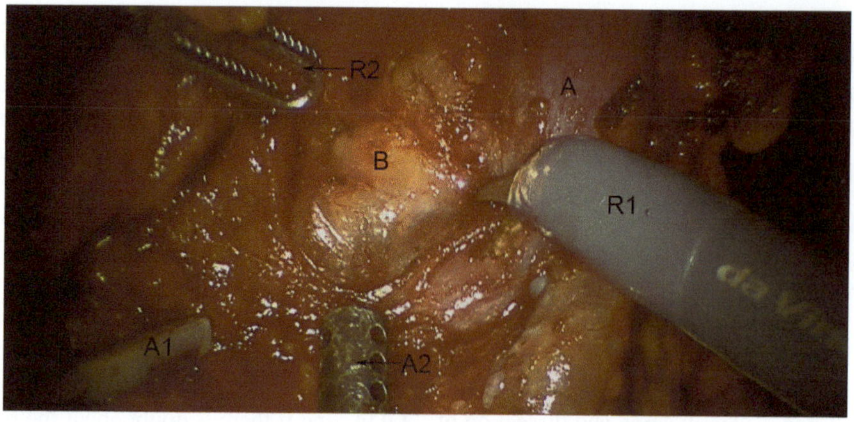


**Fig. 12.5** Hot shears are used for the uncinate dissection off the portal vein. A=superior mesenteric vein, B=pancreas, A1=LigaSure through the assistant port, A2=suction irrigator through the assistant port, R1=hot shears, and R2=fenestrated bipolar

dissection using the suction irrigator like a peanut dissector. Once the length of the neck is traversed, a moistened umbilical tape is placed around the pancreatic neck.

R3 grasps the umbilical tape to lift the pancreas up off the vein and to the right. The A2 port is used for the suction irrigator to protect the SMV-PV during division of the pancreatic neck. Grabbing the inferior edge of the neck of the pancreas with the bipolar and aggressively burning prior to cutting will effectively coagulate the inferior transverse pancreatic artery. The pancreatic neck is divided with monopolar robotic scissors using cautery until reaching the pancreatic duct. The scissors are used "cold" to aid in preservation of the pancreatic duct. The bipolar is used for the superior transverse pancreatic artery superiorly at the neck of the gland. The umbilical tape is removed.

The head of the pancreas is carefully dissected off the right lateral attachments of the SMV by carefully peeling the vein away with scissors—pointing down and jaws spread 1–2 mm (Fig. 12.5). This is done by starting at the top of the neck at the level of the superior pancreaticoduodenal vein moving caudally down to the first jejunal branch entering the SMV. The latter is preserved whenever possible but it is necessary to divide its recurrent tributaries that course back and enter the uncinate. Bipolar cautery is used for these branches as they can bleed.

Once the SMV-PV is exposed anteriorly and laterally, the posterior uncinate dissection and SMA dissection is started. The key to the exposure is placing R3 under the specimen and lifting the pancreas "up and out" analogous to what the surgeon would do with his/her left hand in OPD. Any additional venous tributaries in the mesentery lateral to the first jejunal vein are divided. Once the pancreas is separated and lifted up and away from the first jejunal branch, the SMA will be exposed. As the dissection progresses, so should the adjustment of the R3 retraction of the specimen.

The final and most difficult dissection of the uncinate process off the vascular groove begins. This dissection occurs in 3 layers: (1) anterior most venous layer, (2) middle arterial layer, and (3) posterior lymphatic layer. This dissection may be approached by all three layers from inferior to superior "artery first approach" or layer by layer from anterior to posterior "medial to lateral approach." The latter is often easiest to do with a soft gland, where the former may be better with a hard or thick gland. An energy sealant device through the A1 port is the best to take the posterior lymphatic layer. A combination of the hook and bipolar is best for the anterior venous layer. Without being able to use fingers to palpate the SMA pulse, this dissection should be treated very carefully. Close coordination between the surgeon and assistant is key throughout this dissection. The hook cautery is the best instrument to dissect the SMA and its inferior and superior pancreaticoduodenal arteries (IPDA and SPDA, respectively) since it can be used like the right angle instrument in the open operation. After the SPDA and IPDA are isolated, they are taken with clips in A2 and energy sealant device in A1.

The last move is to ligate the superior pancreaticoduodenal vein with a linear stapler with a gold load. Sometimes, this vessel may be taken earlier to facilitate the uncinate dissection. The specimen is placed into a 15-mm extraction bag and delivered through the LLQ gel port and sent for frozen section evaluation of the pancreas and biliary duct margins. For the sake of safety, we remove all the robotic instruments once the specimen has been passed off the field, since insufflation is lost when the lid is removed from the gel port to extract the specimen.

Robotic cholecystectomy is performed by antegrade or retrograde technique while awaiting the frozen section analysis. The cystic artery is ligated with 5-mm clips and the energy sealant device and the cystic duct are ligated with 5- or 10-mm clips. The specimen is removed in a 10-mm extraction bag.

The resection bed is suctioned and irrigated and inspected for hemostasis. Surgicel (Ethicon, Cincinnati, OH) is used as needed. Three gold fiducials are placed along the vascular groove margin at least 2–3 cm apart and in different planes.

## Robotic Reconstruction

After negative frozen section evaluation, reconstruction is performed. At this point, the divided end of jejunum is oriented so the cut mesentery faces the SMA/SMV without tension. The pancreaticojejunostomy (PJ) is started with three posterior row 2–0 silk sutures, cut to 8 cm length taken full thickness from anterior to posterior, then seromuscular through jejunum in horizontal mattress orientations and back full thickness through the pancreas from posterior to anterior. A Hobbs stent (Hobbs Medical, Stafford Springs, CT) is placed within the PD. The sutures are tied down with the needles attached for later use in the anterior layer. When the middle suture is tied down, the assistant moves the stent in and out of the duct to avoid tying too tight. Next, the duct is aligned against the jejunum and a small full-thickness opening in the jejunum opposite the duct is created with cautery. The PD stent is removed temporarily. A total of four to eight duct-to-mucosa 5–0 absorbable sutures are placed in interrupted fashion depending on duct size, alternating dyed and undyed sutures for easy identification. These are inside-out on the duct and outside-in on the jejunum and tied within the duct. We tie two posterior row sutures, and then replace the pancreatic stent with the self-retained curved end inside the jejunum and the straight end in the pancreatic duct. After completing the anterior row of 5–0 absorbable sutures outside-in on the bowel and inside-out on the duct, the knots are tied on the outside. Then, three seromuscular buttress sutures are placed in the jejunum using the 2–0 silk sutures for the anterior outer layer to complete the PJ.

The hepaticojejunostomy (HJ) is performed approximately 10 cm distal to the PJ allowing for absence of tension between the anastomoses. For normal or large caliber CBDs, two 6 in. 4–0 V-loc sutures (Covidien) are used to create a single running anastomosis. An enterotomy is made on the anti-mesenteric border of the jejunum to match the size of the CBD, and the staple line is removed from the distal CBD with shears. For normal or small CBD, a Hobbs stent is used. The HJ is started laterally at the 9 o'clock position of the CBD; the posterior row is placed first inside-out on the duct and outside-in on full-thickness jejunum. A second 4–0 6 in. V-loc suture is then used anteriorly. This is also sewn lateral to medial but this stitch is outside-in on the duct and inside-out on the jejunum.

Finally, GJ or duodenojejunostomy (DJ) is performed in a 4-layer technique in an antecolic, isoperistaltic fashion. If performing GJ, a corner suture is placed medially which Lamberts the gastric staple line inward and includes the efferent limb of jejunum. R3 port is used to retract this corner suture. The prior Endo Stitch suture is removed.

The first layer is a posterior line of interrupted 2–0 silk Lambert sutures. A true corner suture is placed at the end laterally.

The gastric staple line is removed for a distance of 6 cm. An enterotomy is then created using shears. The second layer is a continuous 3–0 9-in. V-loc (Covidien) posterior full-thickness suture through the stomach and jejunum from medial to lateral and is above the Lambert sutures. This layer continues in Connell fashion anteriorly and another 3–0 9-in. V-loc suture is used medially, taking care not to take big bites at the corners since this may narrow the efferent and afferent lumen. The two V-locs are tied to each other. Finally, the last layer is anterior 2–0 silk Lambert sutures in interrupted fashion completing the anastomosis.

After ensuring adequate hemostasis, we irrigate and place a 19-F Blake drain though R3 anterior to the PJ and GJ and posterior to the GJ/DJ. The robot R3 arm is undocked and R3 is removed keeping the drain in place. The drain is sutured to the skin with 2–0 nylon sutures. The abdominal attachment of the falciform ligament is mobilized and is used as a flap to cover the GDA stump. The robot is undocked and all laparoscopic and robotic ports are removed under visualization. Ports with 12-mm size are closed with previously placed 0-polysorb stitches. The extraction site is closed with #1 Polysorb interrupted sutures. All ports are irrigated and skin is closed with 4–0 absorbable subcuticular stitches and glue.

## Postoperative Management

Management of patients is the same regardless of technique (robotic or open) and pathology. Patients are admitted to the intensive care unit postoperatively. On postoperative day (POD) #1, the NGT is discontinued, the patient is transferred to a regular floor bed, and subcutaneous heparin prophylaxis is resumed. Patients are aggressively ambulated and the Foley catheter is removed by POD #2. The central line and paravertebral pain blocks are discontinued on POD #3 and patients are started on a clear liquid diet. Drain management follows a modified Verona protocol [18]. A drain amylase level is measured on POD #3, and if amylase levels are <3× serum amylase, the drain(s) are removed. Diets are advanced as tolerated on POD #4. Most patients are discharged by POD #7 when the postoperative recovery is uneventful. Patients are seen at 2 and 4 weeks after discharge.

## Acute Complications

Morbidity after pancreaticoduodenectomy is documented to be about 40 % [19–22]. Preliminary studies show that the morbidity and mortality after minimally invasive (laparoscopic and robotic) pancreaticoduodenectomy have been similar to the open approach in specialized centers [7, 11–14, 22–24]. Several series have consistently demonstrated a reduction in estimated blood loss with the robotic approach [12–14, 22–24]. We use the International Study Group of Pancreatic Surgery (ISGPS) grading system for classification of pancreatic fistulas (PF), delayed gastric emptying (DGE), and postoperative pancreatic hemorrhage (PPH) [25–27]. We recently published our pancreatic experience of 250 robotic pancreas cases, including 132 RPD [14]. Clinically significant morbidity (Grade 3–4 Clavien-Dindo scale) [28, 29] after RPD affected 21 % of patients with PF rate of 17 % with only 7.5 % having clinically significant (grade B and C) PFs [14]. We do not routinely place gastric tubes or jejunal feeding tubes. In older patients with poor functional status or patients with malnutrition, we will occasionally place an 18-French gastrojejunal dual port tube. Treatment of DGE varies case by case, but we have found metoclopramide and erythromycin to be largely ineffective. For mild cases, we will sometimes allow oral feeds and manage vomiting with TPN support. For severe cases, nasogastrojejunal tubes or percutaneous gastrojejunal tubes are placed endoscopically to allow for gastric decompression and distal feeds. Our 30 and 90-day perioperative mortality was 1.5 % and 3.8 %, respectively [14].

We treat suspected PPH very aggressively. The typical time window is POD #5–7, however this complication can occur later. PPH typically presents as a decrease in hemoglobin/hematocrit, blood in the drain, or gastrointestinal bleeding. If clinical suspicion is high, patients are managed by interventional radiology (IR) for celiac and SMA angiography. The GDA stump is marked with a 10-mm clip and the RGA stump is marked with a 5-mm clip intraoperatively; we do not leave a stump on these vessels so the clips aid with identification. We manage bleeding with covered stents. If no extravasation is identified, but our suspicion remains high for a sentinel bleed, we will prophylactically use a stent or leave the femoral access catheter in place and watch the patient for evidence of re-bleed. If the clinical suspicion is low, we will obtain a CT angiogram to look for a pseudoaneurysm or extravasation of contrast. If IR and/or CT scan are both negative and they continue with a gastrointestinal bleed, our gastroenterologists perform endoscopic evaluation of the GJ anastomosis and the afferent limb to the HJ and PJ.

## Long-Term Sequelae

Diabetes and pancreatic insufficiency are commonly reported chronic sequelae after pancreaticoduodenectomy [30, 31]. It is uncommon to discharge patients with insulin or pancreatic enzymes. If patients have borderline glucose elevation in the hospital, their sugars are followed on discharge and an endocrinology referral is made. Patients noted on postoperative clinic visits to have diarrhea concerning for steatorrhea have a fecal elastase level tested and are started on pancreatic enzymes accordingly.

## Conclusion

The robotic approach to pancreatic resections has been shown to be safe and feasible with outcomes similar to the open approach. The perceived need for this approach stems from shortcomings of the laparoscopic approach including limited technology and limited training. In the hands of two experienced pancreatic surgeons, the RPD is our preferred approach for pancreatic head resection whenever indicated and feasible.

## References

1. Whipple AO, Parsons WB, Mullins CR. Treatment of carcinoma of the Ampulla of Vater. Ann Surg. 1935;102(4):763–79.
2. Whipple AO. Observations on radical surgery for lesions of the pancreas. Surg Gynecol Obstet. 1946; 82:623–31.
3. Gagner M, Pomp A. Laparoscopic pylorus-preserving pancreatoduodenectomy. Surg Endosc. 1994;8(5): 408–10.
4. Kendrick ML, Cusati D. Total laparoscopic pancreaticoduodenectomy: feasibility and outcome in an early experience. Arch Surg. 2010;145(1):19–23. doi: 10.1001/archsurg.2009.243.
5. Palanivelu C, Rajan PS, Rangarajan M, Vaithiswaran V, Senthilnathan P, Parthasarathi R, et al. Evolution in techniques of laparoscopic pancreaticoduodenectomy: a decade long experience from a tertiary center. J Hepato-Biliary-Pancreat Surg. 2009;16(6):731–40. doi:10.1007/s00534-009-0157-8.
6. Narula VK, Mikami DJ, Melvin WS. Robotic and laparoscopic pancreaticoduodenectomy: a hybrid approach. Pancreas. 2010;39(2):160–4. doi:10.1097/MPA.0b013e3181bd604e.
7. Giulianotti PC, Sbrana F, Bianco FM, Elli EF, Shah G, Addeo P, et al. Robot-assisted laparoscopic pancreatic surgery: single-surgeon experience. Surg Endosc. 2010; 24(7):1646–57. doi:10.1007/s00464-009-0825-4.
8. Gagner M, Gentileschi P. Hand-assisted laparoscopic pancreatic resection. Semin Laparosc Surg. 2001;8(2): 114–25.
9. Gagner M, Pomp A. Laparoscopic pancreatic resection: Is it worthwhile? J Gastrointest Surg. 1997;1(1): 20–5; discussion 5–6.
10. Hanly EJ, Talamini MA. Robotic abdominal surgery. Am J Surg. 2004;188(4A Suppl):19S–26S. doi: 10.1016/j.amjsurg.2004.08.020.
11. Gagner M, Palermo M. Laparoscopic Whipple procedure: review of the literature. J Hepato-Biliary-Pancreat Surg. 2009;16(6):726–30. doi:10.1007/s00534-009-0142-2.
12. Zeh 3rd HJ, Bartlett DL, Moser AJ. Robotic-assisted major pancreatic resection. Adv Surg. 2011;45: 323–40.
13. Zureikat AH, Nguyen KT, Bartlett DL, Zeh HJ, Moser AJ. Robotic-assisted major pancreatic resection and reconstruction. Arch Surg. 2011;146(3):256–61. doi:10.1001/archsurg.2010.246.
14. Zureikat AH, Moser AJ, Boone BA, Bartlett DL, Zenati M, Zeh 3rd HJ. 250 robotic pancreatic resections: safety and feasibility. Ann Surg. 2013;

258(4):554–9. doi:10.1097/SLA.0b013e3182a4e87c; discussion 9–62.
15. Callery MP, Chang KJ, Fishman EK, Talamonti MS, William Traverso L, Linehan DC. Pretreatment assessment of resectable and borderline resectable pancreatic cancer: expert consensus statement. Ann Surg Oncol. 2009;16(7):1727–33. doi:10.1245/s10434-009-0408-6.
16. Abrams RA, Lowy AM, O'Reilly EM, Wolff RA, Picozzi VJ, Pisters PW. Combined modality treatment of resectable and borderline resectable pancreas cancer: expert consensus statement. Ann Surg Oncol. 2009;16(7):1751–6. doi:10.1245/s10434-009-0413-9.
17. Varadhachary GR, Tamm EP, Abbruzzese JL, Xiong HQ, Crane CH, Wang H, et al. Borderline resectable pancreatic cancer: definitions, management, and role of preoperative therapy. Ann Surg Oncol. 2006;13(8):1035–46. doi:10.1245/aso.2006.08.011.
18. Bassi C, Molinari E, Malleo G, Crippa S, Butturini G, Salvia R, et al. Early versus late drain removal after standard pancreatic resections: results of a prospective randomized trial. Ann Surg. 2010;252(2):207–14. doi:10.1097/SLA.0b013e3181e61e88.
19. Cameron JL, Riall TS, Coleman J, Belcher KA. One thousand consecutive pancreaticoduodenectomies. Ann Surg. 2006;244(1):10–5. doi:10.1097/01.sla.0000217673.04165.ea.
20. Hatzaras I, Schmidt C, Klemanski D, Muscarella P, Melvin WS, Ellison EC, et al. Pancreatic resection in the octogenarian: a safe option for pancreatic malignancy. J Am Coll Surg. 2011;212(3):373–7. doi:10.1016/j.jamcollsurg.2010.10.015.
21. Makary MA, Winter JM, Cameron JL, Campbell KA, Chang D, Cunningham SC, et al. Pancreaticoduodenectomy in the very elderly. J Gastrointest Surg. 2006;10(3):347–56. doi:10.1016/j.gassur.2005.12.014.
22. Lai EC, Yang GP, Tang CN. Robot-assisted laparoscopic pancreaticoduodenectomy versus open pancreaticoduodenectomy—a comparative study. Int J Surg. 2012;10(9):475–9. doi:10.1016/j.ijsu.2012.06.003.
23. Chalikonda S, Aguilar-Saavedra JR, Walsh RM. Laparoscopic robotic-assisted pancreaticoduodenectomy: a case-matched comparison with open resection. Surg Endosc. 2012;26(9):2397–402. doi:10.1007/s00464-012-2207-6.
24. Buchs NC, Addeo P, Bianco FM, Ayloo S, Benedetti E, Giulianotti PC. Robotic versus open pancreaticoduodenectomy: a comparative study at a single institution. World J Surg. 2011;35(12):2739–46. doi:10.1007/s00268-011-1276-3.
25. Bassi C, Dervenis C, Butturini G, Fingerhut A, Yeo C, Izbicki J, et al. Postoperative pancreatic fistula: an international study group (ISGPF) definition. Surgery. 2005;138(1):8–13. doi:10.1016/j.surg.2005.05.001.
26. Wente MN, Veit JA, Bassi C, Dervenis C, Fingerhut A, Gouma DJ, et al. Postpancreatectomy hemorrhage (PPH): an International Study Group of Pancreatic Surgery (ISGPS) definition. Surgery. 2007;142(1):20–5. doi:10.1016/j.surg.2007.02.001.
27. Wente MN, Bassi C, Dervenis C, Fingerhut A, Gouma DJ, Izbicki JR, et al. Delayed gastric emptying (DGE) after pancreatic surgery: a suggested definition by the International Study Group of Pancreatic Surgery (ISGPS). Surgery. 2007;142(5):761–8. doi:10.1016/j.surg.2007.05.005.
28. Dindo D, Demartines N, Clavien PA. Classification of surgical complications: a new proposal with evaluation in a cohort of 6336 patients and results of a survey. Ann Surg. 2004;240(2):205–13.
29. Clavien PA, Barkun J, de Oliveira ML, Vauthey JN, Dindo D, Schulick RD, et al. The Clavien-Dindo classification of surgical complications: five-year experience. Ann Surg. 2009;250(2):187–96. doi:10.1097/SLA.0b013e3181b13ca2.
30. Fang WL, Su CH, Shyr YM, Chen TH, Lee RC, Tai LC, et al. Functional and morphological changes in pancreatic remnant after pancreaticoduodenectomy. Pancreas. 2007;35(4):361–5. doi:10.1097/MPA.0b013e3180d0a8d5.
31. You DD, Choi SH, Choi DW, Heo JS, Ho CY, Kim WS. Long-term effects of pancreaticoduodenectomy on glucose metabolism. ANZ J Surg. 2012;82(6):447–51. doi:10.1111/j.1445-2197.2012.06080.x.

## Key Operative Steps

1. *"The Trick Move" (Laparoscopic)*: This is when the lesser sac is exposed and dissection proceeds in the avascular plane that separates the transverse mesocolon from the right gastroepiploic pedicle and then continues laterally to separate the hepatic flexure mesocolon from Gerota's fascia. This step begins the exposure to the head of the pancreas.
2. *"The 'A-Ha' Moment" (Laparoscopic)*: This occurs when the last fibers of the ligament of Treitz are divided and the jejunum comes into view. This allows mobilization of the jejunum into the RUQ.
3. *"Doing Our Homework" (Laparoscopic)*: When the jejunum is stapled and the mesentery of the small bowel is divided, this dissection extends from the mesentery caudally to the duodenal attachments and pancreas cephalad. These maneuvers facilitate the subsequent robotic dissection of the SMV and uncinate.
4. *"Confirming Our Orientation" (Laparoscopic)*: Endo Stitch is used to place sutures to orient the jejunum and secure the bowel to the stomach. This is a critical time saving maneuver to ensure an isoperistaltic orientation of the bowel for the gastrojejunal anastomosis.
5. *"Graduation" (Laparoscopic)*: This step is the closure of the 12-mm camera port with a figure-of-eight Carter Thomason 0-polysorb suture. This step will eliminate the need to reinsert a laparoscope at the end of the robot procedure to close this port site.
6. *Removal of Hepatic Artery Lymph Node (Robotic).*

7. *Robotic Dissection of Porta Hepatis (Robotic)*: These steps allow for identification of a replaced right hepatic artery, initiation of portal lymph node dissection, identification of the right lateral aspect of the portal vein, and creation of a "landing zone" for subsequent common bile duct isolation.
8. *Identifying the Proximal and Distal SMV (Robotic)*: Prior to ligating the right gastroepiploic vein or any other major vein, it is of critical importance to make sure the superior mesenteric vein is safe by visualizing it above and below the gastroepiploic vein.
9. *Umbilical Tape Around Pancreatic Neck (Robotic)*: R3 is used to lift the pancreas and retract it up and to the right, which allows for optimal exposure of the pancreatic neck.
10. *"The First Jejunal" (Robotic)*: This vein is saved whenever possible, but its tributaries that course back and enter the uncinate are divided.
11. *"Up and Out" (Robotic)*: R3 is used to lift the specimen up and out like the left hand of the surgeon during an open case. This is a critical step to provide optimal exposure during the uncinate dissection. R3 may need to be continuously adjusted as the dissection progresses from the inferior to superior.
12. *Pancreaticojejunostomy (Robotic)*: Keeping the needles of the three 2–0 silk stitches on for the final buttress layer.
13. *Hepaticojejunostomy (Robotic)*: The v-lock suture has barbs that do not catch the tissue on the first pass. When this suture is used, the second stitch needs to be placed very close to the first stitch so the barb catches and there is not a gap.
14. *Gastrojejunostomy (Robotic)*: When the corners are sewn using the v-lock, it is important to take full-thickness bites; however, extreme caution must be used to take small bites to avoid kinking or narrowing the efferent or afferent limbs.
15. *Teamwork (Robotic)*: The true key to this technique is a combined understanding, effort, and teamwork between two experienced robotic pancreatic surgeons. To expose key anatomic structures and perform a delicate, vascular dissection requires great coordination between the laparoscopic assistant and robotic surgeon.

# Part III

# Jejunum and Ileum

# Open Technique for Resection of Cancers of the Jejunum and Ileum

13

Gregory C. Wilson and Syed A. Ahmad

## Introduction

The incidence of small bowel cancer has steadily increased over the past two decades [1, 2]. The overall incidence has steadily increased from 11.8 cases per million people in 1973 to 22.7 cases per million people in the most recent decade [1]. In addition, there have only been few advances in the management of these patients and survival for small bowel cancer has remained stagnant [1]. Fortunately, malignancies of the small intestine account for only 1–3 % of gastrointestinal neoplasms and account for less than 1 % of cancer-related mortality [2]. The low relative incidence of malignancy can be attributed to several protective mechanisms specific to the small bowel. Its liquid chyme contents cause less mechanical irritation compared to that of the colon and the rapid transit time minimizes the interaction between enteric carcinogens and bowel mucosa. Additionally, the low bacterial flora prevents the degradation of bile salts by anaerobic bacteria into carcinogenic compounds [3]. High concentrations of mucosal enzymes such as benzpyrene hydroxylase also protect the small bowel through the metabolism of carcinogenic substances [4]. Increased lymphatic tissue and secretory immunoglobulin A provide additional protection to the small bowel [5].

For most small bowel tumors, surgical resection done in a timely manner provides the only potentially curative treatment and therefore remains the foundation of treatment algorithms. Unfortunately, the paucity of early symptoms and lack of effective screening tools result in late presentation and poor overall survival for the majority of patients with small bowel cancer. The four most common tumors of the small intestine include: adenocarcinoma, gastrointestinal stromal tumors (GISTs), lymphomas, and gastrointestinal neuroendocrine (GNET) tumors (formerly referred to as carcinoid tumors). Adenocarcinoma and GNET make up over 70 % of small bowel malignancies while the remainder consist of lymphoma and GISTs [1]. These histologic subtypes confer different tumor biology and therefore have different management algorithms. This chapter will focus on the indications and techniques for open resection of small bowel cancers located in the jejunum and ileum.

## Anatomical Review

The small intestine, consisting of the jejunum and ileum, provides the majority of surface area for nutrient absorption. It is the largest portion of the gastrointestinal tract and spans a total length of approximately 7 m. The jejunum consists of the

G.C. Wilson, M.D. • S.A. Ahmad, M.D. (✉)
Division of Surgical Oncology, Department of Surgery, University of Cincinnati Medical Center, 234 Goodman Street, ML 0772, Cincinnati, OH 45219, USA
e-mail: ahmadsy@uc.edu

J. Kim and J. Garcia-Aguilar (eds.), *Surgery for Cancers of the Gastrointestinal Tract: A Step-by-Step Approach*, DOI 10.1007/978-1-4939-1893-5_13, © Springer Science+Business Media New York 2015

proximal two-fifths of small bowel and begins as a continuation of the duodenum as it traverses from a retroperitoneal structure to an intraperitoneal location. This transition to an intraperitoneal location can be easily identified on surgical exploration by its close approximation with the ligament of Treitz. As the small bowel courses through the abdominal compartment, there is no definitive transition point marking the end of the jejunum and the beginning of the ileum. The ileum consists of the distal three-fifths of small bowel and terminates at the ileocecal junction [6].

The vascular supply of the small intestine comes from the superior mesenteric artery (SMA), which supplies blood to the entirety of the small bowel, right colon, and a majority of the transverse colon. After giving off its first branch, the inferior pancreaticoduodenal artery, the SMA traverses through the mesentery giving off the jejunal and ileal branches. These branches form numerous arcades within the mesentery, which feed the distal vasa recta arteries and directly supply the small bowel with arterial blood flow. This supply of arterial blood originates in the mesenteric side of the bowel and travels circumferentially to the antimesenteric aspect of the bowel wall. The anatomy of this blood supply is particularly important for bowel resection and anastomotic techniques in order to prevent devascularization of bowel segments. Venous drainage mirrors that of the arterial supply and coalesces into the superior mesenteric vein which provides venous flow into the portal system.

## Clinical Presentation

Intestinal tumors as a whole are typically asymptomatic and difficult to detect. Hence, most small bowel lesions are identified only once they have become clinically significant via intestinal obstruction, intussusception, distant metastases, or gastrointestinal hemorrhage. The most frequent presentation of small bowel tumors is nonspecific abdominal discomfort/pain, followed by obstructive symptoms and gastrointestinal hemorrhage [7]. Palpable abdominal masses are rare. GNET tumors can present with the characteristic findings of carcinoid syndrome including diarrhea, flushing, bronchoconstriction, and rarely right-sided heart failure. Carcinoid syndrome, when present, is usually associated with metastatic disease. Intestinal lymphomas typically present with nonspecific abdominal complaints in association with or without constitutional B-symptoms including weight loss, fatigue, intermittent fevers, and night sweats. Occult lower gastrointestinal bleeding with normal colonoscopy and esophagogastroduodenoscopy should alert the clinician to a possible small bowel lesion.

## Preoperative Work-up

Unfortunately due to the nonspecific presentation of small bowel malignancies only 50 % of patients have a correct diagnosis prior to surgical intervention. In patients whom there is a high suspicion of small bowel malignancy, computed tomography with oral and intravenous contrast is the initial diagnostic imaging modality of choice. Findings consistent with small bowel tumor include bowel wall thickening, intraluminal filling defects, or bulky mesenteric lymph nodes. Additional findings concerning for small bowel malignancy include small bowel intussusception or transition point in patients with obstructive symptoms.

Direct visualization of the small bowel with traditional endoscopic techniques is difficult. Emerging new technologies should further advance our capability to evaluate the small intestine. Capsule endoscopy has seen increasing use and allows for visualization of the entire small bowel, however its reliability and accuracy are still being determined and cannot currently be used as a stand-alone modality [8]. Double-balloon enteroscopy has also emerged as a new modality to directly examine the small bowel using conventional endoscopic techniques [9, 10]. This modality provides direct visualization of the small bowel mucosa and biopsy capabilities, however its utilization is limited to select centers [11].

Once small bowel malignancy has been identified additional imaging is necessary to stage the patient and evaluate for metastatic disease. If not already obtained, abdominal and chest computed tomography with oral and intravenous contrast should be obtained to evaluate extent of primary tumor and presence of abdominal and extraabdominal metastatic disease. For GNETs preoperative staging may also include octreotide scanning and serum measurements of chromogranin A and serotonin levels [12].

## Operative Technique

### Indications and Therapeutic Goals of Surgery

#### Adenocarcinoma

The primary treatment modality for patients with small bowel adenocarcinoma without evidence of metastatic disease is surgical resection. Surgical resection must include a mesenteric lymphadenectomy given the predilection for nodal metastases [13]. Resection of the primary tumor should include 6 cm longitudinal margins. Adjacent mesentery and additional adherent structures should be removed en bloc with the primary tumor. Distal ileal lesions may require a right colectomy to achieve adequate margins and nodal clearance. Despite curative intent, 5-year survival remains less than 38 % [1, 14]. Adjuvant therapy with 5-fluorouracil based chemotherapy has demonstrated improved disease-free survival [15].

#### Gastrointestinal Neuroendocrine Tumors

GNETs occur in a number of different locations, however, for the extent of this chapter the focus is on small bowel tumors. The majority of midgut GNETs are located in the distal ileum. Multicentric disease is common and a thorough exploration of the abdominal cavity is imperative. GNETs of the small intestine frequently metastasize and therefore wide en bloc resection is necessary with resection of adjacent mesentery and lymph nodes for locoregional control. The desmoplastic reaction associated with GNETs increases the difficulty of the resection due to mesenteric fibrosis and foreshortening. Almost one-fourth of GNET are unresectable secondary to their involvement of major mesenteric vessels [16].

#### Gastrointestinal Stromal Tumors

For primary, resectable tumors surgery remains the primary treatment. Local en bloc resection with tumor-free margins provides curative treatment for resectable tumors. These tumors rarely metastasize to regional lymph nodes and therefore extensive lymphadenectomy is unnecessary. The role of surgical resection remains unclear for patients with advanced disease or disease progression. Following surgical resection, adjuvant therapy with imatinib results in improved relapse-free survival [17] and improved overall 5-year survival [18].

#### Lymphoma

The small intestine is the second most common location of primary gastrointestinal lymphoma following the stomach. Diffuse, large B-cell lymphoma is the most common subtype. These tumors are typically located in the ileum, where there is a high concentration of lymphoid tissue. Chemotherapy remains the cornerstone of treatment for any lymphoma. Surgical resection does have a role for early local lymphomas of the small intestine [19]. Surgical resection may also be required to treat complications of small intestine lymphoma such as hemorrhage or viscous perforation, which may occur during chemotherapy treatment or as the presenting event. In this case, resection should be performed to grossly healthy bowel in order to treat the complication; any residual disease will be adequately treated with chemotherapy.

### Preoperative Preparation

In preparation for the procedure, patients are instructed to avoid liquids and solids 8 h before the scheduled procedure. Patients are given preoperative antibiotics within 60 min of incision. Once in the operating room, the patient is positioned on the operating table in the supine position (Fig. 13.1). After induction of anesthesia, the patient's arms are protected with gel foam padding and tucked at his/her side.

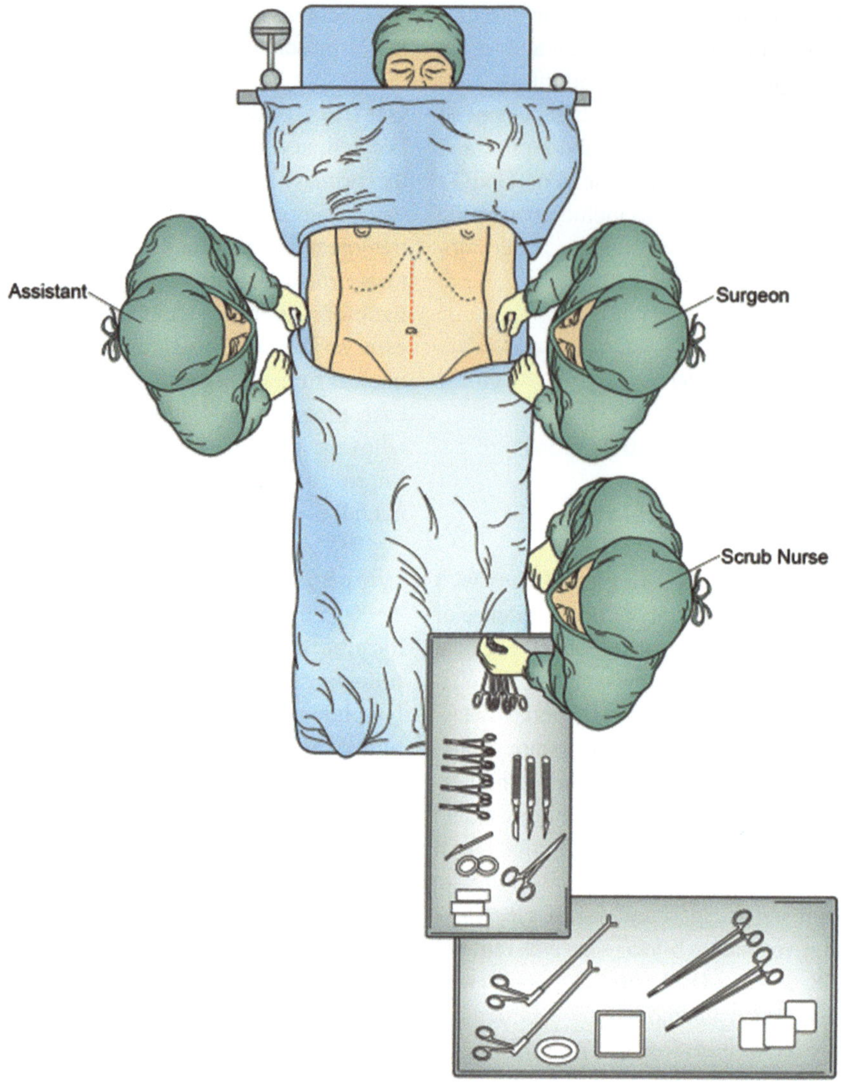


**Fig. 13.1** Proper patient positioning in the operating room. The patient is positioned on the operating table in the supine position. The patient's upper extremities are tucked at the side

## En Bloc Jejunal/Ileal Resection

Exploratory laparotomy is performed through a midline incision. A thorough exploration of the abdomen is imperative to identify any evidence of metastatic disease. Attention should be specifically placed on examining common locations of metastatic disease including the peritoneum, liver, and omentum. The entirety of the small bowel is then examined starting at the ligament of Treitz through the end of the ileum. The area of malignancy is identified and appropriate margins are determined both proximally and distally. The mesentery adjacent to the primary tumor should be palpated for clinically positive lymph nodes, which must be included in the resected specimen. A small window in the adjacent mesentery is created for stapler placement by blunt or electrocautery dissection. The small bowel is then divided with a linear gastrointestinal anastomosis (GIA) stapling device (Ethicon Endo-surgery, Cincinnati, OH). Staple selection is

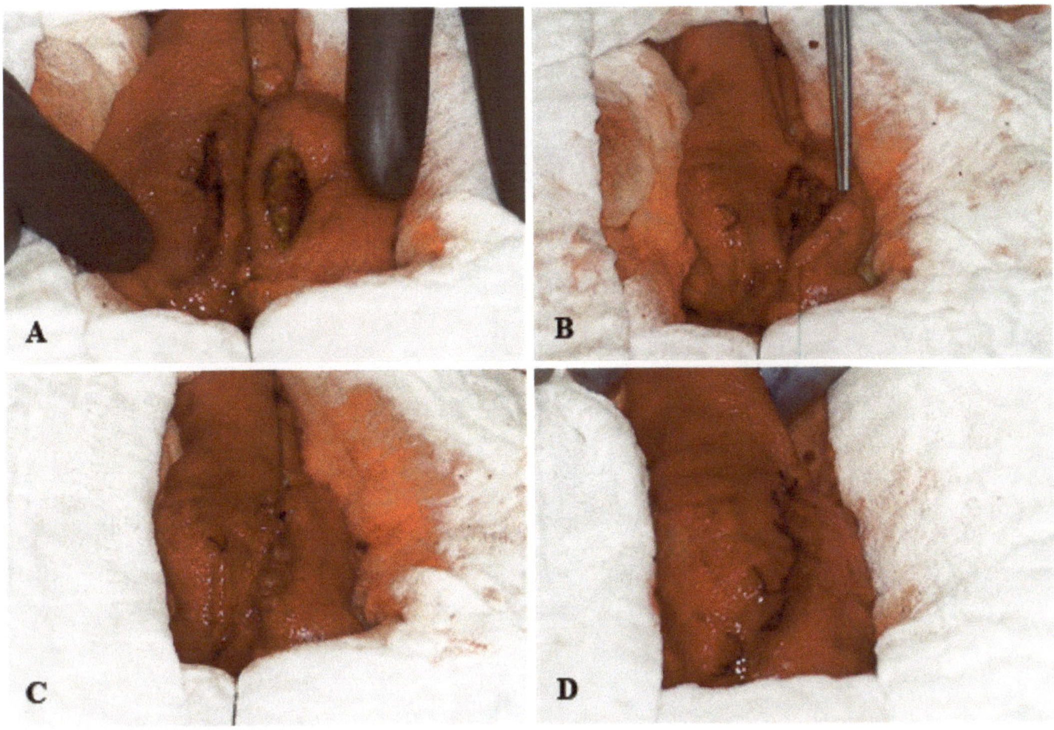


**Fig. 13.2** Hand-sewn anastomosis. (**a**) Full-thickness enterotomies are made for a distance of 5–6 cm. (**b**) The inner layer of the anastomosis is performed with a continuous running suture. This layer is initiated on the posterior aspect of the anastomosis and progresses (**c**) to include entire circumference of the enterotomies. (**d**) The anastomosis is completed with anterior seromuscular sutures

critical and for standard small bowel the staples should have a closed staple height of 1.5 mm (blue load). The mesentery is then divided serially using a clamp and tie technique. Two large Kelly clamps compress the mesentery, which is then sharply divided. The divided portions of mesentery are ligated using 2–0 silk sutures. Energy devices, including ultrasonic vibration instruments such as the HARMONIC FOCUS (Ethicon, Cincinnati, OH) or advanced bipolar devices such as the ENSEAL G2 (Ethicon, Cincinnati, OH), can alternatively be used to divide and ligate the mesentery. This resection is performed to the root of the mesentery with extreme caution to avoid ligation of the superior mesentery artery or one of its main branches supplying the remainder of small bowel. The entire specimen is removed en bloc and prepared for pathologic evaluation. Proximal and distal portions of small bowel are marked using silk suture. Bowel continuity is achieved through an isoperistaltic side-to-side anastomosis. This anastomosis can be performed through one of two techniques: hand-sewn technique or stapled anastomosis technique.

## Hand-Sewn Anastomosis

The first step in utilizing a hand-sewn technique is to align the divided ends of small bowel in an isoperistaltic manner and secure this position by placing anchoring sutures in the mesenteric portion of the serosa. A two-layered technique is utilized. The posterior outer layer is performed first using 3–0 interrupted silk sutures. These sutures should align the two bowel segments for a distance of at least 5–6 cm. Full-thickness enterotomies are made in both of the bowel segments just above the posterior layer (Fig. 13.2a).

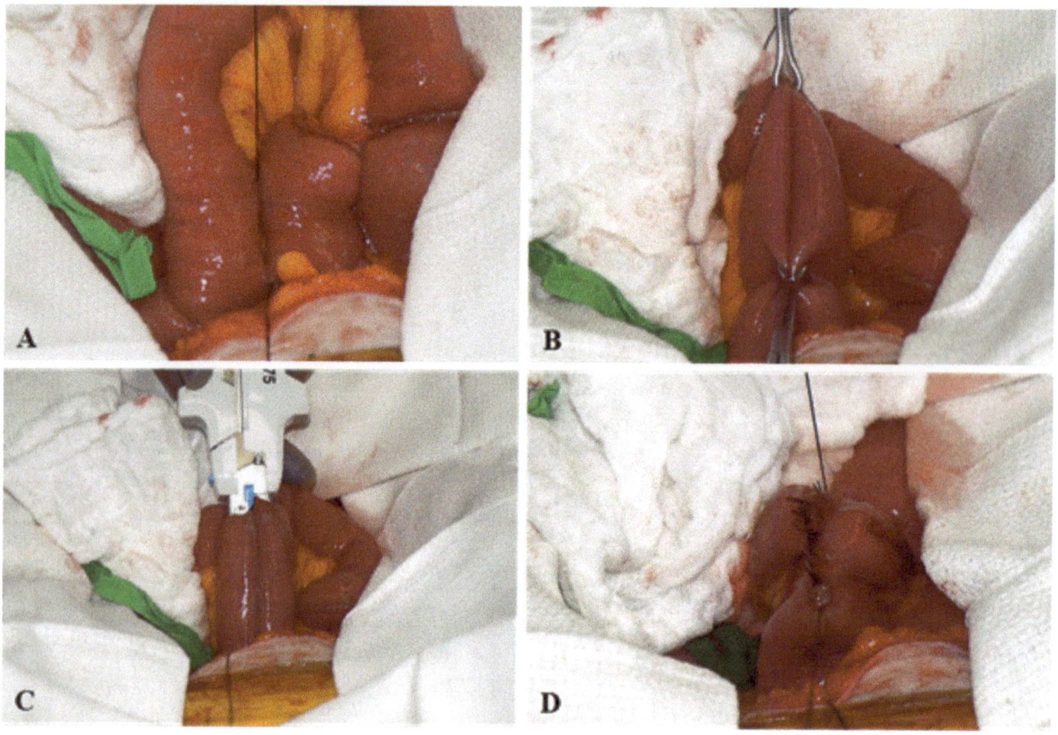


**Fig. 13.3** Stapled anastomosis technique. (**a**) The divided ends are aligned in an isoperistaltic manner. (**b**) Full-thickness enterotomies are made on the antimesenteric bowel wall. (**c**) Side-to-side enteroenterostomy is made with the linear GIA stapling device. (**d**) The remaining defect is then closed with interrupted seromuscular sutures

Next, the inner layer of the two-layer anastomosis is performed as continuous running suture. This inner layer is best completed with a double-armed 3–0 absorbable suture (e.g., Maxon polyglyconate, monofilament synthetic absorbable suture, Covidien, Mansfield, MA) secured initially in the middle of the posterior inner row with full-thickness bites of each bowel segment. Continual full-thickness bites are taken as the running suture continues to each corner of the anastomosis (Fig. 13.2b). This continuous suture is continued on the anterior portion of the anastomosis and secured in the middle of the anterior row completing the inner layer of the anastomosis (Fig. 13.2c). Next, the anterior portion of the outer layer is completed with interrupted, seromuscular bites placed in Lembert fashion using 3–0 silk suture (Fig. 13.2d). The mesenteric defect is closed with interrupted silk sutures to prevent internal herniation.

## Stapled Anastomosis

Similarly, the divided ends of the small bowel are aligned in an isoperistaltic manner. Serosal anchoring sutures are placed in the mesenteric side of the bowel serosa ensuring proper alignment of the divided ends (Fig. 13.3a). Full-thickness enterotomies are made on the antimesenteric surface of both divided ends approximately 1 cm distal to the staple lines (Fig. 13.3b). Side-to-side enteroenterostomy is created along the antimesenteric portion of the divided bowel using a linear GIA stapling device with 3.8 mm staple load (1.5 mm closed staple height) (Fig. 13.3c). The remaining bowel defect is then closed with interrupted, 3–0 silk sutures placed in Lembert fashion (Fig. 13.3d). The mesenteric defect is again closed with simple, interrupted sutures (2–0 silk) to prevent future internal herniation.

## References

1. Bilimoria KY, et al. Small bowel cancer in the United States: changes in epidemiology, treatment, and survival over the last 20 years. Ann Surg. 2009;249(1):63–71.
2. Siegel R, Naishadham D, Jemal A. Cancer statistics. CA Cancer J Clin. 2013;63(1):11–30.
3. Lowenfels AB. Why are small-bowel tumours so rare? Lancet. 1973;1(7793):24–6.
4. Wattenberg LW. Studies of polycyclic hydrocarbon hydroxylases of the intestine possibly related to cancer. Effect of diet on benzpyrene hydroxylase activity. Cancer. 1971;28(1):99–102.
5. Calman KC. Why are small bowel tumours rare? An experimental model. Gut. 1974;15(7):552–4.
6. Moore KL. Clinically oriented anatomy. 5th ed. Baltimore: Lippincott Williams and Wilkins; 2006.
7. Dabaja BS, et al. Adenocarcinoma of the small bowel: presentation, prognostic factors, and outcome of 217 patients. Cancer. 2004;101(3):518–26.
8. Cobrin GM, Pittman RH, Lewis BS. Increased diagnostic yield of small bowel tumors with capsule endoscopy. Cancer. 2006;107(1):22–7.
9. Yamamoto H, et al. Total enteroscopy with a nonsurgical steerable double-balloon method. Gastrointest Endosc. 2001;53(2):216–20.
10. Yamamoto H, et al. Clinical outcomes of double-balloon endoscopy for the diagnosis and treatment of small-intestinal diseases. Clin Gastroenterol Hepatol. 2004;2(11):1010–6.
11. Lo SK, Mehdizadeh S. Therapeutic uses of double-balloon enteroscopy. Gastrointest Endosc Clin N Am. 2006;16(2):363–76.
12. Boudreaux JP, et al. The NANETS consensus guideline for the diagnosis and management of neuroendocrine tumors: well-differentiated neuroendocrine tumors of the jejunum, ileum, appendix, and cecum. Pancreas. 2010;39(6):753–66.
13. Feig BW, Ching CD. The MD Anderson surgical oncology handbook. 4th ed. Philadelphia: Lippincott Williams and Wilkins; 2012.
14. Howe JR, et al. The American College of Surgeons Commission on Cancer and the American Cancer Society. Adenocarcinoma of the small bowel: review of the National Cancer Data Base, 1985-1995. Cancer. 1999;86(12):2693–706.
15. Overman MJ, et al. Is there a role for adjuvant therapy in resected adenocarcinoma of the small intestine. Acta Oncol. 2010;49(4):474–9.
16. Hellman P, et al. Effect of surgery on the outcome of midgut carcinoid disease with lymph node and liver metastases. World J Surg. 2002;26(8):991–7.
17. Dematteo RP, et al. Adjuvant imatinib mesylate after resection of localised, primary gastrointestinal stromal tumour: a randomised, double-blind, placebo-controlled trial. Lancet. 2009;373(9669):1097–104.
18. Joensuu H, et al. One vs three years of adjuvant imatinib for operable gastrointestinal stromal tumor: a randomized trial. JAMA. 2012;307(12):1265–72.
19. Koniaris LG, et al. Management of gastrointestinal lymphoma. J Am Coll Surg. 2003;197(1):127–41.

## Key Operative Steps

1. Exploratory laparotomy to identify primary tumor and assess for multicentric and metastatic disease.
2. Perform wide en bloc resection of primary tumor with 6 cm margins.
3. Resect adjacent mesentery and adherent structures.
4. Reestablish bowel continuity with hand-sewn two-layer anastomosis: outer interrupted layer with 3–0 silk suture and inner running layer with 3–0 absorbable suture.
5. Alternatively, reestablish bowel continuity with stapled side-to-side enteroenterostomy using GIA linear stapler (1.5 mm closed staple height). Close enterotomy with 3–0 silk sutures.
6. Close mesenteric defect with simple interrupted sutures to prevent herniation.

# 14 Minimally Invasive Surgical Techniques for Cancers of the Small Intestine

Bestoun Ahmed, Dilendra H. Weerasinghe, and Michael S. Nussbaum

## Anatomical Highlights

The small intestine is a convoluted tube extending from the pylorus to the ileocecal valve. It is about 7 m long, and gradually diminishes in size from its commencement to its termination. The small intestine is divisible into three portions: the duodenum, the jejunum, and the ileum. In this chapter we will focus on the jejunum and the ileum. The upper 40 % constitutes the jejunum and the remainder is the ileum. There is no morphological line of distinction between the two and the division is arbitrary. However there are subtle changes that make this distinction possible.

Dilendra H. Weerasinghe is supported by a grant from the Foundation for Surgical Fellowships.

Electronic supplementary material: Supplementary material is available in the online version of this chapter at 10.1007/978-1-4939-1893-5_14. Videos can also be accessed at http://www.springerimages.com/videos/978-1-4939-1892-8.

B. Ahmed, M.D., F.A.C.S. • D.H. Weerasinghe, M.D., M.R.C.S.Ed., M.R.C.S. • M.S. Nussbaum, M.D., F.A.C.S. (✉)
Division of General Surgery, Department of Surgery, University of Florida College of Medicine—Jacksonville, 653 West 8th Street, 3rd Floor Faculty Clinic, Jacksonville, FL 32209, USA
e-mail: michael.nussbaum@jax.ufl.edu

The jejunum has a thicker wall and a wider lumen whereas the ileum has a thinner wall and a smaller lumen. Adipose tissue is more abundant in the mesentery of the ileum, thus vessels in the mesentery are not as well visualized. The small intestinal mesentery is fan-shaped with a root of about 15 cm extending obliquely from the left L2 lumbar vertebral transverse process level to the right sacroiliac joint and crossing over the third portion of the duodenum, the aorta, inferior vena cava, and the right ureter. Between the two leaves of the mesentery are the mesenteric vessels and lymph nodes. The superior mesenteric artery (SMA) is the artery of the small intestine. The jejunum has fewer (2–3) series of vascular arcades per segment and the vasa recta are longer; whereas, the ileum has more (4–5) series of arcades and the vasa recta are shorter.

The proximal jejunum and distal ileum are more important for absorption than the rest of the small intestine. Massive resection of small bowel (e.g., in mesenteric vascular disease) or repeated resections (e.g., in Crohn's disease) may result in short bowel syndrome and malabsorption. Resection of a significant portion of the terminal ileum is associated with a loss of absorption of the fat soluble vitamins (i.e., vitamins A, D, E, K, and B12). Major ileal resection also creates changes in cholesterol metabolism and bile acid reabsorption. If undigested fats and bile acids transit directly into the transverse colon, the osmotic pressure of the colon is elevated and diarrhea may result.

J. Kim and J. Garcia-Aguilar (eds.), *Surgery for Cancers of the Gastrointestinal Tract: A Step-by-Step Approach*,
DOI 10.1007/978-1-4939-1893-5_14, © Springer Science+Business Media New York 2015

## Historical Perspective

The first reported small bowel resection was documented in 1727 when the German surgeon Phillip Ramdohr (1694–1755) resected two feet of gangrenous intestine. He inserted the afferent limb into the efferent limb and secured the invagination with two interrupted mucosa-to-serosa sutures [1]. The patient survived and died 1-year later from pneumonia [1]. Vincenz von Czerny in 1882 proposed a two-layered intestinal anastomosis. Only 1-year after it was first published, the technique was widely accepted and became a standard method for performing anastomosis [1]. Later, William Stewart Halsted proved in 1887 using canine experiments that the submucosa provided sufficient strength and he popularized the single layer intestinal anastomosis [1]. With these beginnings nearly 300 years ago, gastrointestinal (GI) anastomosis has been transformed from a life-threatening adventure to a safe and routinely performed procedure [1].

The application of laparoscopy in general surgical practice is attributed to gynecologist Kurt Semm, who is widely regarded as a pioneer of modern laparoscopic surgery for performing the first laparoscopic appendectomy in 1983 [2]. Soon thereafter another German surgeon Eric Muhe performed the first laparoscopic cholecystectomy in 1985 [2]. The acceptance of laparoscopic cholecystectomy in general surgical practice led to its safe application in other minimally invasive gastrointestinal procedures [3, 4]. Such advances were in part due to the development of laparoscopic linear staplers which have allowed the transection of the intestine. Currently, many commonly performed surgical procedures have their own corresponding laparoscopic techniques. Whether the operation is performed in open or minimally invasive fashion, the indications and the principles of each operation remain the same.

## Indications for Operation

Despite the fact that the small intestine occupies a large surface area, it is surprising that neoplasms of the small intestine are exceedingly rare, accounting for approximately 3–6 % of all GI neoplasms [5, 6]. Approximately 75 % of small intestinal tumors tend to be malignant [6]. Despite advances in diagnostic modalities, small intestinal tumors are difficult to diagnose and are often advanced at the time of definitive treatment. These malignancies can cause insidious abdominal pain and weight loss, or create surgical emergencies including hemorrhage, obstruction, or perforation [6–8]. Intestinal obstruction is the most common clinical presentation, followed by bleeding, perforation, and detection of an abdominal mass [6]. Carcinoid is the most frequent histological type, followed by adenocarcinoma, gastrointestinal stromal tumor (GIST), and lymphomas [5]; these account for nearly 98 % of all small bowel tumors. Generally, resection of the small bowel is indicated for primary or metastatic tumors, precancerous conditions, obstruction, ischemia, stricture, bleeding, and trauma.

## Preoperative Work-Up

With the exception of the duodenum and terminal ileum, a direct endoscopic approach to visualize the small intestine is difficult. Therefore, the detection rate of tumors is low and when they are discovered, they are frequently in advanced stages with poor long-term prognosis. Typical work-up begins with routine laboratory studies evaluating serum electrolytes, liver function, complete blood count, nutritional parameters, and tumor markers if a malignancy is suspected. This is followed by plain abdominal X-rays and either upper gastrointestinal series with small bowel follow-through (UGI-SBFT) or flexible endoscopy. Further imaging will follow depending on the initial findings and may include ultrasound, computed tomography (CT) scan, magnetic resonance imaging, positron emission tomography, octreotide scan, enteroscopy, and capsule endoscopy [9–11].

## Carcinoid/Neuroendocrine Tumors of the Small Intestine

Intestinal carcinoids are the most common small intestinal neoplasm with adenocarcinoma in second place [5]. This is largely due to a steep increase in the incidence of this tumor type in the last few decades not only in the US but other parts of the world [5, 12, 13]. Improved diagnostic tools and awareness of GI neuroendocrine tumors may be the reason for this steep rise [12]. Carcinoid tumors of the small intestine arise from the enterochromaffin cells located throughout the crypts of Lieberkuhn, and 50 % of GI carcinoids tend to occur in the small intestine. Patients with mid-gut carcinoids are frequently symptomatic but they may also have only vague abdominal pain or obstructive symptoms. Some patients may present with a palpable abdominal mass. Operation remains the most effective of treatment for carcinoid tumors. For small bowel carcinoids less than 1 cm in size a segmental resection is sufficient. However tumors larger than 1.5 cm require segmental bowel resection with lymphadenectomy.

## Adenoma

These are benign tumors of the small intestine which can undergo malignant transformation. There are three main histologic subtypes: tubular, villous, and tubulovillous. The malignant potential increases with size, degree of villous component, and amount of atypical changes on microscopy. They can present with intussusception, intestinal obstruction, bleeding, or vague abdominal pain; or they may be found incidentally. Sporadic forms of adenomas are usually found as a single lesion while those associated with hereditary polyposis syndromes such as familial adenomatous polyposis coli or Peutz-Jeghers syndrome can present with multiple polyps scattered throughout the entire small intestine. Because of the potential for malignant transformation, operative removal is the mainstay of management for these polyps.

## Adenocarcinoma

Similar to adenocarcinoma of the colon, small bowel adenocarcinoma arises from premalignant adenomas. However, small intestinal adenocarcinomas are only one-fiftieth as common as colonic adenocarcinoma [14]. They commonly occur in the duodenum, followed by the jejunum, and then the ileum. There is a strong positive correlation between Crohn's disease and small intestinal adenocarcinoma, where the significance of the risk tends to increase after ten or more years of active disease. When operating on strictures due to Crohn's Disease, adenocarcinoma must be ruled out. This is particularly pertinent when dealing with multiple strictures with stricturoplasty. Other conditions associated with small intestinal adenocarcinoma include hereditary GI cancer syndromes such as familial adenomatous polyposis, hereditary nonpolyposis colorectal cancer, and Peutz-Jeghers syndrome.

For localized disease, wide segmental resection with regional lymphadenectomy is required. Nodal involvement is one of the strongest predictors of long-term survival and 5-year cancer-specific survival for node-positive small intestinal adenocarcinoma is between 12 and 50 % [14]. Duodenal primary cancers appear to have worse prognosis than tumors arising in the jejunum or ileum [15]. For patients with locally advanced, unresectable, or metastatic small bowel adenocarcinoma, palliative surgical resection of the primary tumor may be needed to prevent bowel obstruction or bleeding. In some instances a palliative bypass may be the only option.

## Small Intestinal Lymphoma

The GI tract is one of the major sites of extranodal lymphomas constituting 10–15 % of all non-Hodgkin's lymphoma cases [10] and 30–40 % of extra-nodal lymphomas overall. Primary gastrointestinal lymphoma (PGL) refers to a tumor that predominantly involves the GI tract with lymph node involvement confined to the drainage area of the primary tumor site with no metastatic spread [16]. Secondary lymphoma is when the GI tract is affected secondarily as part of a broader disease process. PGL accounts for 20 % of all malignant small bowel tumors and the ileum is the most common site. Chemoradiation is the therapy of choice for these neoplasms [17,

18]. When adenopathy and hepatosplenomegaly are absent and there is no evidence of disease on chest CT, the diagnosis of PGL will require histologic confirmation. Only in such cases will surgical exploration with resection of involved segments and regional lymph node dissection be required to confirm the diagnosis. Surgical treatment may also be required when obstruction, bleeding, or perforation occur.

### Gastrointestinal Stromal Tumors

GISTs are rare malignancies of the small intestine and account for 25 % of GISTs in the GI tract. These neoplasms originate from the interstitial cells of Cajal (ICC) and stain positive for the membrane tyrosine kinase receptor c-kit. The ICCs are the pacemaker cells of the intestine, and have features of both smooth muscle cells and mediators of neurotransmitters. The principal therapy for primary GIST is resection. As with other sarcomas, there is usually no nodal spread and a negative margin resection is usually sufficient.

## Perioperative Preparation

A detailed history and physical is obtained when the patient is first seen. Necessary laboratory studies and investigations are carried out for localization and to assess the fitness for operation and anesthesia. Mechanical bowel preparation and oral antibiotics may be administered but are not essential. Chlorhexidine shower is prescribed for the night before and the morning of the operation. The patient is kept nil per os (NPO) overnight. Deep venous thrombosis (DVT) prophylaxis with both sequential compression devices (SCD) and pharmacological (subcutaneous heparin) administration is advisable. Preoperative antibiotics are administered within an hour of initial incision using a first generation cephalosporin and metronidazole; or gentamicin and clindamycin are prescribed in patients with beta-lactam allergies.

## Description of Laparoscopic Small Intestine Resection

The majority of small intestinal neoplasms are amenable to either laparoscopic or laparoscopic-assisted resection. The procedure is carried out under general anesthesia. A nasogastric or orogastric tube and urinary catheter are placed following induction of anesthesia. The patient may be placed in either supine position, split leg, or in low lithotomy position with the arms carefully tucked by the patient's side to allow unfettered access to the operative site and to visualize the pathology clearly. We also use at least two screens with one at the head and one at the foot of the patient as the operating surgeon frequently has to change position during the conduct of the operation. For lesions in the proximal small intestine the surgeon stands on the right side of the patient or between the legs and for lesions in the terminal ileum the surgeon stands on the left side of the patient. The abdomen is prepped with chlorhexidine prep and draped with an iodine impregnated drape.

### Port Placement and Operative Details

We prefer to place a Veress needle in the upper abdomen to create carbon dioxide pneumoperitoneum to 15 mmHg. Following insufflation a right upper quadrant 5 mm optical port is placed using a 5 mm 0° scope. Alternatively, access can be obtained by an open technique with placement of a blunt trocar (Hasson). A 5-mm umbilical camera port, a left lower quadrant 5-mm assistant port, and a 12-mm right lower quadrant port are placed under direct vision (Fig. 14.1). This configuration is for laparoscopic small bowel resection with intracorporeal anastomosis for proximal small bowel pathology with the surgeon standing on the right side of the patient and assistants on the left side (Fig. 14.2). If an extracorporeal anastomosis will be performed, then we place a 12-mm port at the umbilicus or close to where the

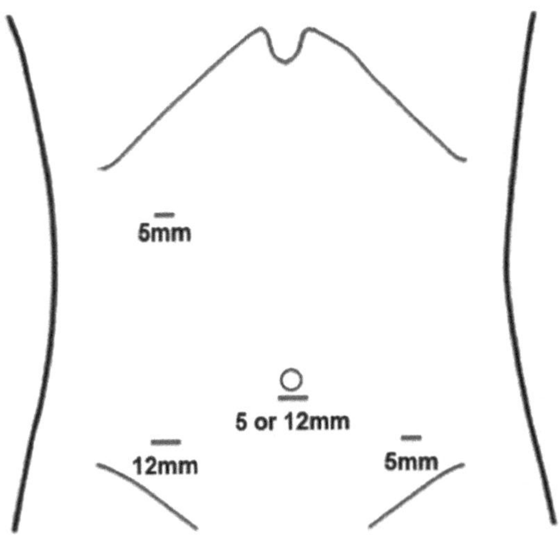


**Fig. 14.1** Port placement for proximal small intestinal resection: right upper quadrant 5-mm port, 5-mm or 12-mm umbilical camera port, a left lower quadrant 5-mm assistant port, and a 12-mm right lower quadrant port

specimen can be easily exteriorized. For resection of distal small bowel lesions, the surgeon stands on the left of the patient with ports placed in the mirror image configuration to the vertical midline position (Fig. 14.3).

Following port placement, we assess the liver and the rest of the abdominal cavity for any significant pathology or metastatic spread. The patient is placed in Trendelenburg position and the transverse colon elevated. The ligament of Treitz is then located. The patient is positioned back in reverse Trendelenburg position. The small bowel is run from the ligament of Treitz to the ileum carefully looking for synchronous pathology. The location of the tumor is identified and confirmed. Next, we identify the proximal and distal resection margins of the tumor. In cases of suspected malignancy we recommend 5 cm distal and proximal margins of resection with a broad mesenteric resection. The mesentery is marked along the site of proposed division. The small bowel mesentery is then elevated and mesenteric windows are created in an avascular plane beneath the bowel using an energy device. We then place a laparoscopic linear stapler through the mesenteric window and across the proximal bowel (Fig. 14.4). Similar transection is performed for the distal margin. The mesentery is then divided using an energy device (Fig. 14.5). The two intestinal ends are held together and two stay sutures are placed to align the bowel. Enterotomies are created and the two jaws of the laparoscopic linear stapler are negotiated carefully into the limbs of the small intestine (Fig. 14.6). The stapler is fired thus creating a side-to-side/functional end-to-end anastomosis. The enteric defect can be closed with a linear stapler or using hand-sewn technique. An important component of the operation is to close the mesenteric defect to prevent the development of an internal hernia. The specimen is extracted using a specimen retrieval bag through either the 12-mm port or natural orifice (transvaginal) in selected cases [19]. After making sure that there is good hemostasis, the 12-mm port fascial incision is closed with an absorbable suture to prevent a port site hernia.

If extracorporeal anastomosis is planned, the initial steps of access and localization of the pathologic segment of intestine are the same. The abdominal incision (and 12-mm port) may be placed at a periumbilical (proximal small intestine), Pfannenstiel (mid to distal intestine), or right lower quadrant (distal intestine) site. A 4-cm incision is made at one of these sites and a wound protector or laparoscopic hand-port is placed. The affected portion of the intestine is exteriorized through the incision, the mesentery is divided with an energy source, the intestine is divided with a linear stapler, and a stapled anastomosis is performed similar to the laparoscopic technique. The mesenteric defect is sutured closed and the intestine is replaced into the abdominal cavity. The abdominal incision is closed.

## Postoperative Management

Postoperatively the patient is extubated and the orogastric or nasogastric tube is usually removed in the operating room. Unless contraindicated, an intravenous dose of ketorolac is given and may be continued every 6 h for 24–48 h. Patients receive a patient controlled anesthesia device for pain control, ondansetron for nausea, and 24 h of parenteral antibiotics. Subcutaneous heparin and SCDs are continued until discharge.

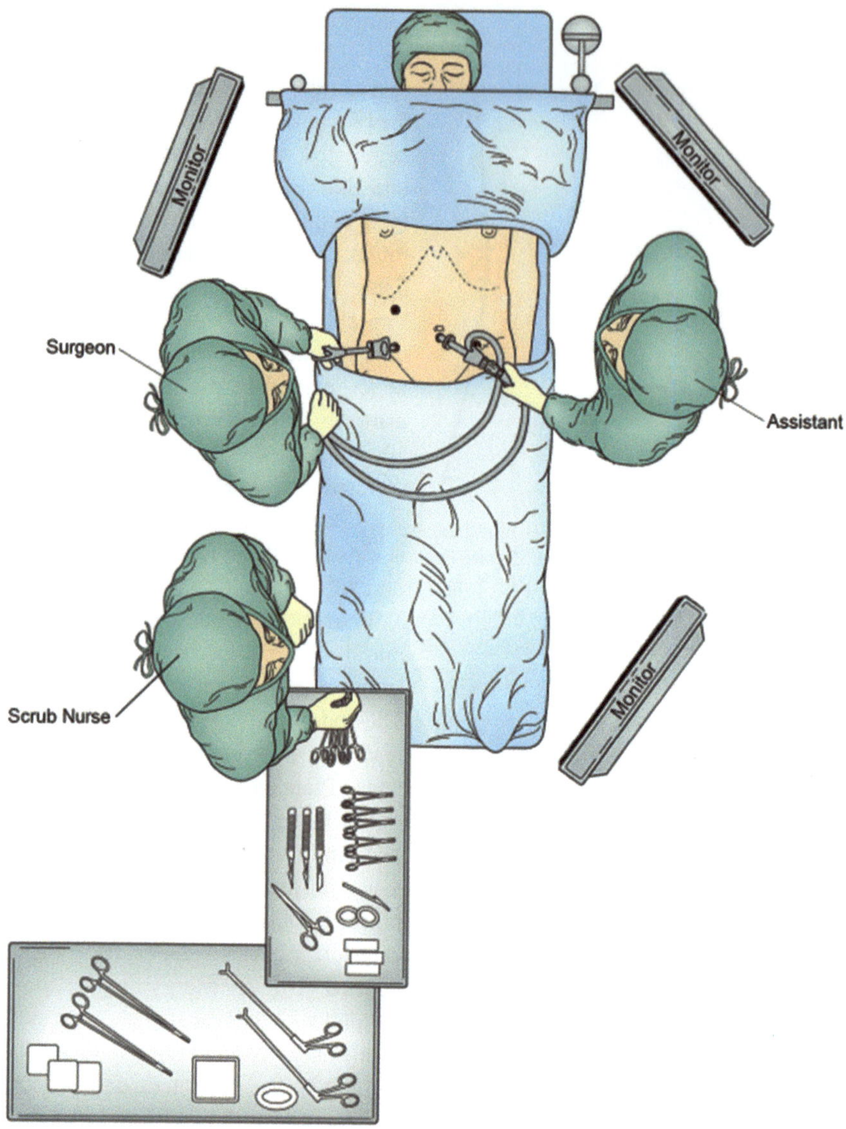


**Fig. 14.2** For proximal small bowel pathology, the surgeon stands on the right side of the patient and the assistant stands on the left side. The monitors are placed at the head and foot of the patient

The patient is ambulated out of bed beginning the evening after operation. If not removed in the operating room, the Foley catheter is removed on postoperative day one. If not nauseated, clear liquids are instituted on the first postoperative day and the diet is advanced to a regular diet by postoperative day two. Once tolerating a regular diet, pain control is continued with oral narcotic analgesics. The patient is usually ready for discharge by postoperative day three or four.

## Complications

Common complications that are seen after laparoscopic small intestinal resection include surgical site infections (superficial and deep), postoperative ileus/ mechanical obstruction, deep venous thrombosis, and bleeding. Anastomotic leak or breakdown occurs in 0.5–1 % of small bowel anastomoses [20–22] and is one of the

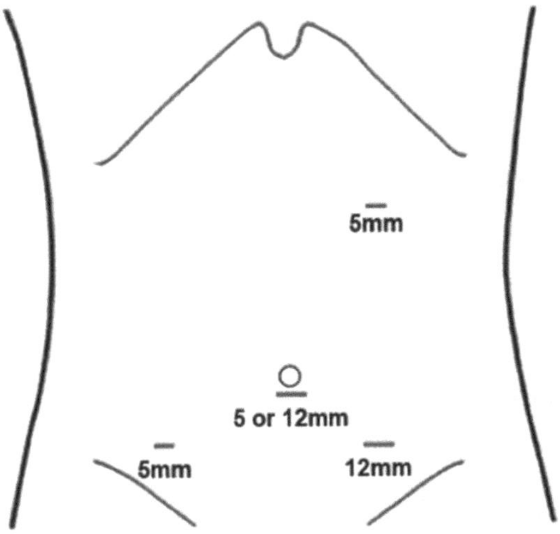


**Fig. 14.3** For resection of distal small bowel the ports are placed in a configuration that is the mirror image of Fig. 14.1. There is a left upper quadrant 5-mm port, 5-mm or 12-mm umbilical camera port, a right lower quadrant 5-mm assistant port, and a 12-mm left lower quadrant port

most dreaded complications of intestinal surgery. Other less common complications include solid organ or viscus injury, anastomotic stricture, and short bowel syndrome when extensive intestinal resection is required.

Prolonged postoperative ileus occurs less frequently following laparoscopic bowel resection compared with open operation [23, 24]. Whenever there is a delay in return of normal bowel function, other complications should be suspected. A mechanical cause for the obstruction, deep space infection, or anastomotic leak all should be excluded before attributing a delay in return of bowel function to postoperative ileus. In cases of true postoperative ileus, management includes NPO (±NGT decompression), hydration, correction of electrolytes, reducing or stopping narcotic medication, sugarless chewing gum, and use of motility agents such as metoclopramide or erythromycin.

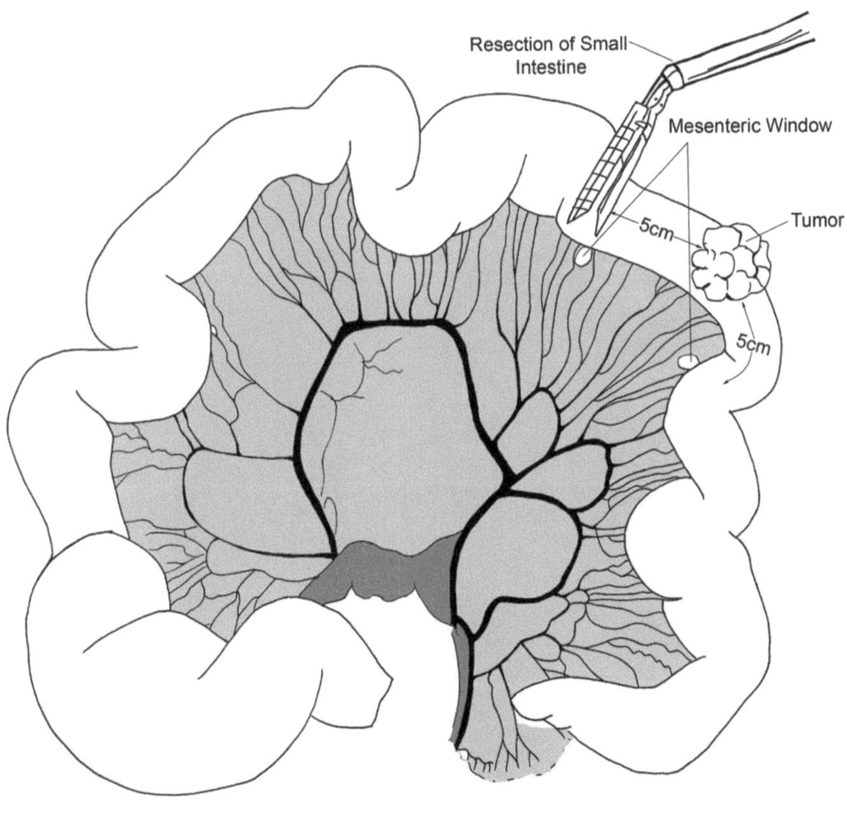


**Fig. 14.4** The location of the tumor is identified and mesenteric windows are created in an avascular plane beneath the bowel using an energy device

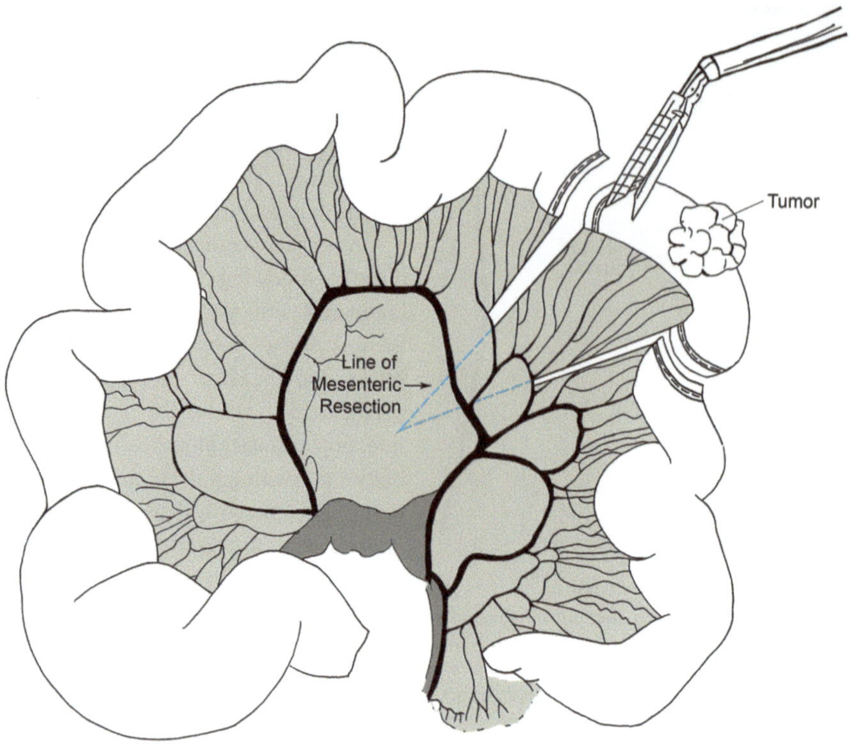


**Fig. 14.5** A laparoscopic linear stapler is placed through the mesenteric window and across the proximal bowel

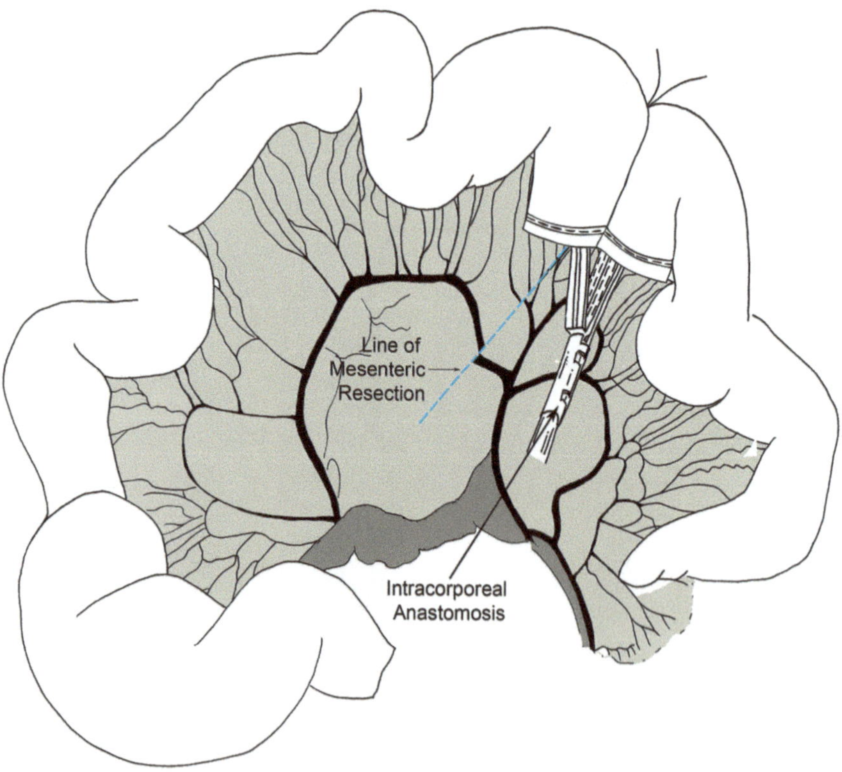


**Fig. 14.6** The two intestinal ends are held together and two stay sutures are placed to align the bowel. Enterotomies are created and the two jaws of the laparoscopic linear stapler are negotiated carefully into the limbs of the small intestine creating a side-to-side/functional end-to-end anastomosis

## Summary

Laparoscopic surgery has gained wide acceptance in the armamentarium of surgeons performing gastrointestinal operations. The potential advantages of the minimally invasive approach to small intestinal neoplasm resection include comparable surgical and oncologic outcomes [3, 25, 26], decreased length of stay [25–28], cosmetically appealing scar, and improved pain scores [24, 28–31]. In addition, when compared with open operations there is a decrease in incisional hernia occurrence, diminished adhesion formation with a presumed lower postoperative bowel obstruction incidence [32]. All of these advantages should translate to improved patient satisfaction with a decrease in overall health care costs [30]. This type of operation will gain more popularity in the coming years as a greater number of surgeons become comfortable with minimally invasive surgical approaches.

## References


1. Dietz UA, Debus ES. Intestinal anastomoses prior to 1882; a legacy of ingenuity, persistence, and research form a foundation for modern gastrointestinal surgery. World J Surg. 2005;29(3):396–401. doi:10.1007/s00268-004-7720-x.
2. Himal HS. Minimally invasive (laparoscopic) surgery. Surg Endosc. 2002;16(12):1647–52. doi:10.1007/s00464-001-8275-7.
3. Fleshman J, Sargent DJ, Green E, Anvari M, Stryker SJ, Beart Jr RW, et al. Laparoscopic colectomy for cancer is not inferior to open surgery based on 5-year data from the COST Study Group trial. Ann Surg. 2007;246(4):655–62. doi:10.1097/SLA.0b013e318155a762; discussion 62–4.
4. Clinical Outcomes of Surgical Therapy Study Group. A comparison of laparoscopically assisted and open colectomy for colon cancer. N Engl J Med. 2004;350(20):2050–9. doi:10.1056/NEJMoa032651.
5. Bilimoria KY, Bentrem DJ, Wayne JD, Ko CY, Bennett CL, Talamonti MS. Small bowel cancer in the United States: changes in epidemiology, treatment, and survival over the last 20 years. Ann Surg. 2009;249(1):63–71. doi:10.1097/SLA.0b013e31818e4641.
6. Kim CH, Kye BH, Lee JI, Kim SH, Kim HJ, Kang WK, et al. Clinicopathological features of primary jejunoileal tumors. J Korean Soc Coloproctol. 2010;26(5):334–8. doi:10.3393/jksc.2010.26.5.334.
7. Catena F, Ansaloni L, Gazzotti F, Gagliardi S, Di Saverio S, De Cataldis A, et al. Small bowel tumours in emergency surgery: specificity of clinical presentation. ANZ J Surg. 2005;75(11):997–9. doi:10.1111/j.1445-2197.2005.03590.x.
8. Han SL, Cheng J, Zhou HZ, Guo SC, Jia ZR, Wang PF. Surgically treated primary malignant tumor of small bowel: a clinical analysis. World J Gastroenterol. 2010;16(12):1527–32.
9. Eliakim R. Video capsule endoscopy of the small bowel. Curr Opin Gastroenterol. 2008;24(2):159–63. doi:10.1097/MOG.0b013e3282f3d946.
10. Gill SS, Heuman DM, Mihas AA. Small intestinal neoplasms. J Clin Gastroenterol. 2001;33(4):267–82.
11. Mustafa BF, Samaan M, Langmead L, Khasraw M. Small bowel video capsule endoscopy: an overview. Expert Rev Gastroenterol Hepatol. 2013;7(4):323–9. doi:10.1586/egh.13.20.
12. Cho MY, Kim JM, Sohn JH, Kim MJ, Kim KM, Kim WH, et al. Current trends of the incidence and pathological diagnosis of gastroenteropancreatic neuroendocrine tumors (GEP-NETs) in Korea 2000–2009: multicenter study. Cancer Res Treat. 2012;44(3):157–65. doi:10.4143/crt.2012.44.3.157.
13. Scherubl H, Streller B, Stabenow R, Herbst H, Hopfner M, Schwertner C, et al. Clinically detected gastroenteropancreatic neuroendocrine tumors are on the rise: epidemiological changes in Germany. World J Gastroenterol. 2013;19(47):9012–9. doi:10.3748/wjg.v19.i47.9012.
14. Overman MJ. Recent advances in the management of adenocarcinoma of the small intestine. Gastrointest Cancer Res. 2009;3(3):90–6.
15. Kelsey CR, Nelson JW, Willett CG, Chino JP, Clough RW, Bendell JC, et al. Duodenal adenocarcinoma: patterns of failure after resection and the role of chemoradiotherapy. Int J Radiat Oncol Biol Phys. 2007; 69(5):1436–41. doi:10.1016/j.ijrobp.2007.05.006.
16. Dawson IM, Cornes JS, Morson BC. Primary malignant lymphoid tumours of the intestinal tract. Report of 37 cases with a study of factors influencing prognosis. Br J Surg. 1961;49:80–9.
17. Beaton C, Davies M, Beynon J. The management of primary small bowel and colon lymphoma—a review. Int J Colorectal Dis. 2012;27(5):555–63. doi:10.1007/s00384-011-1309-2.
18. Koch P, del Valle F, Berdel WE, Willich NA, Reers B, Hiddemann W, et al. Primary gastrointestinal non-Hodgkin's lymphoma: II. Combined surgical and conservative or conservative management only in localized gastric lymphoma—results of the prospective German Multicenter Study GIT NHL 01/92. J Clinical Oncol. 2001;19(18):3874–83.
19. Awad ZT, Qureshi I, Seibel B, Sharma S, Dobbertien MA. Laparoscopic right hemicolectomy with transvaginal colon extraction using a laparoscopic posterior colpotomy: a 2-year series from a single institution. Surg Laparosc Endosc Percutan Tech. 2011;21(6): 403–8. doi:10.1097/SLE.0b013e31823945ac.

20. Lujan JJ, Nemeth ZH, Barratt-Stopper PA, Bustami R, Koshenkov VP, Rolandelli RH. Factors influencing the outcome of intestinal anastomosis. Am Surg. 2011;77(9):1169–75.
21. Pandey R, Kochar R. Management of gastrointestinal stromal tumors: looking beyond the knife. An update on the role of adjuvant and neoadjuvant imatinib therapy. J Gastrointest Cancer. 2012;43(4):547–52. doi:10.1007/s12029-012-9423-0.
22. Telem DA, Sur M, Tabrizian P, Chao TE, Nguyen SQ, Chin EH, et al. Diagnosis of gastrointestinal anastomotic dehiscence after hospital discharge: Impact on patient management and outcome. Surgery. 2010;147(1):127–33. doi:10.1016/j.surg.2009.06.034.
23. Ohtani H, Tamamori Y, Arimoto Y, Nishiguchi Y, Maeda K, Hirakawa K. A meta-analysis of the short- and long-term results of randomized controlled trials that compared laparoscopy-assisted and open colectomy for colon cancer. J Cancer Educ. 2012;3:49–57. doi:10.7150/jca.3621.
24. Schwenk W, Haase O, Neudecker J, Muller JM. Short term benefits for laparoscopic colorectal resection. Cochrane Database Syst Rev. 2005;3, CD003145. doi:10.1002/14651858.CD003145.pub2.
25. Figueiredo MN, Maggiori L, Gaujoux S, Couvelard A, Guedj N, Ruszniewski P, et al. Surgery for small-bowel neuroendocrine tumors: Is there any benefit of the laparoscopic approach? Surg Endosc. 2014;28(5):1720–6. doi:10.1007/s00464-013-3381-x.
26. Ihn K, Hyung WJ, Kim HI, An JY, Kim JW, Cheong JH, et al. Treatment results of small intestinal gastrointestinal stromal tumors less than 10 cm in diameter: a comparison between laparoscopy and open surgery. J Gastric Cancer. 2012;12(4):243–8. doi:10.5230/jgc.2012.12.4.243.
27. Kelly KN, Iannuzzi JC, Rickles AS, Garimella V, Monson JR, Fleming FJ. Laparotomy for small-bowel obstruction: first choice or last resort for adhesiolysis? A laparoscopic approach for small-bowel obstruction reduces 30-day complications. Surg Endosc. 2014;28(1):65–73. doi:10.1007/s00464-013-3162-6.
28. Kim HS, Kim BS, Lee IS, Lee S, Yook JH, Kim BS. Comparison of totally laparoscopic total gastrectomy and open total gastrectomy for gastric cancer. J Laparoendosc Adv Surg Tech A. 2013;23(4):323–31. doi:10.1089/lap.2012.0389.
29. Kaplan M, Salman B, Yilmaz TU, Oguz M. A quality of life comparison of laparoscopic and open approaches in acute appendicitis: a randomised prospective study. Acta Chir Belg. 2009;109(3):356–63.
30. Kuwabara K, Matsuda S, Fushimi K, Ishikawa KB, Horiguchi H, Fujimori K. Community-based appraisal of laparoscopic abdominal surgery in Japan. J Surg Res. 2011;165(1):e1–13. doi:10.1016/j.jss.2010.09.003.
31. Tsui DK, Tang CN, Ha JP, Li MK. Laparoscopic approach for small bowel tumors. Surg Laparosc Endosc Percutan Tech. 2008;18(6):556–60. doi:10.1097/SLE.0b013e3181889d25.
32. Angenete E, Jacobsson A, Gellerstedt M, Haglind E. Effect of laparoscopy on the risk of small-bowel obstruction: a population-based register study. Arch Surg. 2012;147(4):359–65. doi:10.1001/archsurg.2012.31.

## Key Operative Steps

1. Access peritoneal cavity by Veress needle or open (Hasson) approach.
2. Identify the small bowel segment to be resected.
3. Elevate the transverse colon, locate the ligament of Treitz, and run the small bowel.
4. Create a mesenteric window with 5 cm proximal and distal margins.
5. Divide the proximal intestine with a laparoscopic linear stapler.
6. Divide the mesentery with an endoscopic bipolar or ultrasonic energy device.
7. Divide the distal intestine with a laparoscopic linear stapler.
8. Align the two intestinal segments side by side with stay sutures.
9. Create an enterotomy at each end of the intestinal segments.
10. Negotiate the jaws of the linear stapler into the lumen and create a functional end-to-end anastomosis.
11. Close the enterotomy with a linear stapler or with a running suture.
12. Close the mesenteric defect with a running suture.
13. Extract the specimen.

# Part IV

# Colon and Rectum

# 15 Open Right Colectomy

Stephen M. Sentovich

## Surgical Technique

### Preparation

All patients undergoing colectomy have standard preoperative evaluation and laboratory testing. Specialty consultation is obtained for patients with significant cardiac, pulmonary, renal, or other significant organ system dysfunction. While preoperative mechanical bowel preparation is not absolutely necessary, it should be performed in patients who may require intraoperative colonoscopy. Preoperative oral and intravenous antibiotics are mandatory to decrease surgical site infection and all patients are given preoperative deep venous thrombosis prophylaxis by both mechanical (sequential compression stockings) and pharmacologic (heparin or low molecular weight heparin) means.

While the supine position may be adequate for most open right colectomies, lithotomy positioning is never inappropriate. This position allows for both intraoperative colonoscopy and access for rectosigmoid resection or repair if the tumor or inflammatory process of Crohn's disease involves the rectosigmoid colon (Fig. 15.1).

S.M. Sentovich, M.D., M.B.A. (✉)
Department of Surgical Oncology, Colorectal Service, City of Hope National Medical Center, 1500 East Duarte Road, Duarte, CA 91010, USA
e-mail: ssentovich@coh.org

### Incision

A midline incision starting 6–8 cm above the umbilicus and continuing 2–3 cm below the umbilicus is most commonly utilized for open right colectomy (Fig. 15.2a). Alternatively, a transverse incision starting in the midline 2–3 cm above the umbilicus and continuing for 6–8 cm laterally on the right side of the abdomen is another option (Fig. 15.2b). With the transverse incision, the right rectus muscle is divided. In the non-obese patient, the transverse incision is similar in size to a laparoscopic extraction incision and results in minimal postoperative discomfort.

### Exploration

Upon entrance to the abdomen, the peritoneal cavity is explored and the liver is palpated. Biopsy of suspicious lesions should be performed. Particular attention is also directed to the omentum and in women the ovaries are also inspected. Preoperatively, potential oophorectomy should be discussed and a plan developed regarding identification of any ovarian pathology.

### Colon Mobilization

With the assistance of a self-retaining retractor and the patient's right side up, the lateral white line of Toldt is taken down with cautery starting

J. Kim and J. Garcia-Aguilar (eds.), *Surgery for Cancers of the Gastrointestinal Tract: A Step-by-Step Approach*, DOI 10.1007/978-1-4939-1893-5_15, © Springer Science+Business Media New York 2015

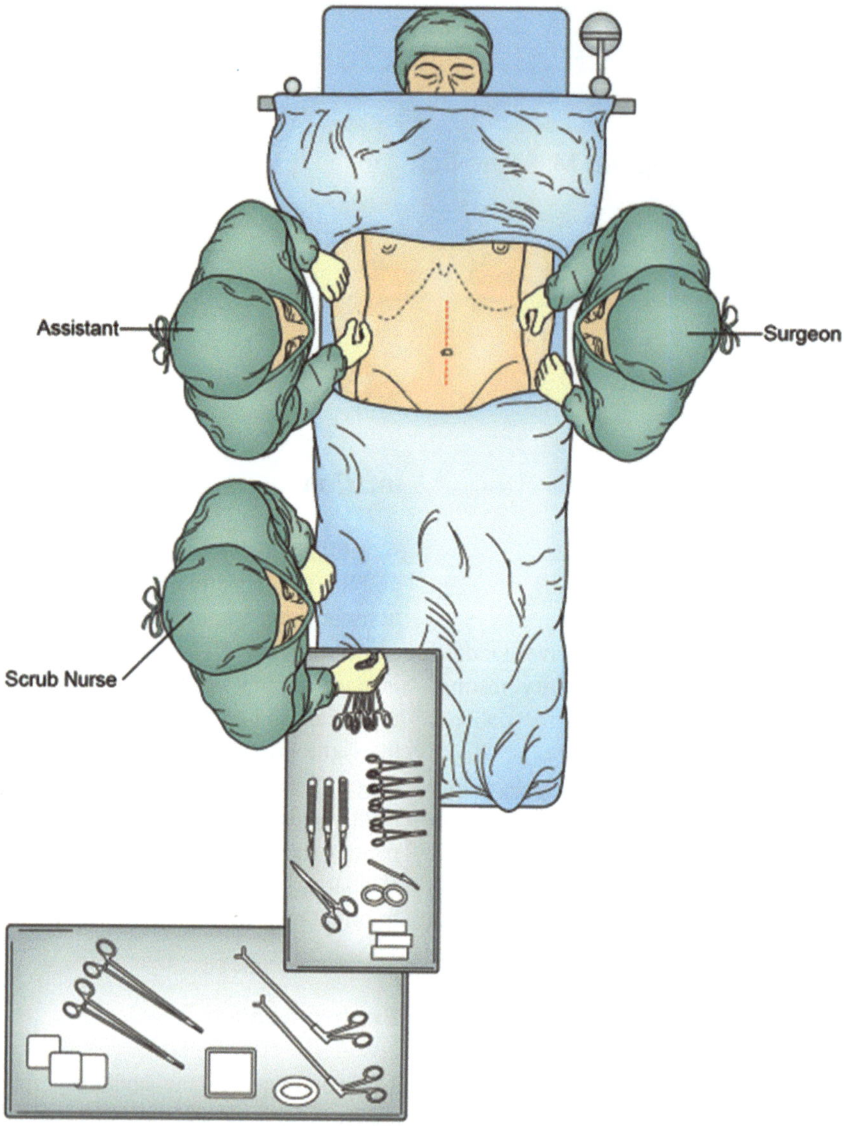


**Fig. 15.1** Operative positioning for open right colectomy. The surgeon stands on the left side of the patient with the assistant on the right side

at the cecum and proceeding superiorly along the ascending colon to the hepatic flexure. Care must be taken to avoid dissecting too deep into the retroperitoneum to avoid injury to the ureter, kidney, and duodenum. If the dissection proceeds in the correct plane, mandatory identification of the ureter is not necessary but in some instances the cecum and terminal ileum can have significant retroperitoneal attachments requiring identification of the ureter in order to avoid injury. The best way to identify the right ureter is to find it as it crosses the external iliac artery at the pelvic inlet and then follow it proximally from this point.

At the level of the hepatic flexure, it is important to identify the duodenum. The surgeon should be aware that the proximal transverse colon attachments are thicker and more vascular than the lateral attachments to the ascending colon. After the omental attachments to the

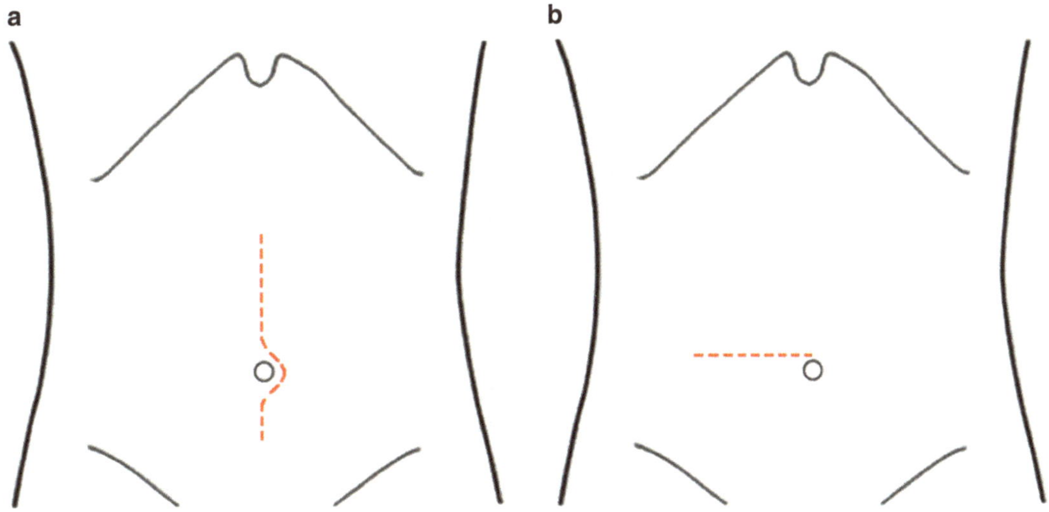


**Fig. 15.2** Abdominal wall incisions for open right colectomy. (**a**) Mid-line peri-umbilical incision. (**b**) Right transverse incision

proximal transverse colon are divided, the entire right colon is now fully mobilized and attached only by its mesentery. The omentum is divided from its free edge to the mid-transverse colon so that it is also resected en bloc with the right side of the colon.

Large cecal or ascending colon cancers can invade the abdominal sidewall requiring an en bloc resection of the tumor and abdominal wall. After en bloc resection, the abdominal wall resection area should be outlined with surgical clips to allow for better localization of the tumor bed for postoperative radiation. Rarely, a bulky tumor at the hepatic flexure or proximal transverse colon may extend into the duodenum and pancreas, requiring a Whipple procedure to complete the en bloc resection. This unusual circumstance should be identifiable on preoperative computed tomography (CT) scans and the operation should be planned accordingly.

## Division of the Mesentery

After complete mobilization of the colon and terminal ileum, the mesentery is sequentially divided with suture ties or an appropriate energy device. My preference during an open right colectomy is to divide the mesentery with 2-0 vicryl ties but possibly use a 2-0 vicryl suture ligature on the ileocolic artery. The mesenteric division usually starts at the terminal ileum approximately 6–10 cm proximal to the ileocecal valve and ends distally at the mid-transverse colon. The mesentery is divided at its base dividing the ileocolic artery and the right colic artery immediately after their take-off from the superior mesenteric artery. The middle colic artery is preserved, but the right branch of the middle colic is divided along with the division of the mesentery (Fig. 15.3). When dividing the proximal transverse colon mesentery, the surgeon should avoid pulling excessively on the colon to expose the often-foreshortened mesentery. Too much tension can result in avulsion of the mesenteric veins and lead to significant bleeding.

## Anastomosis

With the terminal ileum and colon completely devascularized, the antimesenteric border of the proximal, viable terminal ileum is approximated to the antimesenteric border of the distal, viable mid-transverse colon using three to five 3-0 vicryl sutures. Small enterotomies are made in the nonviable terminal ileum and colon (Fig. 15.4a), and a

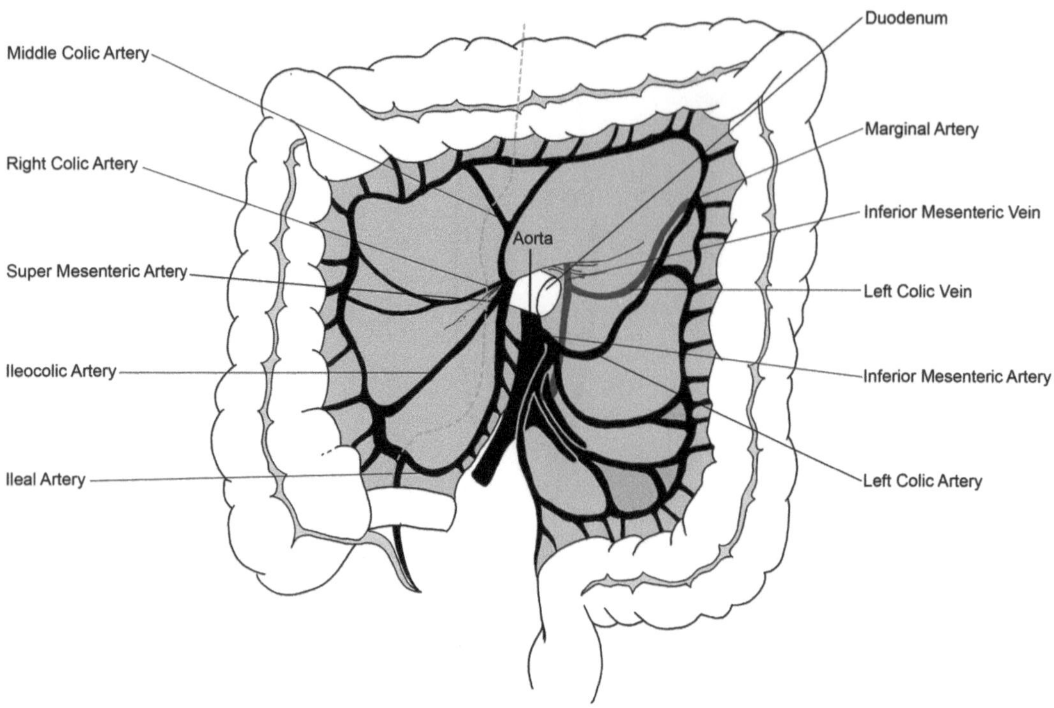


**Fig. 15.3** Anatomic figure of the colon with the dashed line indicating the line of resection from the terminal ileum to the mid-transverse colon

100-mm gastrointestinal anastomosis (GIA) stapler is placed and fired to create a side-to-side, functional end-to-end anastomosis between the viable proximal ileum and mid-transverse colon (Fig. 15.4b). Using three Allis clamps on the edge of the common enterotomy channel, the internal anastomosis is inspected and any sites of significant bleeding are oversewn with 3-0 vicryl sutures. After hemostasis is ensured, the Allis clamps are used to close the common enterotomy channel offsetting the anterior and posterior GIA staple lines. A reload of the 100-mm GIA stapler is then placed transversely across both limbs of the bowel anastomosis, thus closing the enterotomy channel and dividing and closing the ileum and transverse colon to complete the anastomosis (Fig. 15.4c).

Once the ileum and right colon are completely detached, the specimen can be moved to a back table so that it can be opened to check the proximal and distal margins. If there is any concern regarding tumor involvement of the proximal or distal margin, frozen section examination and/or further resection should be performed.

Often the transverse staple line has some oozing that is oversewn with a 3-0 vicryl suture. The anastomosis is checked for patency and leaks, but use of the 100-mm GIA stapler allows for a widely patent side-to-side anastomosis. A 3-0 vicryl suture is often placed at the crotch between the two limbs, and the mesenteric defect can be left wide-open or can be closed. While there are many alternative stapled and hand-sewn ileo-colonic anastomotic techniques, I have preferred the described technique for its simplicity and resulting widely patent anastomosis.

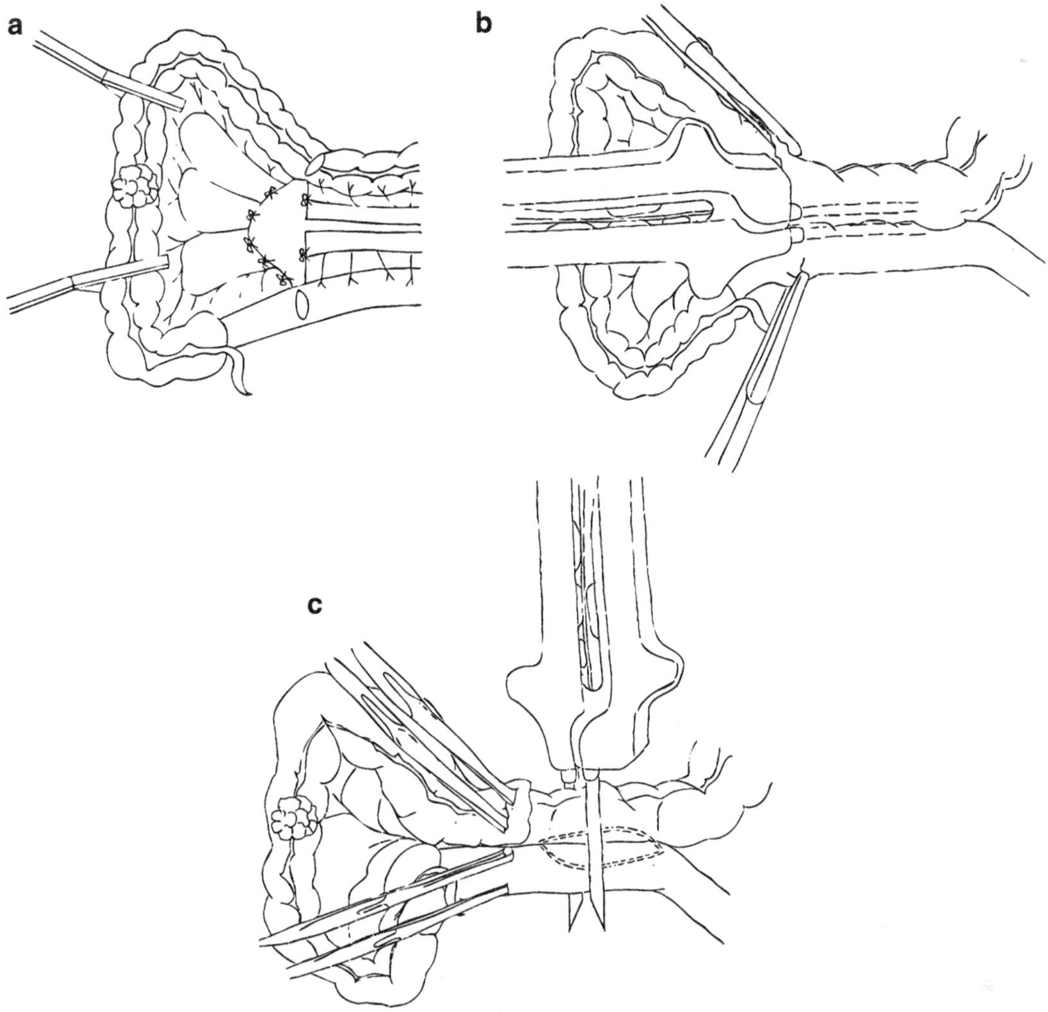


**Fig. 15.4** Diagrams illustrating resection and anastomosis. (**a**) The divided mesocolon. (**b**) Side-to-side anastomosis of the terminal ileum and transverse colon. (**c**) Division of the specimen

## Closure

The abdomen is closed with two looped #1 PDS (Ethicon) sutures that run toward the middle of the incision and then tied together. For patients with previous laparotomy incisions, I use buried interrupted #1 PDS (Ethicon) sutures or full-abdominal wall thickness #2 nylon sutures to prevent evisceration. Patients with transverse incisions have closure of the peritoneum with 0-vicryl suture followed by closure of the anterior rectus sheath with #1 PDS (Ethicon) suture. With either incision, the skin can be closed with staples (preferred) or with a subcuticular suture.

## Suggested Reading

Wolff BG, Wang JY. Right hemicolectomy for treatment of cancer: open technique. In: Fischer JE, Bland KI, Jones DB, Pomposelli FB, Schwaitzberg SD, Upchurch Jr GR, editors. Fischer's Mastery of Surgery. 6th ed. Philadelphia: Lippincott Williams & Wilkins; 2011.

## Key Operative Steps

1. Use a midline or transverse abdominal incision.
2. Explore the abdomen and ensure absence of metastatic disease.
3. Mobilize the colon by incising the white line of Toldt from the cecum to the hepatic flexure.
4. Divide the omental attachments to the proximal transverse colon.
5. Divide the mesentery with sutures or energy device.
6. Align the terminal ileum with the transverse colon.
7. Use a gastrointestinal anastomosis stapler to create an ileocolostomy.
8. Use a second firing of the stapler to close the enterotomy and divide the operative specimen.

# Laparoscopic Technique for Right Colectomy

# 16

Conor P. Delaney, Jeffrey L. Ponsky, and Andrew Russ

## Anatomical Highlights

During medial mobilization of the ileocolic artery for cancer, the surgeon should make the initial peritoneal incision at the base of the ileocolic pedicle, near its origin off the superior mesenteric artery (SMA) to ensure adequate lymph node yield. The incision must be parallel and close to the SMA. The surgeon should take care of the third portion of the duodenum as it courses in the retroperitoneum near the ileocolic pedicle by protecting it while the peritoneal incision is made by gently sweeping the duodenum down to ensure adequate visualization during the dissection.

The colon mesentery should be elevated to create space in loose areolar tissue for safe dissection. During mobilization of the small bowel and separation of its mesentery from the retroperitoneum, attachments to the retroperitoneum should be left undisturbed to protect the ureter, duodenum, and other posterior structures. Medial to lateral mobilization should be continued inferiorly behind the cecum and superiorly over the duodenum and head of pancreas up to the lower border of the liver.

The right branch of the middle colic artery can often be taken intracorporeally or alternatively after specimen extraction in thin patients with a long transverse colon. It is often easier to leave its division until after full mobilization of the hepatic flexure, especially in more obese individuals. The surgeon should be aware of the location of the duodenum, which can be identified inferiorly during hepatic flexure mobilization and should remain close to the colon with lateral mobilization. For patients with cancer near the hepatic flexure or transverse colon, the greater omentum is taken en bloc with the colon. Mobilizing the greater omentum and transverse colon up to or beyond the midline facilitates specimen extraction, especially in obese individuals.

## Historical Perspective

Adoption of laparoscopic techniques by general surgeons was aided by the technique of Hasson and open entrance into the abdomen [1]. Jacobs and colleagues published the first known series

Electronic supplementary material: Supplementary material is available in the online version of this chapter at 10.1007/978-1-4939-1893-5_16. Videos can also be accessed at http://www.springerimages.com/videos/978-1-4939-1892-8.

C.P. Delaney, M.D., M.C.h., Ph.D., F.R.C.S.I., F.A.C.S., F.A.S.C.R.S.
Digestive Health Institute, University Hospitals Case Medical Center, 11100 Euclid Avenue, Cleveland, OH 44106, USA

J.L. Ponsky, M.D.
Surgical Education, Case Western Reserve University, 10900 Euclid Avenue, Cleveland, OH 44106, USA

A. Russ, M.D. (✉)
Department of Surgery, University of Tennessee Medical Center, 1924 Alcoa Highway, Knoxville, TN 37920, USA
e-mail: drewjruss@gmail.com

J. Kim and J. Garcia-Aguilar (eds.), *Surgery for Cancers of the Gastrointestinal Tract: A Step-by-Step Approach*,
DOI 10.1007/978-1-4939-1893-5_16, © Springer Science+Business Media New York 2015

on laparoscopic colectomy in 1991 after successful adoption of laparoscopic techniques for cholecystectomy and appendectomy [2]. However, it was not until the COST trial, which demonstrated equivalent oncologic techniques with improved postoperative outcomes for laparoscopic colectomy compared to open colectomy, did laparoscopic colectomy become the standard of care for colon resection [3]. Progress has been further aided with the advent of laparoscopic stapling devices, as well as more recent innovations in energy devices allowing intracorporeal division of bowel and mesentery. Currently, laparoscopic right colectomy is gaining acceptance as the literature grows regarding its safety and applicability and improved postoperative outcomes. We believe that laparoscopy is the gold standard for colectomy.

Right hemicolectomy is a particularly attractive procedure to perform laparoscopically as it lends itself to a very standardized, reproducible technique based on sound oncologic principles. It is our belief that sound surgical technique and adherence to embryological planes lend itself to improved surgical outcomes. As recently reported by Birkmeyer et al., this concept of surgical proficiency and its relationship to postoperative outcomes has been validated [4]. The importance of a total mesocolic excision can also not be overstated. Our approach to laparoscopic right colectomy is discussed here, emphasizing a structured, stepwise approach.

## Indications for Operation

Classic indications for right colectomy include cancer or colonoscopically unresectable polyps. Patients with inflammatory bowel disease, specifically terminal ileal Crohn's disease, are also often candidates for a laparoscopic approach to the right colon. There are certain relative contraindications to attempt laparoscopic resection of the right colon. The size of the incision itself is directly related to the space necessary to remove the specimen. Thus, a bulky specimen often requires a larger midline incision, which often reduces the benefit of a laparoscopic approach. Disease extension into the retroperitoneum or abdominal wall is also a relative contraindication, as oncologic principles of en bloc resection of associated structures must be upheld. Thus, advanced cases should be performed only by laparoscopic colorectal surgeons who are well past their learning curve.

A previous laparotomy is not a contraindication to laparoscopic techniques. Open access to the abdominal cavity utilizing Hasson technique allows for direct visualization prior to trocar placement and insufflation. Adhesions can often be mobilized using electrocautery or alternative energy devices prior to laparoscopic exploration.

## Preoperative Workup

The preoperative workup generally depends on the indication for the operation. For colorectal cancer, traditional work up should include computed tomographic (CT) imaging of the abdomen and pelvis with oral and intravenous contrast and imaging of the chest (chest X-ray or chest CT) to detect areas of metastasis. For inflammatory bowel disease, work up may require additional evaluation of the small bowel such as small bowel follow-through, CT enterography, or magnetic resonance enterography, which is currently our method of choice. Colonoscopy should also be included with full colonoscopic evaluation with adequate prep to evaluate for additional colonic pathology, synchronous lesions, or extent of colonic disease. If the operative indication is unresectable polyp or another endoscopic finding, then the lesion is ideally tattooed preoperatively. Additional preoperative work up is dictated based on the patient's age and comorbidities, however, generally it should include basic laboratory studies, including CBC, electrolytes, and selective use of EKG. All patients at our institution are screened through preadmission testing, which includes preoperative and preanesthetic evaluation. Anticoagulants and antiplatelet agents are typically held preoperatively, unless there is prohibitive risk to doing so.

## Perioperative Preparation

We utilize oral polyethylene-based bowel prep should the pathology dictate an intraoperative colonoscopic evaluation when the mass is not identifiable on CT or no tattoo has been placed. In patients with a large mass or a well-documented location, oral prep is not required and patients are instructed to take clear liquids the day before surgery. Preoperative subcutaneous heparin (5,000 units) and sequential compression devices are used for deep venous thrombosis prophylaxis. A nonsteroidal antiinflammatory agent is typically given preoperatively and antibiotics are prescribed.

General anesthesia is typically utilized. Abdominal wall relaxation is necessary for effective insufflation and laparoscopic visualization. Postoperative epidural anesthesia is unnecessary as postoperative pain is easily controlled with oral and intravenous analgesia including patient controlled analgesia (PCA) for the first 24 h. In our studies, epidurals have shown no benefit over our standard enhanced recovery pathways [5, 6]. Transversus abdominis anesthetic blocks performed by the surgical team are liberally employed and have been shown to improve pain scores postoperatively [7].

## Surgical Technique

### Patient Positioning

The patient is placed in the supine position on a beanbag on the operating room table. After placement of the endotracheal tube and induction of general anesthesia, an orogastric tube and Foley catheter are inserted. The abdomen is prepped and draped routinely. The legs are then placed in yellow fin stirrups to allow for modified lithotomy position (Fig. 16.1). Both of the arms are tucked at the patient's side and the beanbag is aspirated. In patients who are morbidly obese and both arms do not fit on the table, the arm on the side of the pathology can be left out on an arm board allowing for safety during various positional changes during the operation. The legs are kept low to prevent interference with the instruments. Low lithotomy position is utilized to facilitate handling of the flexures, particularly if mobilization of the splenic flexure is necessary with an extended right colectomy. This also allows the surgeon to move between the legs, if necessary, for the transverse colon.

The primary monitor is placed on the right side of the patient up towards the patient's head. The secondary monitor is placed on the left side of the patient at the same level and is primarily for the assistant during the early phase of the operation and port insertion. The instrument table is placed between the patient's legs. The primary operating surgeon stands on the left side of the patient with the assistant standing initially on the right and moving to the left side once ports have been inserted.

### Port Insertion

Initial entrance into the abdomen is performed utilizing a modified Hasson approach. A vertical 1-cm infraumbilical incision is made with electrocautery using the cut function. This is taken down to the linea alba, which is then grasped on each side of the midline using Kocher clamps. Electrocautery is then used to open the fascia between the Kocher clamps and forceps are used to open the peritoneum bluntly. It is important to keep this opening small (<1 cm) to minimize air leak. After confirming entry into the peritoneal cavity, a purse string suture is fashioned around the fascial defect and a rumel tourniquet is applied. A 10-mm reusable port is inserted through this port site allowing the abdomen to be insufflated with $CO_2$ to a pressure of 12–15 mmHg.

A 10-mm zero-degree camera lens is used and inserted into the abdomen and an initial inspection is performed carefully to evaluate the liver, small bowel, and peritoneal surfaces. A 5-mm port is inserted in the left lower quadrant approximately 2–3 cm medial and superior to the anterior superior iliac spine. This is carefully inserted lateral to the inferior epigastric vessels keeping the tract of the port going as perpendicular as

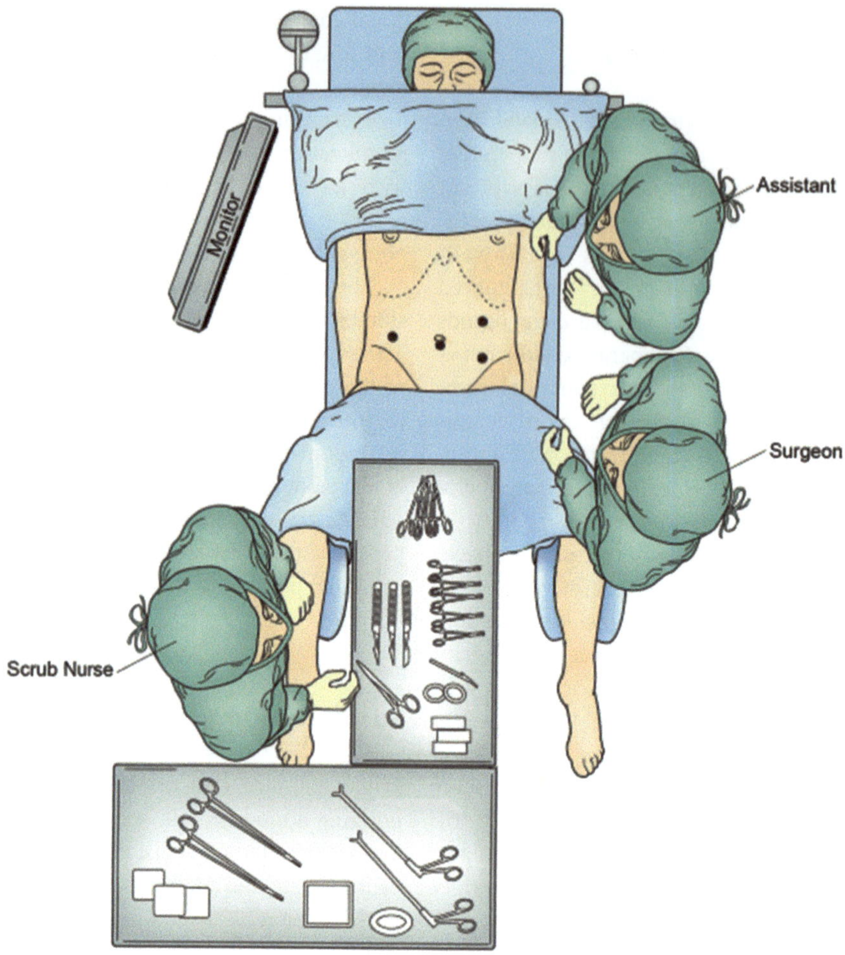


**Fig. 16.1** Patient positioning with both arms at the patient's side and the legs in lithotomy position

possible through the abdominal wall. If significant intraabdominal adhesions are encountered, they can usually be taken down through this lateral 5-mm port, with electrocautery scissors or an energy device. All additional ports are placed lateral to the epigastric vessels, which can be identified laparoscopically or additionally with transillumination. A 5-mm port is inserted in the left upper quadrant at least a hands breath superior to the lower quadrant port. Particularly when teaching, a right lower quadrant 5-mm port is also inserted (Fig. 16.2). Very rarely, in the case of a difficult hepatic flexure, a 5-mm right upper quadrant port may also be inserted.

In patients with extensive adhesions, a 5-mm 30-degree camera may be inserted away from adhesions to permit lysis of adhesions adequate

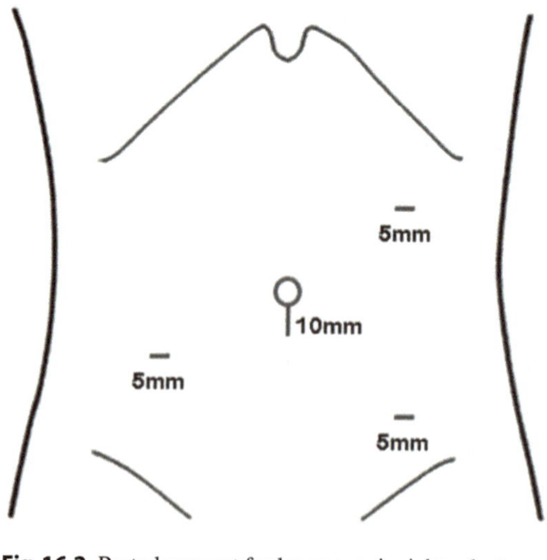


**Fig. 16.2** Port placement for laparoscopic right colectomy

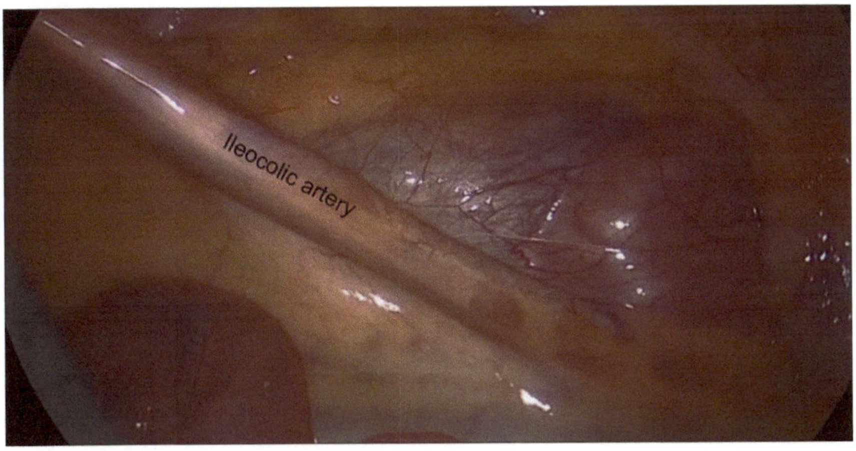


**Fig. 16.3** Elevation of the ileocolic pedicle in preparation for its ligation

to insert midline ports and adequate to mobilize the omentum and colon. In patients who are morbidly obese, the left sided ports can be moved closer to or even with the midline, so that instruments can reach the right colon. If standard left sided ports are used in morbidly obese patients, the instruments simply do not reach.

## Definitive Laparoscopic Set-Up

The assistant now moves to the patient's left side, standing to the left of the surgeon. The patient is placed in slight Trendelenburg position and then rotated left side down as far as the table permits. This helps to move the small bowel over to the left side of the abdomen and allows for gravitational migration of the small bowel away from the operative field. The operating surgeon then inserts two noncrushing bowel clamps through the two left sided abdominal ports. The greater omentum is reflected over the transverse colon. Appropriate orogastric tube placement is essential to allow for gastric decompression and appropriate omental retraction. The small bowel is moved to the patient's left side with one-third in the pelvis, one-third laterally, and one-third in the upper abdomen. The tumor is assessed for size and fixation to surrounding structures as an initial assessment of resectability. The ileocecal mesentery is then grasped with a noncrushing bowel clamp and retracted to the right lower quadrant to visualize the ileocolic pedicle.

## Defining and Dividing the Ileocolic Pedicle

A noncrushing bowel clamp is placed on the mesentery at the ileocecal junction. This area is then stretched up towards the right lower quadrant port, stretching the vessel and also lifting it up from the retroperitoneum (Fig. 16.3). This demonstrates a sulcus between the medial side of the ileocolic pedicle and the retroperitoneum. Electrocautery scissors are then used to open the mesenteric peritoneum along the ileocolic vessel. Blunt dissection with noncrushing bowel clamps is then used to lift the vessel away from the retroperitoneum, opening the plane cranially up to the origin of the ileocolic artery as it branches from the SMA. Electrocautery is then used to open a window in the peritoneum to isolate the vessel. Meticulous dissection ensures that the plane of dissection is anterior to the congenital layer of peritoneum lying over the retroperitoneum and its structures (duodenum and ureter). Preservation of this layer precludes the absolute need to visualize the ureter. After we have isolated the ileocolic pedicle, the vessel is then divided often with an energy device,

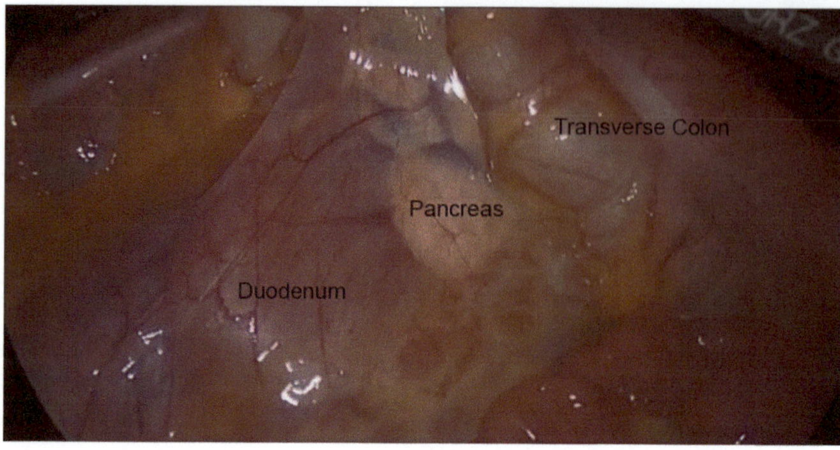


**Fig. 16.4** Retroperitoneal dissection of the right colon revealing the duodenum and pancreas

while maintaining proximal control at its origin with a noncrushing bowel clamp. Laparoscopic staplers or other energy sources may also be used, although this requires upsizing the left iliac fossa port to accommodate a 12-mm trocar. After division of the ileocolic pedicle, the plane between the ascending colon mesentery and the retroperitoneum is developed in a medial to lateral approach out to the lateral attachment of the colon, and superiorly dissecting the bowel off the anterior surface of the duodenum and pancreas up to the level of the hepatic flexure (Fig. 16.4).

## Mobilization of the Hepatic Flexure

The proximal transverse colon is then grasped with a noncrushing bowel clamp and drawn inferiorly. The omentum is then grasped and elevated superiorly and cranially to allow for tension on the gastrocolic ligament. This is then incised with electrocautery scissors to gain entrance into the lesser sac. The operating surgeon continues to progress along this mobilization plane to draw the hepatic flexure inferiorly and medially. Care must be taken to avoid injury to the gallbladder and second portion of the duodenum that is encountered inferiorly as the hepatic flexure is mobilized. The line of traction as the gastrocolic ligament is divided changes to more elevation of the transverse colon by the assistant and medial rotation of the proximal colon by the surgeon. It is important to keep the plane of dissection near the colon in the appropriate plane to minimize blood loss and injury to retroperitoneal vessels.

As the plane of dissection continues, one encounters the area of prior retroperitoneal dissection during division of the ileocolic pedicle. The lateral peritoneal attachments are then divided along the white line of Toldt with electrocautery scissors. This line is divided right down to the base of the cecum, and it may be possible to completely mobilize the appendix and base of the cecum to the midline from this direction. The colon is then completely dissected free from the underlying duodenum and retroperitoneum and the specimen is reflected entirely to the midline.

In patients who are morbidly obese, the release of the hepatic flexure can sometimes be facilitated by turning the patient to a reverse Trendelenburg position, and placement of an additional right upper quadrant 5-mm port to apply additional traction on the hepatic flexure.

## Division of Middle Colic Vessels

After mobilizing the hepatic flexure, attention is turned to the transverse colon mesentery. We prefer to take the right branch of the middle colic

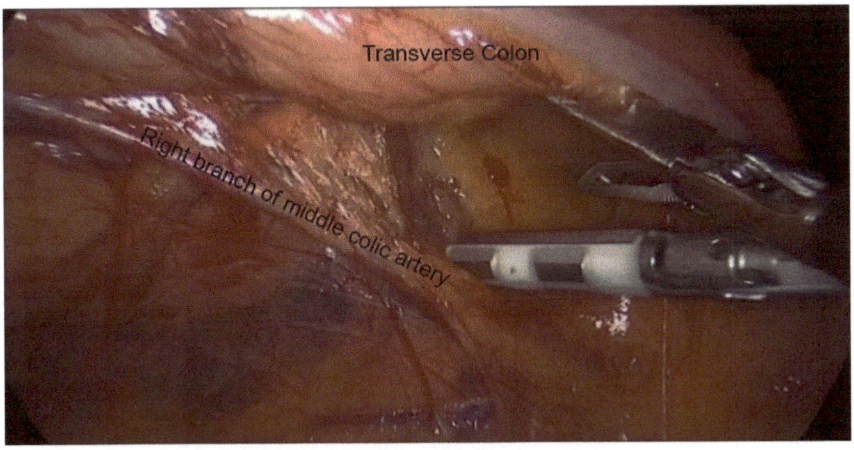


**Fig. 16.5** Division of the right branch of the middle colic artery

intracorporeally, specifically in obese individuals and those with foreshortened mesentery. Attempts at extracorporeal ligation can often be extremely difficult.

The transverse colon is then elevated by two noncrushing bowel clamps and retracted towards the hepatic and splenic flexures. Initially, an opening is made above the transverse colon to the lesser sac through the avascular window. It is easy to be more posterior than expected and care must be taken not to damage the pancreas or fourth part of duodenum.

The right branch of the middle colic vessels is identified and ligated with an energy device or between clips (Fig. 16.5). It is essential that the vascular pedicle is confirmed prior to division as the SMA and vein lie deep to the dissection line and the pancreas is fully exposed as dissection progresses.

An extended right colectomy may be performed for more distal ascending or proximal transverse lesions taking further branches of the middle colic vessels and entering the lesser sac. Additionally, the greater omentum is taken en bloc with the transverse colon for transverse colon cancers. This dissection may be facilitated by moving the surgeon between the patient's legs. The splenic flexure may also require mobilization for more distal lesions.

## Mobilization of the Ileocecal Junction

The patient is placed into steep Trendelenburg position and the small bowel is reflected superiorly. The base of the attachment between the small bowel and terminal ileal mesentery and retroperitoneum is then exposed. The mesentery of the terminal ileum is then elevated to expose the junction of the visceral peritoneum and the retroperitoneum. Electrocautery scissors are used to dissect the terminal ileum off the retroperitoneum. This line of dissection extends from the ileocecal junction towards the origin of the SMA (Fig. 16.6). As the dissection proceeds more proximally, mobilization should be performed with scissors alone in order to avoid injury to the third part of the duodenum, which appears near the end of the dissection. The plane between the retroperitoneum and the terminal ileum is developed and the terminal ileum reflected medially and cephalad. It is important to complete the medial dissection to the level of the third part of the duodenum in order to facilitate eventual delivery of the complete specimen at the end of the case.

Prior to extracting the specimen the surgeon should grasp the right colon and draw it to the midline. In some cases there are remnant areolar attachments that may be divided. It is essential

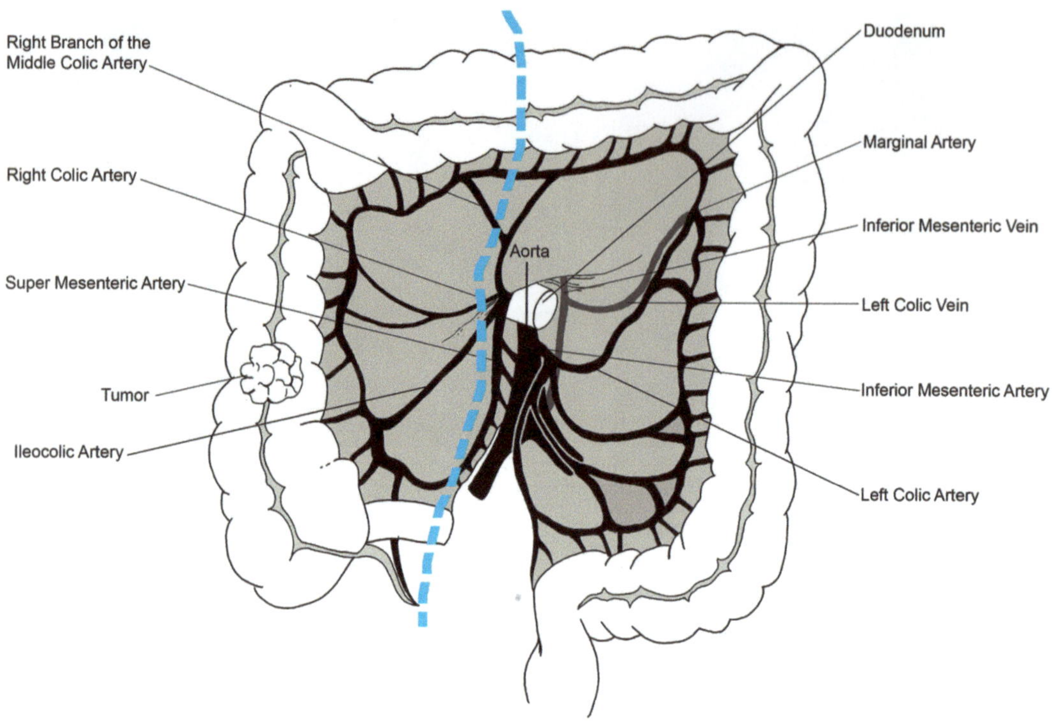


**Fig. 16.6** Major arteries and line of resection for laparoscopic right colectomy

that the root of the ileal mesentery is as mobile as possible to permit easy extraction of the small bowel through the midline incision. A final check on complete mobility of the entire specimen and hemostasis is ensured before extracting the specimen.

## Specimen Extraction

If placed, the 12-mm port site is closed using an endoclose instrument prior to specimen extraction. The appendix or cecum is now grasped firmly through the right lower quadrant port site with a noncrushing bowel clamp. The pneumoperitoneum is deflated through the ports. The umbilical port is removed and this port site is extended into a 3–4 cm midline incision. This may be made larger if necessary to remove larger phlegmons or tumors. Next, a wound protector is inserted to reduce the risk of skin infection or tumor implantation in the wound. In patients who are morbidly obese or have a pendulous abdomen, the extraction site can be made in the epigastrium with a transverse incision.

The right colon is then exteriorized. The distal small bowel is assessed and the small bowel mesentery divided extracorporally using 0 polyglactin sutures for hemostasis. In cases of bulky ileal mesentery suture ligation of the mesentery may be used. The bowel is divided with a gastrointestinal (GIA) stapler and clamps are applied.

Attention is now turned to the area for division of the colon. The colonic mesentery is divided with electrocautery or between clamps and 0 polyglactin ties. The colon is then divided with the GIA stapler. The specimen is then removed from the field and examined to confirm the pathological findings and the adequacy of proximal and distal margins. Care is taken to ensure the mesenteric defect is straight and there is no twisting of the bowel ends prior to proceeding with anastomosis. A side-to-side, functional end-to-end anastomosis is fashioned with a GIA stapler. The crotch is then buttressed with an interrupted 3-0 polyglactin suture. The resulting opening from the GIA stapler insertion site is then closed with a thoraco-abdominal (TA) stapler after lining up the staple lines and offsetting the GIA staple line with clamps. The TA staple line is then oversewn with 3-0 polyglactin suture in a continuous fashion. The anastomosis is checked for hemostasis and returned to the abdomen.

The mesenteric window is not closed. The fascia is closed with interrupted figure of eight #1 polydioxanone sutures. The subcutaneous space is irrigated and the wounds are closed with subcuticular 4-0 polyglactin sutures. The patient is awakened, extubated, and transferred to recovery to follow the standard postoperative care plan.

## Postoperative Management

A standardized perioperative care plan is used. Orogastric tubes are removed before completion of the operation. Intravenous fluids are minimized both intraoperatively and postoperatively. Urinary catheters are discontinued on postoperative day one. Patients are ambulated immediately postoperatively and an active walking program is encouraged. Intravenous opioids are limited and an oral regimen is encouraged as soon as liquids are tolerated. Acetaminophen is given intravenously during or immediately after surgery, and 1 g is administered orally every 6 h starting the morning after surgery. Additional nonsteroidal antiinflammatory medications are used in patients without gastrointestinal or renal contraindications. Oral opioids are given for breakthrough pain. Deep venous thrombosis prophylaxis is given postoperatively, typically with subcutaneous unfractionated heparin (5,000 units three times per day). A liquid diet is offered immediately with advancement to a soft diet the morning after surgery. Discharge criteria include tolerance of liquids with passage of flatus or stool, adequate home support, and patient wish to be released to home. Many patients are well enough to be discharged 1–2 days after surgery.

Standard algorithms are utilized through all aspects of patient care. Perioperative care pathways are utilized from the clinic until hospital discharge. This standardization helps to decrease communication difficulties, reduce errors, and ensure consistent and reproducible high-quality and efficient outcomes [8].

## Complications

Complications related to laparoscopic right hemicolectomy can be described in a stepwise manner through the steps of the operation. Initial operative complications can include those related to initial entrance into the abdomen. These may include inadvertent bowel injury or bleeding. Although exceedingly rare, bowel injury may require conversion to an open incision for full mobilization and injury identification and repair. Bleeding is usually controlled with electrocautery, but clips or an energy device may be used. Additional complications can stem from trocar placement laterally, which can include injury to the epigastric vessels. This is usually controlled upon placement of the trocar by tamponade, however it can lead to potentially catastrophic bleeding upon desufflation of the abdomen and trocar removal. Bleeding is usually controlled with electrocautery for minor port site bleeding, however may require control laparoscopically either with electrocautery or an energy device. Alternatively, a suture passer can be used to ligate the vessel both above and below the trocar for effective suture ligation.

Ureteral injury has been reported and should be carefully avoided; but it has not been an issue in our experience even with a large number of reoperative and inflammatory cases. When operating in the correct plane, the retroperitoneal attachments are left undisturbed, which precludes the need for definite identification of the ureter. Injury to the ureter should mandate urologic consultation.

Duodenal injury may take place upon division of the ileocolic pedicle as the third portion of the duodenum lies in the retroperitoneum close to the origin of the SMA. This is especially pertinent during oncologic resection, as one attempts to take the ileocolic pedicle at its origin in order to maximize lymph node yield. Additionally, as medial-to-lateral dissection continues up to the level of the middle colic vessels, the duodenum must always be in view and away from your dissection with gentle blunt retraction. Immediate identification can often allow for laparoscopic repair or imbrication if necessary.

Bleeding from the ileocolic pedicle can also occur, especially in obese individuals, patients with inflammatory bowel disease, or patients with calcified vessels. The pedicle is often taken with an energy device or vascular stapler. If bleeding is encountered proximally it can either be regrasped with an energy device or can be controlled with careful application of clips. It may be safer with clips, as the duodenum is often coursing just beneath. Care must be taken not to inadvertently injure the SMA, specifically with high ligation of the ileocolic pedicle. One can often control the distal bleeding with energy, however this can also be managed with clips once the vessel is isolated. Sometimes a vessel loop is required for proximal vascular control.

Anastomotic leak is uncommon in our experience, with an approximate 0.8 % leak rate and a 0.8 % rate of intraabdominal abscess distant from the anastomosis [9]. Patient factors often contributing to leak may include use of immunosuppressants, poor nutritional status, and additional comorbidities. However, meticulous dissection, appropriate blood supply, and tension-free anastomosis are paramount. We typically utilize a side-to-side, functional end-to-end stapled anastomosis imbricating the corners and buttressing the crotch. A leak after a right colectomy is intraperitoneal by definition and should be managed as such. If a leak is identified radiographically without untoward clinical deterioration, management should be expectant and can include bowel rest with serial abdominal exams and broad-spectrum intravenous antibiotics.

For patients demonstrating focal peritonitis and clinical stability, CT with oral, intravenous, and rectal contrast should be obtained. Small contained (<3 cm) abscesses without clinical deterioration can be managed with bowel rest and broad-spectrum antibiotics. Those with larger (<3 cm) or complicated collections should have attempt at percutaneous drainage. Those patients with clinical instability regardless of size or location should be resuscitated and brought to the operating theater emergently. Intraoperative options include resection of the anastomosis with creation of end stoma and mucus fistula, and resection with reanastomosis and proximal diversion. Rarely, in patients with minor defects with good tissue quality and hemodynamic stability, primary repair with drain placement and proximal diversion may be considered [10].

## References

1. Hasson HM. Open laparoscopy vs. closed laparoscopy: a comparison of complication rates. Adv Plan Parent. 1978;13(3–4):41–50.
2. Jacobs M, Verdeja JC, Goldstein HS. Minimally invasive colon resection (laparoscopic colectomy). Surg Laparosc Endosc. 1991;1(3):144–50.
3. Clinical Outcomes of Surgical Therapy Study Group. A comparison of laparoscopically assisted and open colectomy for colon cancer. N Engl J Med. 2004;350(20):2050–9. doi:10.1056/NEJMoa032651.
4. Birkmeyer JD, Finks JF, O'Reilly A, Oerline M, Carlin AM, Nunn AR, et al. Surgical skill and complication rates after bariatric surgery. N Engl J Med. 2013;369(15):1434–42. doi:10.1056/NEJMsa1300625.
5. Delaney CP, Brady K, Woconish D, Parmar SP, Champagne BJ. Towards optimizing perioperative colorectal care: outcomes for 1,000 consecutive laparoscopic colon procedures using enhanced recovery pathways. Am J Surg. 2012;203(3):353–5. doi:10.1016/j.amjsurg.2011.09.017; discussion 5-6.
6. Adamina M, Kehlet H, Tomlinson GA, Senagore AJ, Delaney CP. Enhanced recovery pathways optimize health outcomes and resource utilization: a meta-analysis of randomized controlled trials in colorectal surgery. Surgery. 2011;149(6):830–40. doi:10.1016/j.surg.2010.11.003.
7. Favuzza J, Delaney CP. Laparoscopic-guided transversus abdominis plane block for colorectal surgery. Dis Colon Rectum. 2013;56(3):389–91. doi:10.1097/DCR.0b013e318280549b.
8. Delaney CP. Outcome of discharge within 24 to 72 hours after laparoscopic colorectal surgery. Dis Colon Rectum. 2008;51(2):181–5. doi:10.1007/s10350-007-9126-y.
9. Delaney CP, Chang E, Senagore AJ, Broder M. Clinical outcomes and resource utilization associated with laparoscopic and open colectomy using a large national database. Ann Surg. 2008;247(5):819–24. doi:10.1097/SLA.0b013e31816d950e.
10. Phitayakorn R, Delaney CP, Reynolds HL, Champagne BJ, Heriot AG, Neary P, et al. Standardized algorithms for management of anastomotic leaks and related abdominal and pelvic abscesses after colorectal surgery. World J Surg. 2008;32(6):1147–56. doi:10.1007/s00268-008-9468-1.

## Key Operative Steps

1. The patient is positioned and ports are placed.
2. The patient is rotated to left side down and placed in Trendelenburg position.
3. The omentum is placed over the transverse colon into the upper abdomen and the small bowel is moved to the left side to give adequate operative space.
4. Dissection and division of the ileocolic pedicle, protecting the ureter and duodenum.
5. Perform a medial-to-lateral dissection of the colonic mesentery.
6. Mobilize the hepatic flexure.
7. Mobilize the terminal ileum off the retroperitoneum.
8. Confirm full mobilization of the right colon to the midline.
9. Divide the right branch of the middle colic artery before the specimen is exteriorized.
10. Extension of the umbilical incision, placement of a wound retractor, and exteriorization of the specimen.
11. Extracorporeal resection and anastomosis.

# Robotic Technique for Right Colectomy

17

Gemma Gossedge and David Jayne

## Introduction

The da Vinci® surgical system (Intuitive) is the only commercially available robotic system. It consists of three components: the operating console, the vision stack, and the robotic cart supporting the robotic arms. The operating console is remotely situated from the operating table and is where the surgeon sits to control the robotic arms and instruments. A pseudo-three-dimensional (3-D) operative view is provided by a binocular imaging system. Movements of the robotic arms and instruments are controlled by the surgeon's fingers in the master controls and through a series of foot pedals. The robotic cart supports a laparoscopic camera and two (da Vinci) or three (da Vinci-S, da Vinci-Si) robotic arms. This system is ideally suited to operating within the abdomen. Its advantages over conventional laparoscopy include a stable camera platform under direct surgeon control, a 3-D operative field, intuitive instrument handling with 6-degrees of freedom and an ergonomic operating position for the surgeon.

G. Gossedge, M.B.Ch.B., M.R.C.S.
Leeds Institute for Biological and Clinical Sciences, University of Leeds, Leeds, UK

D. Jayne, B.Sc., M.B.B.Ch., M.D., F.R.C.S. (✉)
St. James's University Hospital, Level 7 Clinical Sciences Building, Leeds LS9 7TF, UK
e-mail: d.g.jayne@leeds.ac.uk

Since its introduction into clinical practice in 1999, this robotic system has been gaining increasing popularity, particularly in urology, gynecological oncology, and colorectal surgery. Initial reports have confirmed the feasibility and safety of robotic colorectal surgery with a variety of totally robotic and hybrid robotic techniques being described for benign and malignant disease. However, just because a procedure can be performed robotically does not mean that it should be the default operative technique. The robotic approach needs to be justified in terms of patient benefit and cost-effectiveness. Efforts are being directed to determine the benefit of the robotic approach in colorectal disease with multicenter, randomized clinical trials currently recruiting [1].

The purpose of this chapter is to discuss robotic right colectomy, providing a brief overview of the literature, describing the operative technique, and exploring potential advantages and disadvantages as compared to conventional laparoscopic approaches.

## Historical Perspective

The Food and Drug Administration (FDA) approved the da Vinci Robotic System (Intuitive) for intraabdominal surgery in 2000 and the first robotic-assisted colectomy was performed by Weber in 2001 [2]. Since then, there have been a number of publications, consisting mainly of

J. Kim and J. Garcia-Aguilar (eds.), *Surgery for Cancers of the Gastrointestinal Tract: A Step-by-Step Approach*, DOI 10.1007/978-1-4939-1893-5_17, © Springer Science+Business Media New York 2015

single institution series and including a mix of benign and malignant disease [3–13]. The most notable of these case series for right colectomy is from D'Annibale and colleagues [11]. They evaluated surgical and oncological short-term outcomes of robotic-assisted right colectomy for malignant disease in 50 consecutive patients. Surgery-related morbidity was 2 %, disease-free survival was 90 %, and overall survival was 92 % at a median follow-up of 36 months, with stage II–IV disease included in the analysis. The authors concluded that robotic assistance facilitates oncological dissection of the right colon [11].

A number of reports have compared robotic to laparoscopic colectomy. The only study specific to right colectomy was reported by De Souza et al., who retrospectively compared 40 robotic-assisted to 135 laparoscopic right colectomies, performed at a single institution [14]. The results failed to show a difference in conversion rate, resection margin positivity, lymph node yield, length of stay, or morbidity. The robotic procedure was associated with significantly longer operative times (laparoscopic, 118 min vs. robotic, 159 min; $P<0.001$) and significantly higher total costs (median, total laparoscopic cost $12,362 vs. total robotic cost $15,192; $P=0.003$). The authors concluded that robotic right colectomy was safe and feasible and, despite the longer operative time and higher cost, right colectomy was as an ideal procedure to begin the learning curve in robotic colorectal surgery. Rawlings et al. again provided a subgroup analysis of right colectomies in their retrospective case series and compared 17 right robotic resections with 15 right laparoscopic resections [15], with intracorporeal anastomosis in the robotic cases and extracorporeal anastomosis in the laparoscopic cases. The total operative time was significantly longer for the robotic as compared to the laparoscopic cases (219 min vs. 169 min, $P=0.002$), which was attributed to the time for robotic setup and intracorporeal anastomosis. Hospital costs were higher for the robotic cases ($9,225 vs. $8,073, $P=0.43$), including total operative cost, operating personnel cost, and operating room time.

The only case-matched study comparing robotic and open surgery for right-sided colon cancers is from Luca et al. [16], who performed extracorporeal anastomosis in all cases. Despite this, the mean operative time was significantly longer in the robotic group (robotic, 192 min vs. open, 136 min; $P>0.001$). The median length of hospital stay was significantly shorter in the robotic group (robotic, 5 days vs. open, 8 days; $P=0.001$) and significantly more patients in the robotic group had 15 or more lymph nodes retrieved from resection specimens (robotic, 100 % vs. open, 88.2 %; $P=0.038$).

The only randomized, controlled trial comparing robotic with laparoscopic right colectomy was performed by Park et al. [17]. In this single center study, a total of 70 patients were equally assigned to either robotic or laparoscopic surgery. No difference was observed in length of stay, complications, completeness of excision, and postoperative pain. Mean operative times for robotic cases were significantly longer than laparoscopic surgery (robotic, 195 min vs. lap, 135 min), but more intracorporeal anastomoses were performed robotically ($n=30$) than laparoscopically ($n=7$).

In 2009, Ostrowitz et al. [18] reported a series of three robotic single-incision (SILS) right colectomies using the da Vinci-S robotic system, through a single 4-cm incision at the umbilicus, with three robotic arms, a 12-mm camera, and two 8-mm robotic ports. There are theoretical advantages for the robot in SILS given the ability to cross instruments yet realign operator control to maintain intuitive manipulation. The da Vinci single site platform® subsequently received FDA approval in 2011. Morelli et al. [19] reported a robotic single-incision right colectomy through a 2.5-cm umbilical incision and concluded the technique was safe and feasible and that right colectomy was ideally suited to single site techniques due to the small incision required for specimen extraction. They also felt the procedure was easier than standard laparoscopic SILS as the curved instruments help to restore normal triangulation.

On the basis of the limited available data it appears that robotic right colectomy is feasible and safe, but is associated with longer operative times and increased costs, although it is not clear what effect, if any, the learning curve had on operative times. In addition, hospital costs are subject to large variation depending on the surgeon's operative preferences and the logistics of individual healthcare systems. The authors would argue that operative times are not dissimilar to conventional laparoscopy as docking times can be reduced to around 5 min with experience, and the costs of the robotic instruments can be offset against the expensive energy devices routinely used in laparoscopic surgery.

## Indications

Right colectomy is performed for a variety of benign and malignant conditions, but the most common indication is for carcinoma of the right colon. Indications for robotic right colectomy are no different to those for the laparoscopic approach. Care should be taken in patients with a multiply scarred abdomen or locally advanced disease with either a large tumor mass or invasion of neighboring structures necessitating multivisceral resection. Obesity is not a contraindication for use of the robot and indeed there is circumstantial evidence that the laparoscopic or robotic approach may be beneficial in terms of reduced wound complications. There are no reports of robotic right colectomy performed in the emergency setting.

Several techniques have been described for robotic right colectomy. The principal differences relate to port placement, operative approach (medial-to-lateral vs. lateral-to-medial), and whether an extracorporeal or intracorporeal anastomosis is undertaken. To maximize the benefits of the robot, a totally robotic approach is often preferred. This has facilitated conventional laparoscopic techniques, including medial-to-lateral dissection with "vessel-first division" of the ileocolic pedicle.

## Preoperative Considerations

Preoperative evaluation is no different to standard workup for colon cancer surgery. Investigations include a colonoscopy with biopsy and India ink tattooing, or computed tomographic (CT) colonography if colonoscopy is not possible or is incomplete. Radiological staging includes CT scan of the chest, abdomen, and pelvis to assess local disease and the presence of distant metastatic spread.

Perioperative preparation is the same as for open and laparoscopic surgery. The principles of enhanced recovery after surgery (ERAS) are adopted to maximize patient recovery and include the avoidance of bowel preparation (even when intracorporeal anastomosis is planned), preoperative carbohydrate loading, and free fluids until 2 h prior to surgery. The patient is provided with venous compression stockings and broad-spectrum antibiotics are administered on induction of anesthesia.

## Surgical Techniques

### Patient Position

The patient is placed supine on the operating table with the legs held in stirrups in the modified Lloyd-Davies position. The arms are secured by the patient's sides and all pressure points protected with gel pads and cotton wool padding. A vacuum beanbag or retaining strap over the chest is used to prevent patient slippage. The use of shoulder supports is discouraged because of reported cases of upper limb neuropraxia.

### Robotic Setup

A number of factors need to be considered when planning robotic setup and port placement. In particular, it is important to consider not only access to the abdominal pathology but also potential external clashes of the robotic arms. Placement of the camera port should take into account the magnified view provided by the robot, with sufficient distance of the camera from the operating field to enable a panoramic view to be obtained. Adequate access should be provided for the assistant to manipulate instruments though an additional 10-mm port without restriction by the robotic arms.

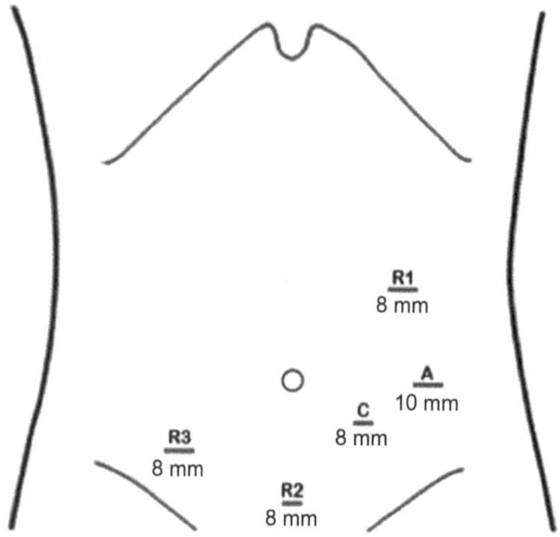


**Fig. 17.1** Operative port placement for robotic right hemicolectomy

A number of techniques can be used to create pneumoperitoneum and aid insertion of the first camera port. It is the authors' preference to establish pneumoperitoneum using a Veress needle inserted below the left subcostal margin in the mid-clavicular line (Palmer's point). A 10/12-mm disposable camera port is then inserted under laparoscopic vision in the left iliac fossa, ensuring airtight port placement, using a conventional laparoscopic stack. An extralong 12-mm Optiview port (Ethicon Endosurgery, Cincinnati, OH, USA) can be used if the patient is obese. Using a marking pen, the remaining port sites are marked out taking care to leave sufficient space between the ports to avoid clashing of the robotic arms; generally, a hands breadth of space between ports is sufficient. It is our philosophy to maximize the benefits of the robot by utilizing all four arms. Three additional robotic 8-mm ports are placed: an 8-mm port for a robotic left hand (arm #3) 1 cm superior to the right anterior superior iliac spine, an 8-mm port for a second robotic left hand (arm #2) in the suprapubic region, and an 8-mm port for a robotic right hand (arm #1) in the left upper quadrant. All ports are placed under direct laparoscopic vision. A 10-mm disposable assistant port is placed between the camera port and the left upper quadrant robotic port in the left flank (Fig. 17.1). Once all ports are in place, a preliminary laparoscopy is performed and the operative field prepared. The patient is placed in slight Trendelenburg position, with 5–10° of left-sided downward tilt. The peritoneal cavity is inspected for metastatic disease and feasibility of resection confirmed. Any abdominal adhesions are divided, the omentum displaced cephalad, and the small bowel retracted into the pelvis and left upper quadrant. The terminal ileum and cecum are displayed by retracting the ileocecal junction, enabling visualisation of the ileocolic vessels. The robotic system is now ready to be docked and the laparoscopic stack is removed from the vicinity of the operating table.

The robotic cart is positioned on the same side as the pathology. For right colectomy this means maneuvering the robotic cart and approaching the operating table over the patient's right shoulder. The vision stack is also located on the patient's right side, by his right foot (Fig. 17.2). The bedside assistant and the scrub nurse are situated to the patient's left side. Once the robot is docked, there can be no change to the patient's or robot's position, without first undocking the robotic arms. The camera arm is attached to the left iliac fossa port and adjusted to point towards the ileocolic pedicle. The remaining robotic arms are secured to their respective ports. The robotic camera is inserted along with a robotic bowel grasper for arm #3 and a second robotic bowel grasper for arm #2. The monopolar scissors is inserted into arm #1 in the left upper quadrant. The scene is now set for the robotic operation to begin.

## Robotic Procedure

Robotic right colectomy does not differ in any way from its laparoscopic counterpart. We routinely perform medial-to-lateral dissection with early division of the ileocolic pedicle close to its origin from the superior mesenteric vessels. Arm #3 provides traction to the cecum/terminal ileum to give tension and to lift the ileocolic vessels. The retroperitoneal space immediately below the vessels is entered and a retroperitoneal "cave" is developed, making maximum use of the pneumoperitoneum

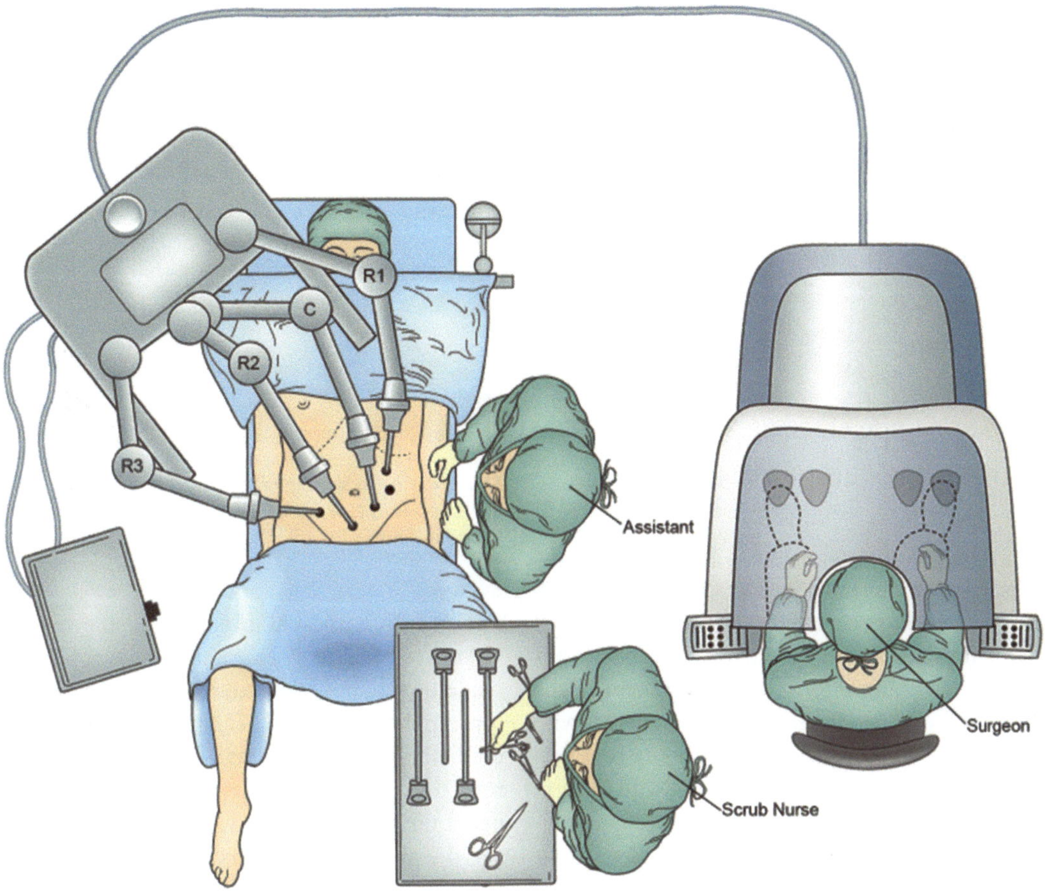


**Fig. 17.2** Operating room set-up. The robotic cart is located on the patient's right with the vision stack located inferiorly. The scrub nurse is located near the patient's left foot. The assistant is located on the patient's left. The console is also located on the left

(Fig. 17.3). The duodenum is identified and displaced posteriorly and the ileocolic vessels are skeletonized and ligated/divided with clips, endovascular linear stapler, or energy source (Fig. 17.4). Arm #3 then grasps the divided ileocolic pedicle and retracts it toward the anterior abdominal wall. The retroperitoneal "cave" is further developed with identification of the right ureter. Gerota's fascia is displaced posteriorly and the retroperitoneal dissection is completed out to the lateral parietal attachments and to the underside of the hepatic flexure.

The mesentery of the terminal ileum is divided up to the point of division of the small bowel. The assistant then divides the terminal ileum using a

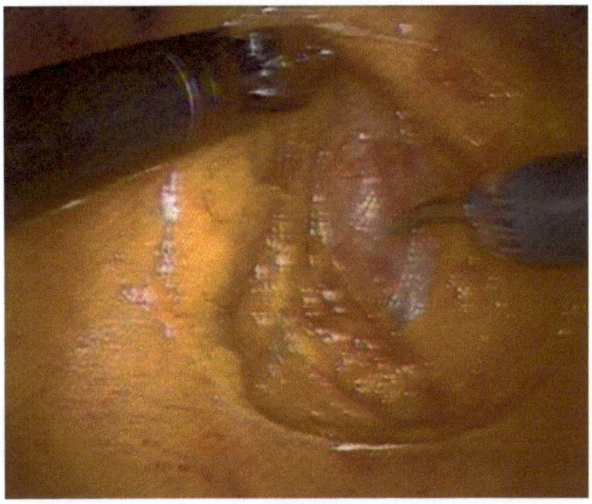

**Fig. 17.3** Dissection of the retrocolic "cave" with posterior displacement of the duodenum

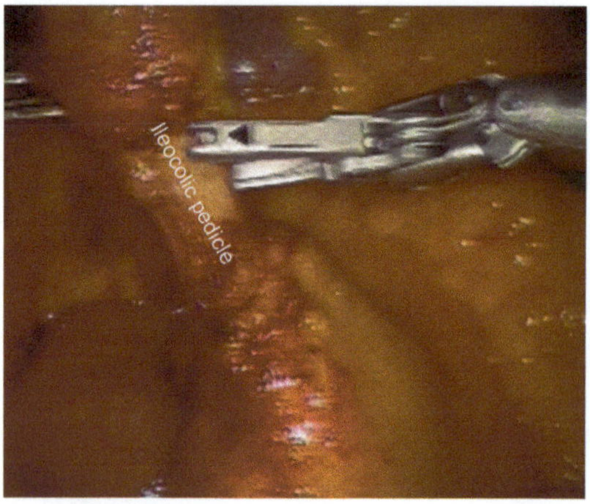


**Fig. 17.4** Ligation of the ileocolic vessels with clips

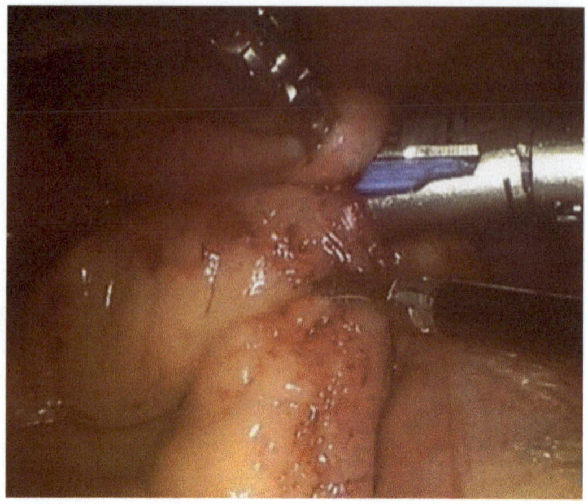

**Fig. 17.5** A linear stapler is passed through one of the upper ports and is used to create the ileocolostomy anastomosis

laparoscopic linear stapler. Division of the remaining peritoneal adhesions holding the inferior pole of the cecum and appendix is performed and extended up the right paracolic gutter, thus freeing the entire inferior and lateral part of the right colon. The dissection is completed with division of the hepatic flexure. This is best performed by retracting the right colon with the arm #3 grasper, retracting the transverse colon caudally by the assistant, and opening up the greater sac along the proximal transverse colon.

Once the hepatic flexure has been fully mobilized extending past the origin of the middle colic vessels, consideration is given to whether the middle colic vessels should be divided. This is a decision based upon the location of the tumor in the right colon. For proximal cancers it is usual to take the right branch of the middle colic artery. For hepatic flexure tumours the entire middle colic blood supply may be sacrificed. Division of the middle colic vessels may take either an infracolic or supracolic approach, depending on the ease of access. Vessel division and ligation is performed by the assistant using either clips or the laparoscopic linear stapler with a vascular cartridge. The right colon is now fully mobilized and resection is completed by division of remaining mesocolon up to the point of resection of the transverse colon.

The next decision is whether to perform an extracorporeal or intracorporeal anastomosis. For an extracorporeal anastomosis, the robot is undocked and a 5-cm umbilical incision is made to accommodate an Alexis wound retractor (Applied Medical). The right colon is delivered through the wound retractor and the resection and anastomosis completed in the usual fashion. For an intracorporeal anastomosis, the proximal transverse colon is divided by the assistant with a laparoscopic stapler and the mobilized right colon placed out of the way in the pelvis. Two sutures are used to approximate and orientate the divided ends of the terminal ileum and transverse colon. An enterotomy and colotomy are made at the distal proposed anastomotic site using diathermy scissors. A laparoscopic stapler is placed into the lumen of the bowel ends by the assistant with tension provided by a robotic grasper on the orientating sutures. The stapler is fired and carefully removed to prevent spillage of enteric contents (Fig. 17.5). The resulting entero-colotomy is closed by robotic suturing to complete the anastomosis (Fig. 17.6). The resected right colon is retrieved and extracted through a convenient site, but usually in the suprapubic region for best cosmesis. A final laparoscopic inspection is performed to ensure good hemostasis and the wounds closed taking care to prevent port-site herniation.

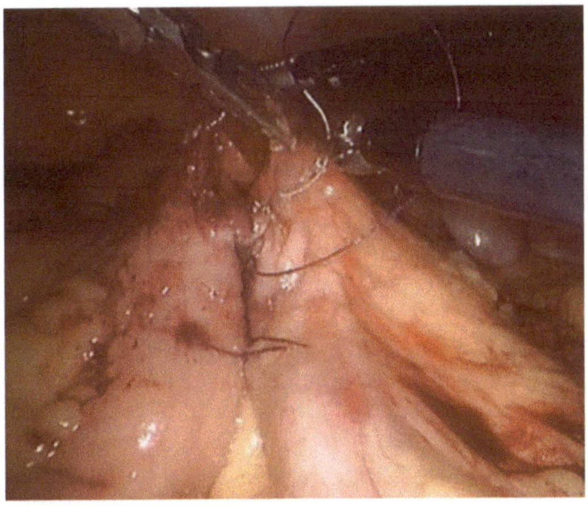

**Fig. 17.6** The entero-colotomy is closed with two layers of absorbable suture to complete the anastomosis

## Postoperative Management

Postoperatively, patients are managed according to an enhanced recovery protocol [20]. Fluids are given as tolerated including dietary supplements and soft diet is commenced as tolerated from postoperative day #1. Patient controlled analgesia (PCA) is used until fluids and oral analgesia are tolerated. Early mobilization is encouraged with physiotherapy support. Thromboprohylaxis with fractionated subcutaneous heparin and anti-embolism stockings is continued in the early postoperative period and continued for 1 month. Further antibiotics are avoided, unless there is a clinical indication. Patients are discharged when they are tolerating normal diet, mobile, and comfortable on oral analgesia.

## Complications

The potential complications following robotic right colectomy include those related to any major abdominal operation with general anesthesia and those specific to a laparoscopic or robotic approach.

## Conclusions

The technical advantages of the robot over conventional laparoscopy have been well-documented. In our opinion, the main advantages in right colon surgery include the stable camera platform, the additional dexterity of the Endowrist (Intuitive) instruments allowing precise dissection at the root of the ileocolic and middle colic vessels, and the ease of formation of an intracorporeal anastomosis.

In summary, the main benefits arising from robotic colorectal surgery are likely to be oncological, particularly when performing right colectomy with radical lymphadenectomy, due to the improved accuracy of dissection. However, these differences will be subtle and will not be apparent in small series with short-term follow-up. It is likely that more advanced robotic systems will be developed in the future and that market competition will reduce costs. If this is the case, the use of robotic systems for right colectomy will become more commonplace.

## References


1. Collinson FJ, Jayne DG, Pigazzi A, Tsang C, Barrie JM, Edlin R, et al. An international, multicentre, prospective, randomised, controlled, unblinded, parallel-group trial of robotic-assisted versus standard laparoscopic surgery for the curative treatment of rectal cancer. Int J Colorectal Dis. 2012;27(2):233–41. doi:10.1007/s00384-011-1313-6.
2. Weber PA, Merola S, Wasielewski A, Ballantyne GH. Telerobotic-assisted laparoscopic right and sigmoid colectomies for benign disease. Dis Colon Rectum. 2002;45(12):1689–94. doi:10.1097/01.dcr.0000037657.78153.a8; discussion 95-6.
3. Delaney CP, Lynch AC, Senagore AJ, Fazio VW. Comparison of robotically performed and traditional laparoscopic colorectal surgery. Dis Colon Rectum. 2003;46(12):1633–9. doi:10.1097/01.dcr.0000098941.42470.d9.
4. Corcione F, Esposito C, Cuccurullo D, Settembre A, Miranda N, Amato F, et al. Advantages and limits of robot-assisted laparoscopic surgery: preliminary experience. Surg Endosc. 2005;19(1):117–9. doi:10.1007/s00464-004-9004-9.
5. Braumann C, Jacobi CA, Menenakos C, Borchert U, Rueckert JC, Mueller JM. Computer-assisted laparoscopic colon resection with the Da Vinci system: our first experiences. Dis Colon Rectum. 2005;48(9):1820–7. doi:10.1007/s10350-005-0121-x.
6. Spinoglio G, Summa M, Priora F, Quarati R, Testa S. Robotic colorectal surgery: first 50 cases experience. Dis Colon Rectum. 2008;51(11):1627–32. doi:10.1007/s10350-008-9334-0.
7. Buchs NC, Pugin F, Bucher P, Morel P. Totally robotic right colectomy: a preliminary case series and an overview of the literature. The International Journal of

Medical Robotics + Computer Assisted Surgery: IJMRCAS. 2011. doi:10.1002/rcs.404.
8. Huettner F, Pacheco PE, Doubet JL, Ryan MJ, Dynda DI, Crawford DL. One hundred and two consecutive robotic-assisted minimally invasive colectomies–an outcome and technical update. J Gastrointest Surg. 2011;15(7):1195–204. doi:10.1007/s11605-011-1549-z.
9. Park SY, Choi GS, Park JS, Kim HJ, Choi WH, Ryuk JP. Robot-assisted right colectomy with lymphadenectomy and intracorporeal anastomosis for colon cancer: technical considerations. Surg Laparosc Endosc Percutan Tech. 2012;22(5):e271–6. doi:10.1097/SLE.0b013e31826581bd.
10. Witkiewicz W, Zawadzki M, Rzaca M, Obuszko Z, Czarnecki R, Turek J, et al. Robot-assisted right colectomy: surgical technique and review of the literature. Wideochir Inne Tech Malo Inwazyjne. 2013;8(3):253–7. doi:10.5114/wiitm.2011.33761.
11. D'Annibale A, Pernazza G, Morpurgo E, Monsellato I, Pende V, Lucandri G, et al. Robotic right colon resection: evaluation of first 50 consecutive cases for malignant disease. Ann Surg Oncol. 2010;17(11):2856–62. doi:10.1245/s10434-010-1175-0.
12. Zimmern A, Prasad L, Desouza A, Marecik S, Park J, Abcarian H. Robotic colon and rectal surgery: a series of 131 cases. World J Surg. 2010;34(8):1954–8. doi:10.1007/s00268-010-0591-4.
13. Rawlings AL, Woodland JH, Crawford DL. Telerobotic surgery for right and sigmoid colectomies: 30 consecutive cases. Surg Endosc. 2006;20(11):1713–8. doi:10.1007/s00464-005-0771-8.
14. deSouza AL, Prasad LM, Park JJ, Marecik SJ, Blumetti J, Abcarian H. Robotic assistance in right hemicolectomy: is there a role? Dis Colon Rectum. 2010;53(7):1000–6. doi:10.1007/DCR.0b013e3181d32096.
15. Rawlings AL, Woodland JH, Vegunta RK, Crawford DL. Robotic versus laparoscopic colectomy. Surg Endosc. 2007;21(10):1701–8. doi:10.1007/s00464-007-9231-y.
16. Luca F, Ghezzi TL, Valvo M, Cenciarelli S, Pozzi S, Radice D et al. Surgical and pathological outcomes after right hemicolectomy: case-matched study comparing robotic and open surgery. The International Journal of Medical Robotics + Computer Assisted Surgery: IJMRCAS. 2011. doi:10.1002/rcs.398.
17. Park JS, Choi GS, Park SY, Kim HJ, Ryuk JP. Randomized clinical trial of robot-assisted versus standard laparoscopic right colectomy. Br J Surg. 2012;99(9):1219–26. doi:10.1002/bjs.8841.
18. Ostrowitz MB, Eschete D, Zemon H, DeNoto G. Robotic-assisted single-incision right colectomy: early experience. The International Journal of Medical Robotics + Computer Assisted Surgery: IJMRCAS. 2009;5(4):465–70. doi:10.1002/rcs.281.
19. Morelli L, Guadagni S, Caprili G, Di Candio G, Boggi U, Mosca F. Robotic right colectomy using the Da Vinci Single-Site(R) platform: case report. The International Journal of Medical Robotics + Computer Assisted Surgery: IJMRCAS. 2013;9(3):258–61. doi:10.1002/rcs.1488.
20. Lassen K, Soop M, Nygren J, Cox PB, Hendry PO, Spies C, et al. Consensus review of optimal perioperative care in colorectal surgery: enhanced recovery after surgery (ERAS) group recommendations. Arch Surg (Chicago, IL: 1960). 2009;144(10):961–9. doi:10.1001/archsurg.2009.170.

## Key Operative Steps

1. Establish pneumoperitoneum with a Veress needle.
2. Mark out the robotic port sites.
3. Insert a conventional laparoscopic camera port in left iliac fossa and perform initial diagnostic laparoscopy.
4. Insert additional ports under direct vision in the right iliac fossa, suprapubic region, right flank, and right upper quadrant.
5. Position patient securely in Trendelenburg and left side down.
6. Position the robotic cart over the patient's right shoulder and dock the robotic arms.
7. Perform medial-to-lateral dissection with high ligation of the ileocolic pedicle.
8. Extend the retroperitoneal "cave" while protecting the duodenum and right ureter.
9. Divide the terminal ileum and mesentery.
10. Mobilize the hepatic flexure.
11. Divide the remaining vessels (right colic vessels and right branch of the middle colic artery).
12. Perform intracorporeal or extracorporeal anastomosis.
13. Retrieve the specimen and check for hemostasis.

# Open Left Colectomy

# 18

Robert D. Madoff and Mark Y. Sun

## Introduction

Surgical resection remains the foundation for curative treatment of colon cancer. A proper oncologic resection comprises: (1) a complete en bloc removal of the tumor along with any extracolonic involvement, (2) clear proximal, distal, and radial margins, and (3) an adequate clearance of locoregional lymph nodes. The manner in which the resection is performed may vary, e.g., laparoscopic vs. robotic vs. open, but the principles remain the same.

This chapter will specifically focus on open left hemicolectomy with emphasis on mobilization of the left colon, determination of an adequate lymphadectomy, and various reconstructive techniques to restore bowel continuity. We will highlight proper anatomic understanding of the vasculature and lymphatic drainage when approaching surgery in order to ensure a proper oncologic resection.

R.D. Madoff, M.D., F.A.C.S., F.A.S.C.R.S. (✉)
Division of Colon and Rectal Surgery,
Department of Surgery, University of Minnesota,
MMC 450, 420 Delaware St. SE, Minneapolis,
MN 55455, USA
e-mail: Madoff@umn.edu

M.Y. Sun, M.D.
Division of Colon and Rectal Surgery,
Department of Surgery, University of Minnesota
1055 Westgate Drive, Suite 190, Saint Paul,
MN 55114, USA
e-mail: msun@crsal.org

## Indications

A left hemicolectomy is most commonly indicated for: (1) biopsy-proven malignancy, (2) endoscopically unresectable polyps, and (3) recurrent/high-risk polyps. In each of these circumstances an oncologic resection should be performed. In situations involving endoscopically unresectable polyps or high-risk polyps, a formal resection is still recommended because of the risk that the lesion may harbor an underlying malignancy.

## Anatomic Considerations

The left colon can present unique surgical difficulties due to its inconsistent vascular supply. In general, the mid/distal transverse colon is supplied by the left branch of the middle colic artery, which is the first branch off the superior mesenteric artery. The descending colon is supplied by the left colic artery, which is the first branch off the inferior mesenteric artery. The sigmoid colon is perfused by multiple branches arising from the superior hemorrhoidal artery, which is the terminal branch of the inferior mesenteric artery. The area of the splenic flexure is supplied by a vascular arcade known as the marginal artery of

J. Kim and J. Garcia-Aguilar (eds.), *Surgery for Cancers of the Gastrointestinal Tract: A Step-by-Step Approach*,
DOI 10.1007/978-1-4939-1893-5_18, © Springer Science+Business Media New York 2015

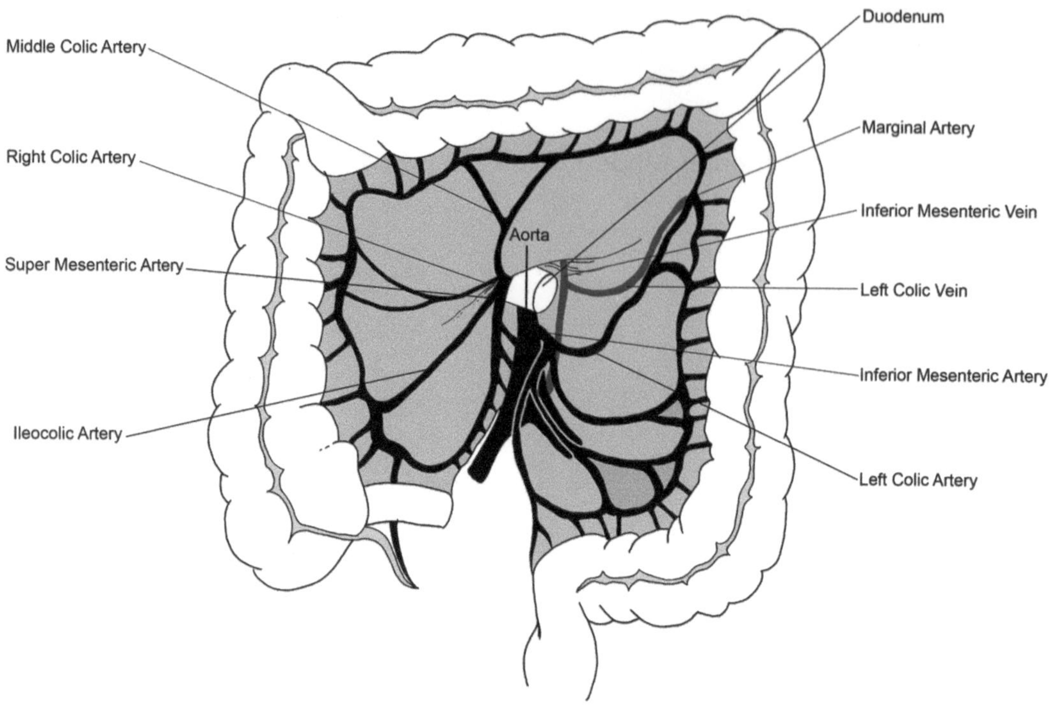


**Fig. 18.1** This figure shows the major vessels of the colon that must be identified during open left colectomy. The marginal artery of Drummond is the collateral vessel between the superior and inferior mesenteric arteries

Drummond that acts as a collateral bridge between the superior and inferior mesenteric circulations (Fig. 18.1). Unfortunately, the marginal artery can be insufficient or absent in 4–20 % of cases, which is the reason this area of the colon is considered a watershed area [1]. This anomaly can become of clinical significance when the left colic or inferior mesenteric artery is ligated and one is planning to perform an anastomosis using the splenic flexure or descending colon. In this case, the absence of a marginal artery will lead to an inadequate blood supply to the proximal colon. Under these circumstances, an extended left hemicolectomy or a subtotal colectomy would be warranted.

The venous drainage mirrors the arterial supply. The small and intermediate veins eventually join to become the inferior mesenteric vein. The inferior mesenteric vein courses within the mesentery just lateral to the duodenum and eventually drains into the splenic vein. The splenic and superior mesenteric veins then merge to create the portal vein.

Lymphatic drainage follows the vascular supply. Colonic resection is often determined by the margins of devascularized colon following an adequate lymphadenectomy. As the lymphatics are thought to be an early site of tumor metastasis, it is imperative to have an appropriate sampling of paracolic and intermediate lymph nodes to be considered an adequate oncologic resection. A minimum retrieval of 12 lymph nodes has been adopted as a quality measure by many groups. However, node count is influenced not only by surgical technique, but also by adequacy of pathologic assessment, patient-related factors (e.g., age) and tumor-related factors (e.g., tumor location, T stage, or microsatellite status).

There is debate as to the extent of lymphadenectomy required for optimal oncologic clearance. Several authors have advocated the widespread adoption of "complete mesocolic excision" (CME) with anatomic dissection of the mesocolon along its embryological fascial planes and high ligation of the vascular pedicle (e.g., for left colon cancer, the origin of the inferior mesenteric artery and vein). While excellent results have been reported by experienced CME surgeons, randomized trials comparing CME to conventional resection have not been performed.

## Preoperative Management

A thorough preoperative workup is necessary to afford patients the greatest chance for a positive outcome following surgery. All patients should undergo a complete history and physical exam. All medical comorbidities should be optimized prior to surgery and any further cardiovascular or pulmonary workup should be performed when deemed appropriate.

If a complete colonoscopic evaluation was not previously performed, it should be done to rule out synchronous tumors and polyps. The tumor should be tattooed in at least 3 and preferably 4 quadrants to aid in intraoperative identification of the area in question. Tattooing becomes especially important when operating for smaller lesions or endoscopically unresectable/high-risk polyps. Basic lab work including hemoglobin, platelet count, comprehensive metabolic panel to check for renal and hepatic function, and carcinoembryonic antigen (CEA) should be performed. Not all colon malignancies will secrete CEA, but for those that do it is helpful in the surveillance of patients postoperatively as it is usually one of the first signs of recurrence.

A complete metastatic workup should also be performed consisting of a computed tomographic (CT) scan of the chest, abdomen, and pelvis with oral and intravenous (IV) contrast. If the tumor is found to be locally invasive, i.e., involving any surrounding organs or structures, preoperative consultation with surgical specialists would be beneficial to ensure that an en bloc, curative resection could be performed at the time of surgery. If there is any question to the resectability of a locally invasive lesion or if there are indeterminate hepatic lesions, a magnetic resonance imaging (MRI) scan can be helpful in aiding preoperative decision making.

If distant disease is identified and the patient is otherwise asymptomatic from the primary lesion, consideration should be given to systemic therapy with chemotherapy prior to surgery. In the situation of distant disease, overall survival will be tied to the effectiveness of systemic treatment and not to the resection of the primary tumor. After treatment with chemotherapy, restaging should be performed. For patients with resectable metastases, options include resection of the metastases first, resection of the primary first, or in patients with hepatic metastases, minimal medical comorbidities, and good performance status, a synchronous procedure to remove both the primary and metastatic lesions. Resection of the primary tumor in the face of unresectable metastases is a controversial issue, but in general, resection should be avoided unless the patient is symptomatic from the primary lesion or if there is clear evidence of impending obstruction.

The day prior to surgery the patient should be maintained on a clear liquid diet and consideration of a mechanical bowel preparation. There have been numerous studies to demonstrate the safety and potential benefits of performing elective colon resections without prior mechanical bowel preparation. However, in cases involving small tumors or malignant polyps, consideration should be given to mechanical bowel preparation to allow the possibility of performing intraoperative colonoscopy for possible localization of the lesion.

## Perioperative Preparation

Prior to the patient being transferred into the operating room, a prophylactic dose of antibiotic as well as 5,000 units of subcutaneous heparin should be administered within 1 h of incision. Various antibiotic regimens are acceptable, but our preference is to use 1 g of IV ertapenem (Merck, Whitehouse Station, NJ) as it is a single dose that will last for 24 h. In addition, patients should be maintained with an active warming device in the preoperative area to achieve normothermia (>36 °C).

After the induction of general anesthesia, the patient is placed into a modified low lithotomy position. The arms are abducted in such a position to allow for future placement of a self-retaining retractor. Care must be taken to ensure that both shoulders, elbows, and calves are appropriately positioned/padded to avoid positional neuropathies. A sterile Foley catheter and an orogastric tube are placed. The abdomen is then prepped with a chlorhexidine solution and towels are used to square off the operative field. A plastic adhesive is then placed over the abdomen to secure the towels in place. A "time out" is performed to confirm the patient's identity and the planned operation.

## Incision

A midline laparotomy incision is made (Fig. 18.2). The extent of the incision will vary depending on the portion of the left colon being removed. For distal lesions, a lower midline incision down to the pubic bone may be sufficient. For proximal lesions near the splenic flexure, extension of the incision to the xiphoid process may be required. Once an adequate incision has been made, a plastic wound protector is placed

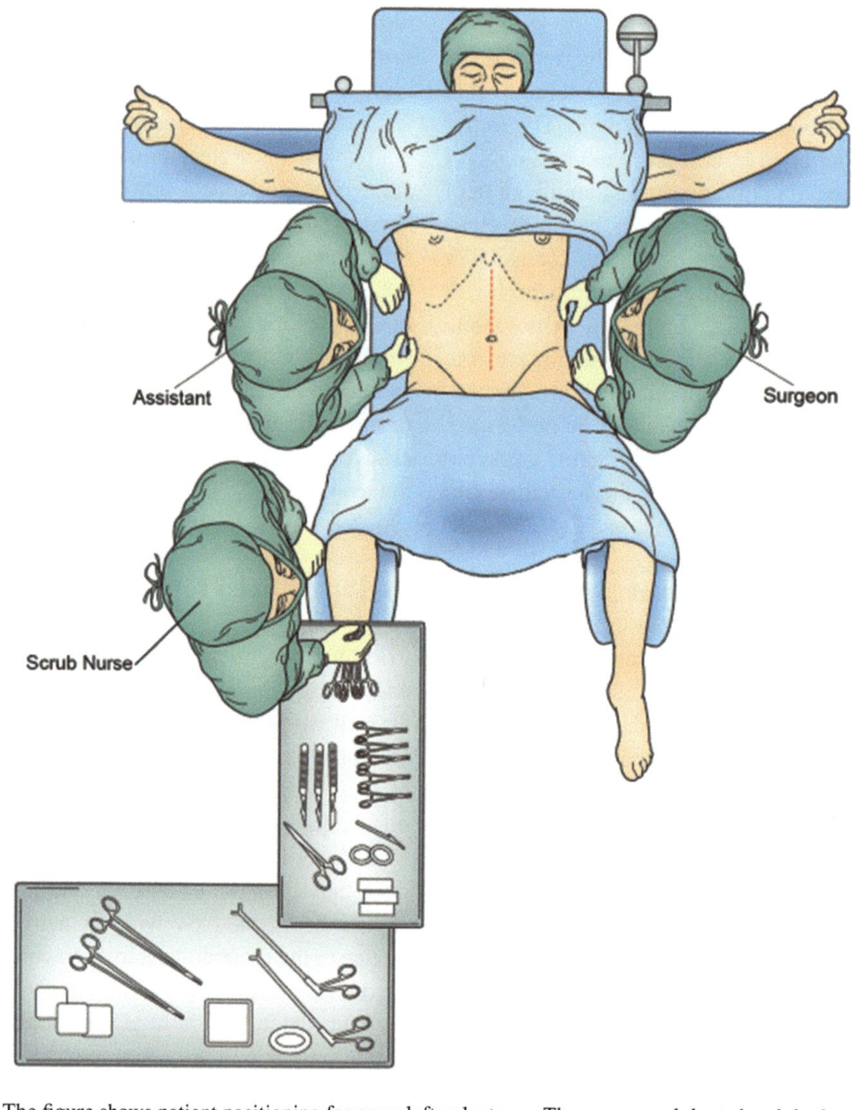


**Fig. 18.2** The figure shows patient positioning for open left colectomy. The arms are abducted and the legs are placed in lithotomy position

into the wound to not only aid in prevention of contamination of the wound itself, but also to aid in maximizing the exposure for any given incision.

## Examination of the Peritoneal Cavity

A complete abdominal exploration should then be undertaken to rule out the presence of metastatic disease as well as to confirm the location of the lesion in question. Both lobes of the liver should be palpated and the peritoneal surfaces visually inspected. Both ovaries should be inspected for possible metastatic disease. Unexpected masses/nodules should be biopsied and sent for frozen section. If carcinomatosis is encountered, closure of the abdomen and referral for either systemic therapy or heated intraperitoneal chemotherapy and tumor debulking may be warranted.

Once distant disease has been ruled out, a self-retaining retractor should be placed to maintain exposure. For distal lesions it is advantageous to keep the ring of the retractor close to the patient's skin and center the ring at the lower portion of the incision. For proximal lesions and splenic flexure mobilization it is helpful to position the ring more cephalad and to the left. It is often helpful during splenic flexure mobilization to place the ring at an angle, with the left/superior aspect of the ring elevated several inches off the abdominal wall to provide anterior retraction and improve visualization of the flexure. The surgeon should not hesitate to move the ring and reset the retractors to optimize exposure during various phases of the case. The small bowel is then packed into the right upper quadrant with moist laparotomy pads.

## Extent of Resection

Once proper exposure has been established, it is necessary to determine the extent of resection that will be required. The lymphadenectomy will often times dictate the margins of resection. For splenic flexure lesions, proper lymphadenectomy will require ligation of the left branch of the middle colic artery at its base as well as ligation of the left colic artery as it takes off from the inferior mesenteric artery. For left colon cancers the left branch of the middle colic, left colic, and possibly the first sigmoidal branch need to be ligated depending on the location of the tumor. For sigmoid lesions the superior hemorrhoidal artery is ligated distal to the take-off of the left colic artery and the distal extent will be within the proximal rectal mesentery (Fig. 18.3). We do not advocate routine ligation of the inferior mesenteric artery itself, as there have been no studies to prove an oncologic benefit to a high ligation. Occasionally this may be necessary if a concerning lymph node is identified or to obtain adequate length for a tension-free

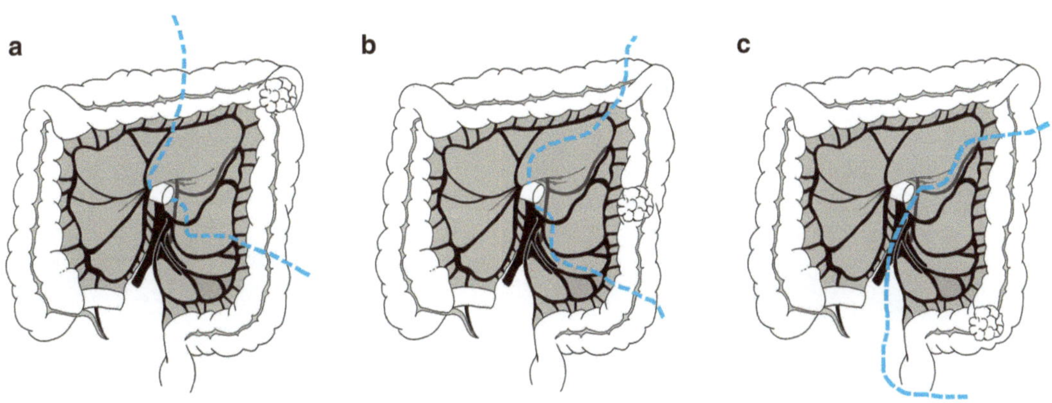


**Fig. 18.3** The figure illustrates the extent of resection for (**a**) splenic flexure lesion, (**b**) descending colon lesion, and (**c**) sigmoid colon lesion

anastomosis. High ligation is also easier when the entire left side of the colon (including sigmoid) is being removed, such as in the case of synchronous lesions, uncertain location of a previously resected malignant polyp, or the presence of significant diverticular disease when operating for descending colon cancer.

## Mobilization

The operating surgeon should stand on the patient's left side with the assistant either on the right side or between the legs. Mobilization should begin with separating the sigmoid colon from the retroperitoneum and left pelvic sidewall. The assistant begins by retracting the sigmoid colon medially while the operating surgeon dissects the sigmoid colon from the peritoneum using electrocautery. When performed properly, this will expose the peritoneal reflection along the sigmoid mesentery and lead to the avascular plane that will be carried up along the descending colon and eventually the splenic flexure. It is imperative to enter into the proper avascular plane as dissecting too deeply into the retroperitoneum could lead to troublesome venous bleeding or injury to the ureter. Once the gonadal vessels and left ureter are identified in the retroperitoneum, the peritoneum is then incised medially along the white line of Toldt to separate the lateral attachments of the left colon (Fig. 18.4).

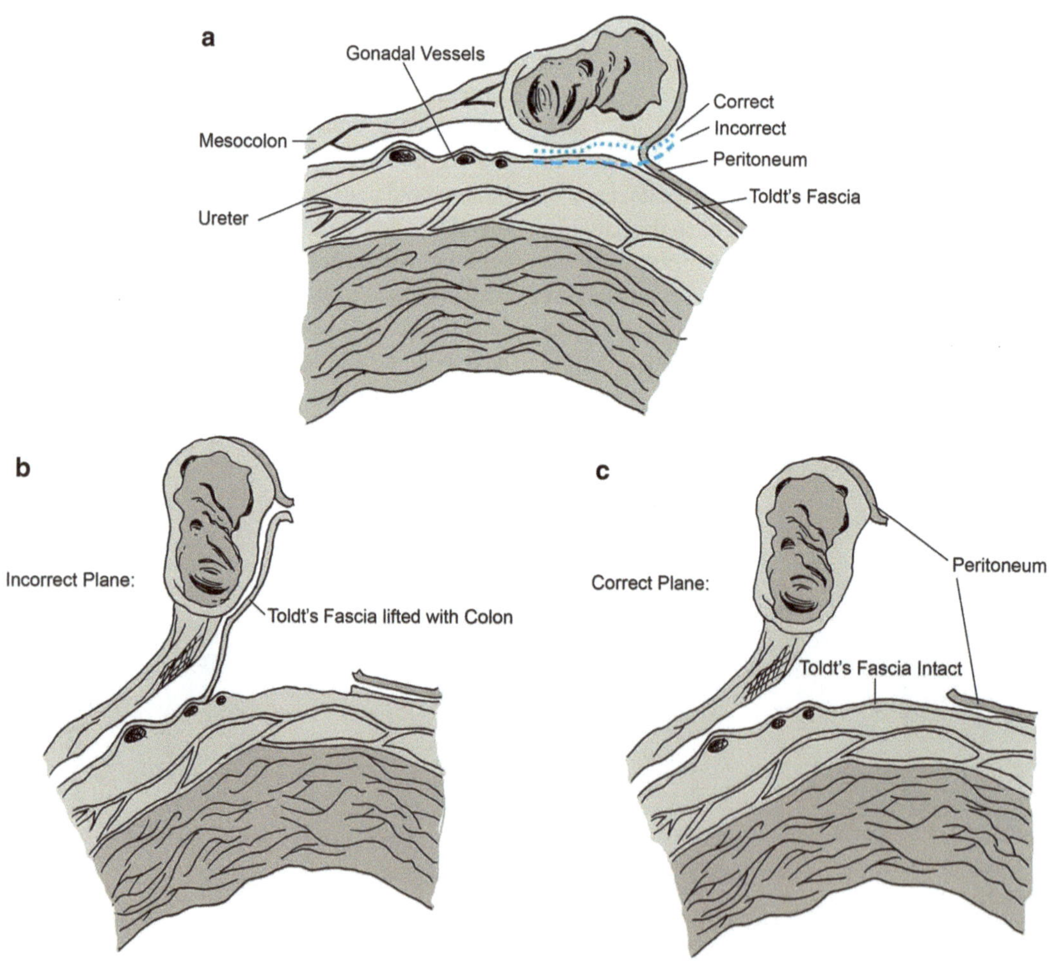


**Fig. 18.4** Proper lateral dissection of the left colon requires careful dissection of the peritoneum from Toldt's fascia. (**a**) Correct and incorrect planes of resection. (**b**) The result of incorrect plane of resection. (**c**) The result of correct plane of resection

Once the peritoneum is incised, the mesentery of the sigmoid colon and left colon can often be dissected anterior to Toldt's fascia using a combination of gentle blunt dissection with a sponge stick and cautery. One should be aware when dissecting the left colon mesentery off of the retroperitoneum that it becomes quite thin at its base and it is easy to make a hole through the mesentery. Care must be taken that if a mesenteric defect is made that the small bowel is not injured on the other side. The gonadal vessels and left ureter should constantly be gently swept laterally to keep them out of the operative field. Once the mesenteries of the sigmoid and left colon are appropriately medialized, it can then be used as a fan retractor to keep the small bowel out of the way while mobilizing the splenic flexure.

After the sigmoid and left colon have been mobilized, the self-retaining retractor should be moved to the left upper quadrant to expose the splenic flexure. The separation of the lateral attachments is carried superiorly to the tip of the spleen. The operating surgeon then follows the wall of the colon using blunt finger dissection, exposing the splenocolic attachments for division by electrocautery or with a vessel sealing energy device. This maneuver is best performed with the surgeon positioned between the patient's legs and the first assistant on the patient's right side. The surgeon must take great care to avoid excessive traction on the colon, which can lead to splenic injury. If difficulty is encountered during the distal-to-proximal dissection, it is often helpful to work in the proximal-to-distal direction. The omentum is separated from the distal transverse colon to enter into the lesser sac. The remainder of the splenocolic attachments is then divided and the mesentery completely mobilized off the retroperitoneum. Full mobilization of the splenic flexure occurs once the tail of the pancreas is visualized at the base of the dissected mesentery.

## Anastomosis: Colo-colonic

In all cases, we advocate complete mobilization of the colon along with division of the necessary mesentery prior to any division of the bowel wall. Once the mesentery and all the major vascular pedicles have been divided on both the proximal and distal ends, this will allow for demarcation of the colon prior to creation of the anastomosis. Once the proximal and distal resection margins have been chosen, those sites are then completely cleared of their remaining mesentery all the way down to the bowel wall. A decision for reconstructive technique of the anastomosis must then be made with the options being stapled vs. hand-sewn.

If a stapled anastomosis is chosen, our preference is to use an in-line technique to create a side-to-side functional end-to-end anastomosis (Fig. 18.5). Fully dividing the mesentery of the specimen first, and then aligning the bowel walls of the anastomosis obviates the risk of placing a twist into the remaining mesentery once the anastomosis is completed. Towels are then laid around the bowel to be resected to minimize contamination. Colotomies are then made along the antimesenteric taeniae of the proximal and distal colon, and positioned so that they will be eventually resected with the specimen. A gastrointestinal anastomosis (GIA) 75-mm stapler is then placed through the colotomies into both limbs of the proximal and distal bowel. The stapler is then fired to create the common channel of the anastomosis. On withdrawal of the stapler, the staple line is inspected for hemostasis. Allis clamps are then used to offset the staple lines as well as close the edges of the common colotomy in a transverse fashion. A thoraco-abdominal (TA) 90-mm stapler is then placed below the common colotomy in the area of the bowel that had been previously cleared of mesentery. The stapler is then fired and the specimen separated from the newly created anastomosis. Hemostasis of the transverse staple line is then controlled with suture ligatures. A 3-0 absorbable suture is then used to reinforce the crotch of the anastomosis.

Our preference is to use a hand-sewn end-to-end anastomosis unless there is a significant size discrepancy between the proximal and distal bowel. A hand-sewn anastomosis can be performed in either a 1-layer or 2-layer fashion. Our favored technique is a modified 1-layer anastomosis. The mesentery is completely cleared

a

b

c

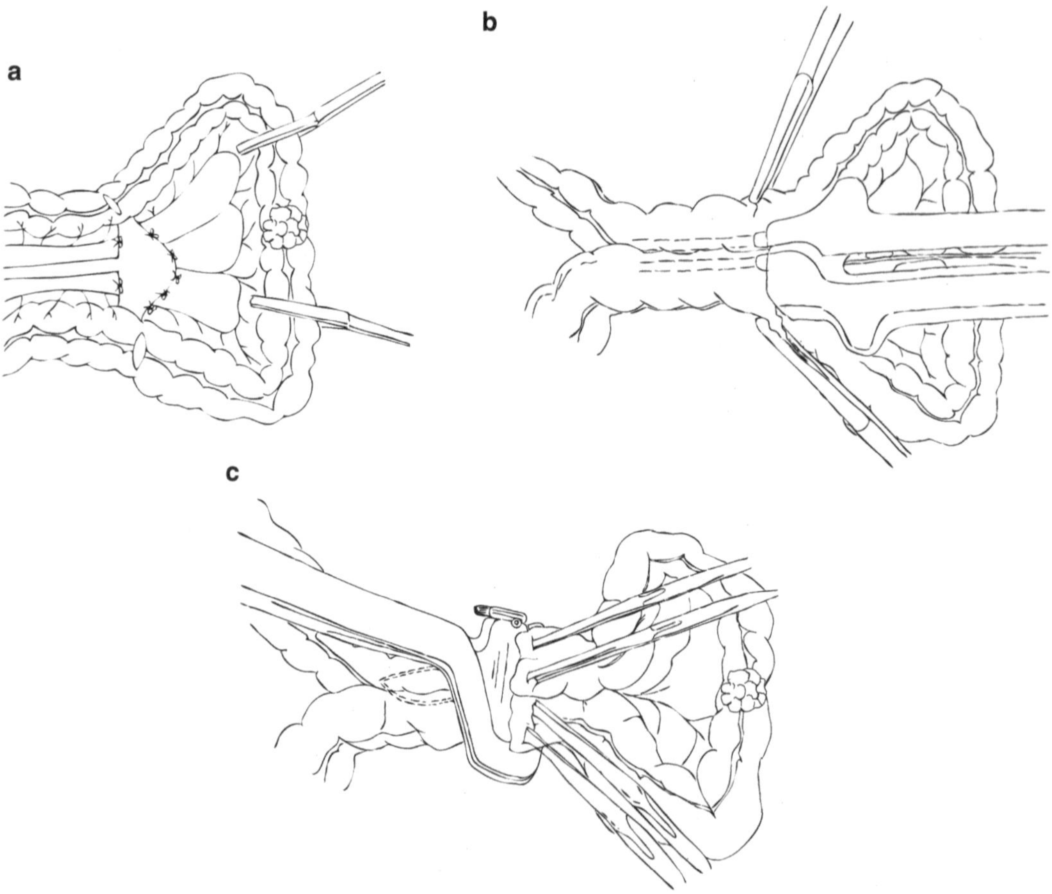

**Fig. 18.5** The technique for stapled anastomosis. (**a**) The mesentery is fully divided and colotomies are made along the anti-mesenteric taeniae of the proximal and distal colon. (**b**) A linear stapler is placed through the colotomies and fired to create the anastomosis. (**c**) A TA stapler is used to divide and close the colon

down to the bowel wall at the site of the proximal and distal resection just like with a stapled anastomosis. At both the proximal and distal resection sites, the bowel wall is clamped on the patient side with a noncrushing clamp (e.g., Dennis clamp) and with a crushing clamp (e.g., Kocher clamp) on the specimen side. The Dennis clamp is closed only 1-click to minimize trauma to the bowel wall. The specimen is then separated from the patient by cutting between the Dennis and Kocher clamps with a knife. It is important not to cut directly on top of the Dennis clamp but instead to leave a small 1–2 mm cuff of colon on top of the clamp so that the bowel does not slip through. The Dennis clamps are then arranged to approximate the two ends of the bowel to be anastomosed (Fig. 18.6). A seromuscular Lembert stitch of 4-0 silk is then placed on either corner of the bowel and secured, untied, with a hemostat to maintain orientation. Interrupted 4-0 silk Lembert stitches on a small (i.e., RB-1) needle are then placed along the antimesenteric side of the bowel. When placing this row of stitches, it is suggested to serially bisect the anastomosis to ensure that the stitches are all evenly spaced. The stitches are placed 6–8 mm apart and all of these stitches are left untied. Once the antimesenteric side is completed, the Dennis clamps are rotated 180° to expose the mesenteric side of the anastomosis. At this point the small 1–2 mm cuff of colon that was previously left on the Dennis clamp is

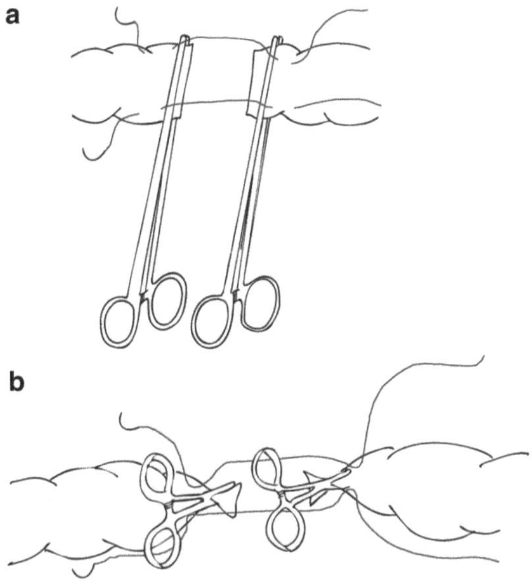

**Fig. 18.6** The technique for handsewn one-layer anastomosis. (**a**) Dennis clamps are used to align the two ends of the colon and seromuscular interrupted sutures are placed. (**b**) Transverse view of the alignment of the Dennis clamps and placement of sutures

trimmed flush to the clamp so that the eventual anastomosis is well opposed. We then place another row of 4-0 interrupted silk stitches in the same manner. Once the mesenteric side is completed, the Dennis clamps are then removed and the lumen of both sides of the colon are opened to make sure none of the stitches caught the back wall. All of the 4-0 silk stitches are then tied down and the tails are left long. We then use a 4-0 double-armed absorbable stitch to sew around the entire anastomosis in a full-thickness running fashion, using the silk suture tails to elevate the portion of bowel being sewn. The use of a double-armed stitch allows the surgeon to sew in both directions along the anastomosis. When placing this stitch, the previously placed silk stitches are essentially ignored and the running stitch is placed as if one were performing a routine 1-layer anastomosis. Our rationale for this modified 1-layer approach is that the first layer of 4-0 silk stitches inverts the bowel ends and lines them up to make it easier to perform an even, well-spaced 1-layer anastomosis.

## Anastomosis: Colo-rectal

For tumors in the mid to distal sigmoid colon, an end-to-end stapled anastomosis is our reconstruction method of choice. Again, the entire mesentery of the specimen is divided prior to transecting the bowel wall, and the bowel ends are cleared of fat. We find it is generally easier to eventually pass the circular stapler if the upper portion of the rectum is mobilized. Once the resection margins have been cleared, a decision must be made to either perform a double-stapled end-to-end anastomosis or a double-purse-string end-to-end anastomosis. Our preference is to perform a double-purse-string anastomosis to avoid crossing staple lines. However, if the anastomosis sits too low in the pelvis to comfortably sew a purse-string stitch or there is significant size mismatch of the proximal colon and the distal rectum, then a double-stapled technique is employed.

In order to perform a double-purse-string anastomosis, the proximal resection margin is clamped with a Dennis clamp on the patient side and a Kocher clamp on the specimen side. The specimen is then cut between the two clamps with a knife. Two right-angled Glassman clamps are then placed on the distal resection margin. Prior to division of the distal resection margin, a dilute betadine solution is used to irrigate the rectum to clear it of any remaining fecal material. Once the rectum is cleared, the specimen is then removed by cutting between the two Glassman clamps. The distal Glassman clamp is then removed and a 2-0 double-armed prolene stitch is then used to create a purse-string stitch around the rectum in a running baseball fashion. The purse-string is then pulled tight to help prevent contamination and the two ends of the stitch are secured with a hemostat. Attention is then turned to the proximal portion of the anastomosis. A second 2-0 double-armed prolene suture is again used to create another purse-string stitch in the proximal bowel in the same manner. The purse-string is again pulled tight to prevent fecal contamination. The assistant then goes between the legs in order to pass the circular stapler up the rectum. We recommend passing the entire stapler up the rectum intact with the anvil attached. The smooth edges of the anvil help ease the stapler to the top of the rectal stump without getting caught on the rectal valves. If there is difficulty advancing the stapler all the way to the top of the rectal stump, the operating surgeon can place a finger into the rectum from the top of the rectal stump to help guide the stapler into proper position. Once it is at the top of the rectal stump, the stapler is then opened by the assistant and the anvil is advanced into the abdomen under direct vision. The operating surgeon then removes the anvil from the post of the stapler and secures the distal purse-string stitch around the stapler. The anvil is then placed into the proximal bowel and secured in place with the other previously placed purse-string stitch. The anvil and the post of the stapler are then reunited and then closed under direct vision. Care must be taken that the orientation of the proximal bowel is such that the proximal mesentery is not twisted and no epiploicae are pulled into the anastomosis. In women, it is also important to ensure the vagina is free of the stapler prior to firing. The stapler is then fired, released, and removed. The integrity of the anastomotic donuts is then inspected to ensure that they are complete. A rigid proctoscopy is then performed to check the anastomosis for hemostasis as well as to perform a leak test.

A double-stapled anastomosis is performed in a similar fashion. Once the proximal and distal resection sites have been cleared of mesentery, the proximal margin is again clamped between a Dennis clamp on the patient side and a Kocher clamp on the specimen side. The proximal margin is then cut between the two clamps with a knife. A TA 45-mm stapler is then used to secure the distal resection margin and fired to completely separate the specimen. A 2-0 double-armed prolene stitch is then used to create the purse-string in the proximal bowel and the anvil of the circular stapler is secured in place. The assistant then goes between the patient's legs and the stapler is passed to the top of the rectal stump under the guidance of the operating surgeon. Once the stapler is felt to be flush and centered with the transverse staple line, the post of the stapler is advanced through the top of the rectal stump. The anvil is then reunited with the stapler and the anastomosis completed in the same fashion as previously described.

## Postoperative Care

The orogastric tube is removed prior to extubation. If there were previous signs of obstruction, the orogastric tube can be converted to a nasogastric tube. The patient should then be maintained on a crystalloid fluid for the first 24–48 h until the initial resuscitation is completed. Strict monitoring of both intake and output is vital to ensure adequate tissue perfusion. Intravenous fluids should be minimized as much as possible to avoid bowel edema and the chances of postoperative ileus. Prophylactic subcutaneous heparin (5,000 units Q8h) is continued on the day of the operation as long as bleeding is not a major concern. Postoperative pain can be managed with either an epidural or a patient-controlled analgesia (PCA) pump. Use of nonnarcotic analgesics can also be helpful to minimize the chances of postoperative ileus. Ambulation as well as incentive spirometry is encouraged to begin on postoperative day #0. If a beta-blocker was used preoperatively, this should be continued intravenously until intestinal function returns. No further antibiotic prophylaxis is warranted 24 h postsurgery.

On postoperative day #1, the diet is advanced to clear liquids as long as there is no nausea or vomiting. The urinary catheter is also removed as long as the urine output is adequate; the presence of an epidural is only a relative indication for continuation of the catheter. Urinary retention rates remain <10 % even in the presence of a thoracic epidural [2]. Once the patient begins passing flatus, the diet can be advanced to a soft mechanical/low-fiber diet. Medications are all transitioned to the oral route and the patient is prepared for discharge home.

A postoperative fever must always raise concern for abdominal abscess or possible anastomotic leak. Urinary, pulmonary, and wound complications are certainly more common causes of fever, but an anastomotic leak is always something to be considered due to the potential severity of its consequences. If there is suspicion for a leak, a CT of the abdomen/pelvis or a water-soluble contrast enema should be performed. Performing a CT prior to postoperative day 5 is generally not recommended as the postsurgical artifact is such that it makes interpretation difficult, though we do not hesitate to obtain an earlier scan if clinical circumstances warrant it. The grade of anastomotic leak will determine management. If the patient remains hemodynamically stable and tissue perfusion remains adequate, consideration to bowel rest, IV antibiotics and possibly a percutaneous drain can be a reasonable alternative. If fevers persist, abdominal pain worsens, or hemodynamic instability develops, immediate operative reexploration should be undertaken and most often results in a diverting stoma along with wide abdominal drainage. The type of diversion depends upon the size and location of the leak. Complete or near-complete disruptions at any level generally require complete takedown of the stoma with Hartmann closure and proximal end colostomy. Minor leaks, especially in the low pelvis, are often best treated with washout, drainage, and proximal loop ileostomy.

## References

1. The ASCRS Textbook of Colon and Rectal Surgery. 2nd ed. New York: Springer; 2011.
2. Basse L, Werner M, Kehlet H. Is urinary drainage necessary during continuous epidural analgesia after colonic resection? Reg Anesth Pain Med. 2000;25(5): 498–501. doi:10.1053/rapm.2000.9537.

## Key Operative Steps

1. A midline laparotomy incision is made.
2. Begin mobilization by separating the sigmoid colon from the retroperitoneum and left pelvic sidewall. Expose the peritoneal reflection leading to the avascular plane that runs from the sigmoid mesentery up to the splenic flexure.
3. Once the gonadal vessels and left ureter are identified, then incise the white line of Toldt to separate the lateral attachments of the left colon.
4. The mesentery of the sigmoid and left colon can be dissected anterior to Toldt's fascia.
5. Perform takedown of the splenic flexure and visualize the tail of the pancreas.
6. The extent of resection will depend on the location of the tumor. For splenic flexure lesions, ligate the left branch of the middle colic artery and left colic artery. For left colon cancers, the left branch of the middle colic, left colic, and first sigmoidal branch are ligated. For sigmoid lesions, the superior hemorrhoidal artery is ligated distal to the takeoff of the left colic artery.
7. Divide the mesentery prior to division of the bowel wall to allow for demarcation.
8. Perform stapled anastomosis by dividing the mesentery first. Align the bowel walls and create colotomies along the antimesenteric taeniae of the proximal and distal colon. Use a GIA stapler for the anastomosis. Use a TA stapler to divide and close the colon.
9. Perform hand-sewn anastomosis in a 1-layer fashion. Align the ends of the colon with Dennis clamps and use interrupted seromuscular sutures to create the anastomosis.
10. For distal tumors consider using a circular stapler for the anastomosis.

# Laparoscopic Left Colectomy 19

Tushar Samdani and Julio Garcia-Aguilar

## Introduction

The laparoscopic approach to colon resection for cancer has several advantages over the open approach, such as shorter hospital stay, reduced postoperative ileus, earlier resumption of oral nutritional intake, reduced pain, and improved cosmesis [1–3]. Despite initial reluctance to perform laparoscopic colectomy for colon cancer due to concerns over port-site recurrence and substandard oncologic outcomes, multiple studies have established the oncologic equivalence of laparoscopy with open surgery [4–7]. In the United States, approximately half of all colon cancer resections are performed via laparoscopy [8]. There are no absolute contraindications for laparoscopic colon cancer surgery; however, patients with intestinal obstruction, patients with previous multiple abdominal surgeries and extensive abdominal adhesions, and patients who cannot tolerate lengthy pneumoperitoneum may be better served with an open surgical approach. In this chapter, we review the essential technical steps involved in optimal laparoscopic left colectomy for cancer.

Electronic supplementary material: Supplementary material is available in the online version of this chapter at 10.1007/978-1-4939-1893-5_19. Videos can also be accessed at http://www.springerimages.com/videos/978-1-4939-1892-8.

T. Samdani, M.D.
Department of Surgery, Memorial Sloan Kettering Cancer Center, 1275 York Avenue, New York, NY 10065, USA
e-mail: tushar.samdani@googlemail.com

J. Garcia-Aguilar, M.D., Ph.D. (✉)
Department of Surgery, Benno C. Schmidt Chair in Surgical Oncology, Memorial Sloan Kettering Cancer Center, 1275 York Avenue, Room C-1067, New York, NY, USA
e-mail: garciaaj@mskcc.org

## Historical Perspective

Dennis Fowler reported the first two laparoscopic sigmoid resections in 1991 [9]. That same year Jacobs reported his experience with 20 laparoscopic colectomies, primarily for treatment of benign conditions [10]. Monson and colleagues were the first to report a larger series of colon cancer patients treated laparoscopically [11]. They described successful completion of laparoscopy in 33 of 40 patients with a median hospital stay of 8 days. Since then, laparoscopic colectomy has become more widely accepted for treatment of malignant as well as benign disease.

## Indications

As with other segmental colon resections, a left colectomy is most commonly indicated in the setting of colon cancer and colonic polyps that are too large for endoscopic resection. The left colon, extending from the middle of the transverse colon

J. Kim and J. Garcia-Aguilar (eds.), *Surgery for Cancers of the Gastrointestinal Tract: A Step-by-Step Approach*, DOI 10.1007/978-1-4939-1893-5_19, © Springer Science+Business Media New York 2015

to the rectosigmoid junction, is the most common location for colon cancer. However, a true left hemicolectomy is indicated only for tumors that are located in the portion of colon situated between the splenic flexure and the beginning of the descending colon; that is, the portion of colon located between the left colic vessels and the first sigmoidal branches. A left hemicolectomy may also be indicated in patients with synchronous tumors or polyps located between the rectosigmoid junction and the splenic flexure. Individual tumors located in the left side of the transverse colon can be treated with a segmental splenic flexure resection, which requires division of the left branch of the middle colic and the left colic vessels, or even by an extended right hemicolectomy. In contrast, tumors located in the sigmoid colon can be treated with a sigmoid colectomy [12].

## Anatomic Considerations

Laparoscopic left hemicolectomy requires a good understanding of the relationship of the mesentery and vascular supply of the left colon to the retroperitoneal structures. The left colon receives its blood supply from the superior mesenteric artery though the left branch of the middle colic artery, and from the inferior mesenteric artery (IMA) through the left colic artery and sigmoidal branches. The venous drainage follows the course of the arteries, except in the case of the inferior mesenteric vein (IMV), which has a longer course than its corresponding artery. The IMV forms from the junction of the superior rectal vein and the sigmoidal branches and drains into the splenic vein behind the pancreas. From its origin near the bifurcation of the IMA to where it joins the left colic vein the IMV runs parallel to the left colic artery. From until its junction with the splenic vein, the IMV travels without an accompanying artery.

The mesentery of the left colon overlies the iliac vessels, the left ureter, the left gonadal vessels, Gerota's fascia covering the left kidney, and the left side of the pancreas. The mesentery of the left side of the transverse colon is attached to the inferior border of the pancreas. The splenic flexure of the colon is anatomically related to the lower pole of the spleen and is anchored to the retroperitoneal structures by the phrenicocolic ligament. Preoperative computed tomographic (CT) scan imaging should be reviewed before surgery to identify all of the important anatomical structures mentioned above. Review of the CT scan also helps in planning the surgical approach and intraoperative dissection.

## Patient Preparation

Although the value of mechanical bowel preparation before colon resection is debatable, we recommend it for all patients undergoing laparoscopic colectomy. Patients are maintained on a clear liquid diet and given oral antibiotics on the day prior to surgery. Thromboembolic prophylaxis with low molecular weight heparin is started in the holding area. Intravenous antibiotics (usually a second-generation cephalosporin) are delivered before the surgical incision is made.

## Surgical Technique

### Required Instruments

- Veress needle
- Trocars: 5 mm × 2, 12 mm × 2
- Camera: endoscope 5-mm and 10-mm (our preference is a 30° or flexible tip camera)
- Laparoscopic bowel graspers
- Laparoscopic scissors
- Laparoscopic needle holder
- Laparoscopic bipolar vessel sealer device
- Small wound protector
- Laparoscopic linear stapler
- Circular stapler for end-to-end anastomosis (sizes 28-mm and 31-mm)

### Operating Room Configuration

The operating room should be spacious enough to accommodate surgeon, assistants, scrub nurse, laparoscopic tower with insufflation equipment, energy devices, and a colonoscope. As the surgeon will be working from the right side of the patient, the laparoscopic tower should be located on the

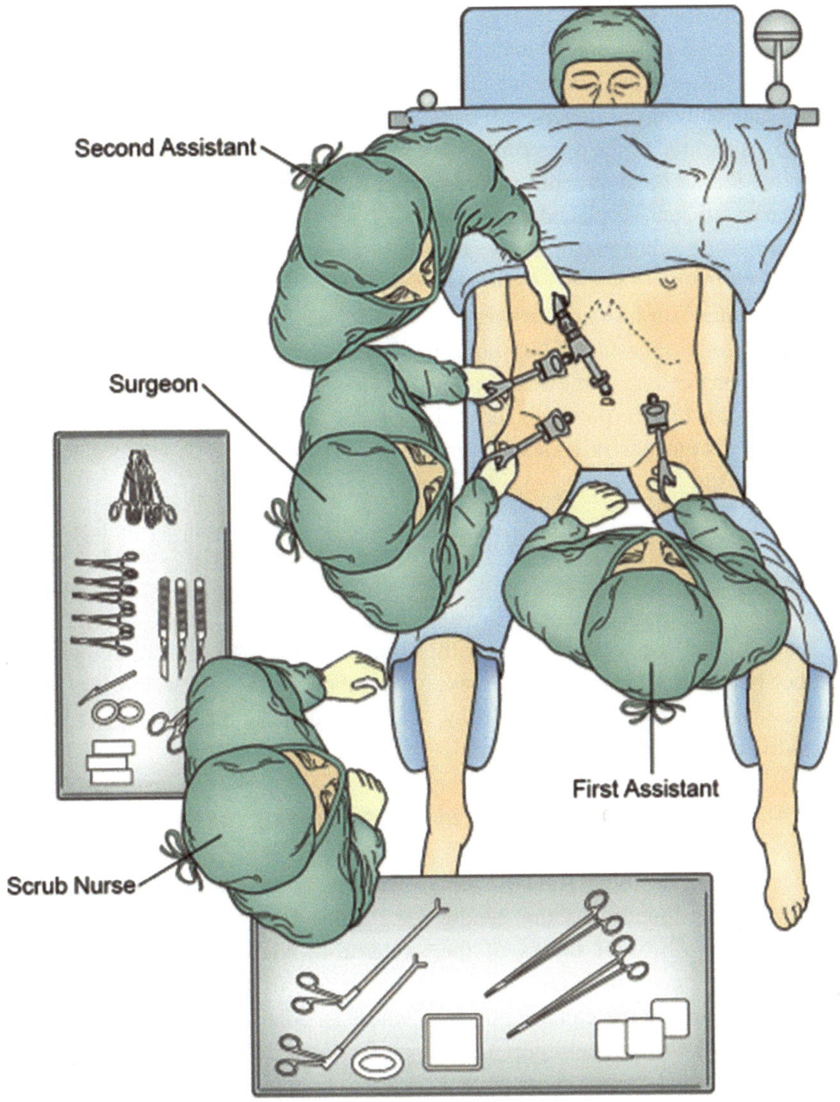


**Fig. 19.1** Operating room configuration for laparoscopic left colectomy

left side, toward the head of the table. The scrub nurse and the instrument table should also be on the right side, toward the foot of the OR table. The camera holder should be on the right side, toward the head of the table. The first assistant usually starts between the patient's legs, but he/she may change position with the operating surgeon during some portions of the procedure. Before starting, it is important to adjust video monitors and the overhead lights. Figure 19.1 shows a view of the recommended operating room configuration for laparoscopic left colectomy.

## Patient Positioning

The patient is placed in the Lloyd Davis position, with the buttocks protruding slightly over the end of the table; the thighs are abducted and aligned in a direction pointing to the contralateral shoulder. The hips, particularly on the left side, should be fully extended, and the knees flexed at 45°, so as not to interfere with the operating surgeon. Both legs should be gently rotated internally to avoid lateral pressure on the peroneal nerve. The patient's arms are placed alongside the body to lessen the possibility of shoulder injury, and provide sufficient space for the surgeon and assistant to move freely around the operating table. Pressure points and bony prominences are padded, and the body is secured to the operating table with straps around the legs and vacuum-mattress device. A urinary catheter is placed, whereas nasogastric or orogastric tubes are optional. The patient is covered with a body warmer to prevent hypothermia. Sequential compression devices are applied to the legs for deep venous thrombosis prophylaxis. Before proceeding to the next step, it is advisable to make sure that the patient is secured to the table and does not move with Trendelenburg position and left side tilt.

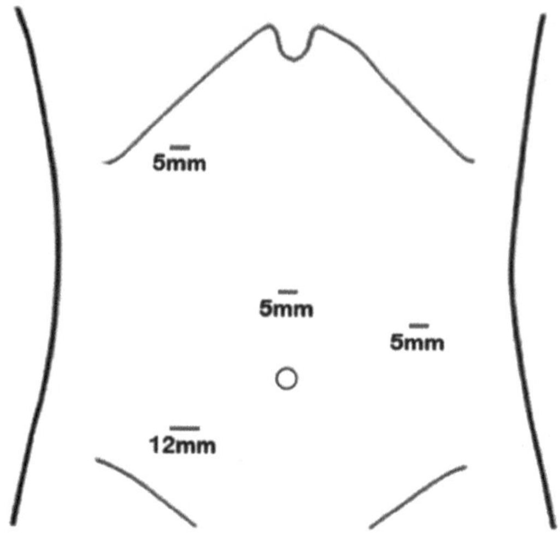


**Fig. 19.2** Trocar placement for laparoscopic left colectomy. Four trocar sites are utilized

## Port Placement

Pneumoperitoneum can be established with open technique, but we prefer to use a Veress needle because it is safe and technically easy, even in morbidly obese patients. We create a small stab incision with a 15-blade knife at Palmer's point (below the left costal margin in the mid-clavicular line). With careful insertion of the Veress needle it is possible to feel the rectus sheaths and the peritoneum as the needle penetrates through the different layers of the bowel wall. Once the pneumoperitoneum has reached 15 mmHg, we place the camera port in the umbilical region using a semiopen technique. Next, the peritoneal cavity is inspected before placing additional trocars.

The positioning of additional ports is adjusted based on the patient's body habitus (abdominal wall surface area), site of the lesion, scars, proximity to bony structures, and abdominal wall vessels. For standard left hemicolectomy, a 12-mm port is placed in the right lower quadrant on the line between the umbilicus and the anterior superior iliac spine (ASIS) (approximately 4–5 cm medial to the ASIS). A 5-mm port is placed in the right upper quadrant along the mid-clavicular line, more than a fist-length away from the 12-mm port and at least two fingerbreadths below the right costal margin. One additional 5-mm port is placed on the left side of abdomen, two fingerbreadths medial to the left ASIS (Fig. 19.2). Ports are placed under direct vision, only after the abdominal cavity has been inspected to exclude contraindications to surgery.

## Surgical Approach

The operation can be performed by mobilizing the colon first and then controlling the vessels (lateral-to-medial approach), or by controlling the vessels first and mobilizing the colon afterwards (medial-to-lateral approach). The authors prefer the medial-to-lateral approach because it allows easy visualization and control of the vascular structures, immediate delineation of the plane between the mesentery and the retroperitoneum, early identification of the left ureter and other retroperitoneal structures, and quick access to the splenic flexure.

The operating table is tilted left side up and in slight Trendelenburg position, allowing the small bowel to fall to the right upper quadrant of the abdomen. The goal is to expose the ligament of Treitz and the origin of the mesentery on the left side of the colon. This sometimes requires dividing adhesions between the small bowel and the colon mesentery. The omentum and the left side of the transverse colon should be retracted cephalad over the stomach.

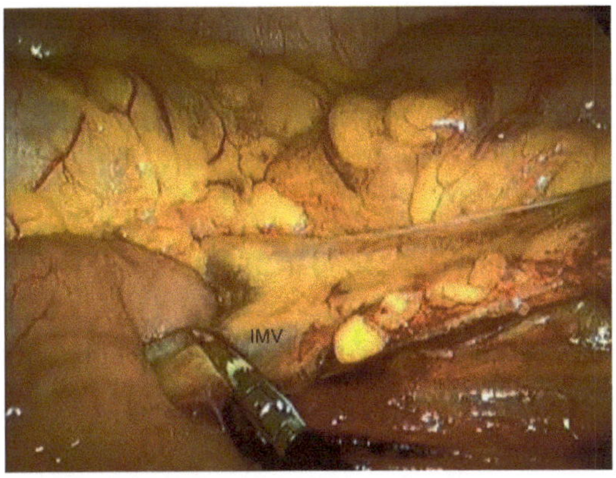


**Fig. 19.3** Division of the inferior mesenteric vein proximal to the junction of the left colic vein. The inferior mesenteric artery has been already divided

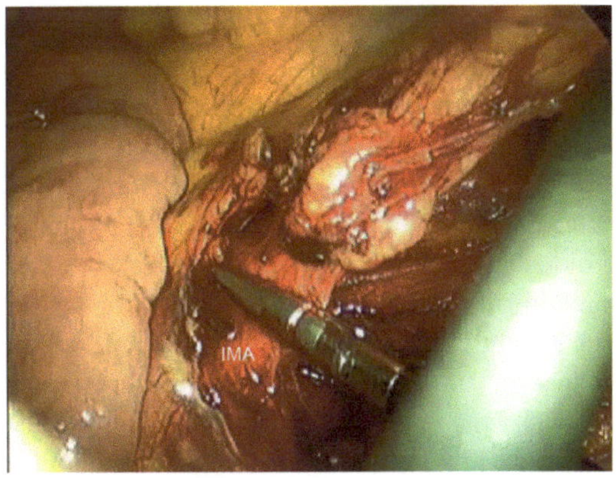


**Fig. 19.4** Division of the inferior mesenteric artery close to its origin

## Division of Inferior Mesenteric Vessels

When performing a left hemicolectomy, we prefer to identify and divide the IMV first, close to the ligament of Treitz (Fig. 19.3). This provides easy access to the retroperitoneum by creating a cave, by blunt dissection, along the inferior border of the pancreas and Gerota's fascia in the direction of the splenic flexure. The attachment of the mesentery of the transverse colon to the inferior border of the pancreas is opened, entering the lesser sac. The peritoneum along the inferior border of the IMV is incised in the direction of the origin of the IMA, as the mesentery of the descending colon is lifted from the retroperitoneal structures laterally and inferiorly. The IMA is identified and dissected close to the bifurcation by extending the peritoneal incision toward the promontory. The origin of the mesentery of the sigmoid colon is lifted using a grasper, and the space behind the superior rectal vessels is entered, exposing the left ureter and the hypogastric plexus. The superior rectal artery is traced to its origin from the IMA. The IMA is isolated, sealed, and divided close to its bifurcation and away from the aorta, to prevent injury to the hypogastric plexus. Alternatively, the IMA can be approached, dissected, and divided before the IMV (Fig. 19.4). In any case, the mesentery of the sigmoid colon is dissected bluntly from the retroperitoneum exposing the left ureter and left gonadal vein in their course over the iliac vessels (Fig. 19.5).

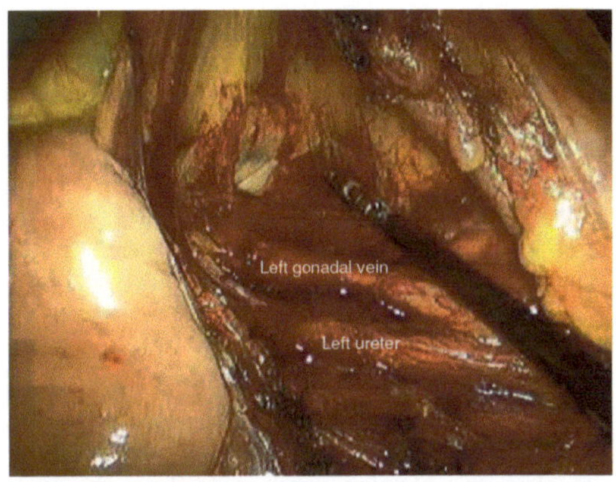


**Fig. 19.5** Intraoperative view of the left ureter and left gonadal vein in the retroperitoneum after lifting the mesentery of the left colon

## Identification and Division of the Middle Colic Vessels

We also prefer to approach the left branch of the middle colic vessels from the inferior aspect of the transverse mesocolon. Division of the IMV close to the ligament of Treitz and entrance into the lesser sac from the retroperitoneum makes finding the origin and the bifurcation of the middle colic vessels quite easy. However, the left branch of the middle colic vessels can also be divided once the gastrocolic omentum has been divided and the mesentery of the transverse mesocolon exposed from the lesser sac.

## Lateral Colon Mobilization

Once the vessels have been divided and the mesentery lifted from the retroperitoneal attachments, we proceed to divide the lateral attachments of the colon along the white line of Toldt. During this part of mobilization it is convenient for the operating surgeon to stand between the patient's legs and use the bipolar vessel sealer device or the laparoscopic monopolar scissors through the left lower quadrant port. The descending colon is mobilized up to the splenic flexure along the avascular plane.

## Splenic Flexure Takedown

The division of the gastrocolic omentum and the completion of the splenic flexure mobilization is facilitated by changing the operating table to reverse Trendelenburg position. The surgeon should be working again from the left side, holding the proximal portion of the gastrocolic omentum with a grasper introduced though the right upper quadrant port. The assistant, who is now between the patient's legs, should provide gentle traction from the transverse colon while the surgeon is dividing the omentum and gastrocolic vessels with a bipolar vessel sealer from the mid-transverse colon to the direction of the splenic flexure. If removal of the omentum is not necessary, the surgeon should retract the omentum over the stomach and open the avascular attachment of the omentum to the transverse colon with his right-hand instrument, while the assistant retracts the colon inferiorly. In either case the omentum is divided or detached from the midline to the splenic flexure.

## Dividing the Colon

Now the entire left colon is mobilized and attention is directed to transection at the rectosigmoid junction. The operating table is again placed in the Trendelenburg position. The mesentery at the level of the rectosigmoid junction is divided at the chosen site, using the bipolar vessel sealer device introduced through the right lower quadrant port. It is important to mobilize the upper rectum along the avascular plane to facilitate the anastomosis. The colon and the rectosigmoid junction are then divided using a laparoscopic stapler introduced through the right lower quadrant 12-mm port. The sigmoid colon is transected with a laparoscopic stapler at the proposed site.

## Proximal Colon Resection and Specimen Extraction

A small Pfannenstiel or periumbilical incision is made to deliver the specimen. A small wound protector is placed and the descending colon is delivered through the incision. Proximal descending colon transection depends on the distance from the tumor and the blood supply. The marginal vessels are then divided at the proposed site of transection with a bipolar vessel sealer. A purse-string suture is placed around the divided end of the colon creating a baseball stitch with 2-0 polypropylene suture. The anvil of a circular stapler is then secured with the purse-string and the descending colon is returned to the peritoneal cavity.

## Anastomosis

The pneumoperitoneum is reestablished by closing the wound protector with clamps. The circular stapler is introduced through the anus and an end-to-end anastomosis is done under laparoscopic vision. The anastomotic rings are checked and the integrity of the anastomosis proven with an air leak test. Once the specimen is removed and the anastomosis completed, hemostasis is confirmed, particularly at the site of the vascular pedicles. The ports are removed under direct vision and the fascial defect of the 12-mm port site is closed with a suture passer. The skin is closed with subcuticular absorbable suture.

## Postoperative Care

Most patients undergoing laparoscopic colectomy are managed according to enhanced recovery pathways [13]. Patients ambulate the day of or the day after surgery. The goal is to minimize the use of narcotics in order to shorten the postoperative ileus. Patients are started on clear liquid diet on the first postoperative day, and the diet is advanced as tolerated. The Foley catheter is removed on the first or second postoperative day. Postoperative pain is managed with patient-controlled analgesia until oral analgesics can be given. In a recent review of the US Nationwide inpatient database, the average length of stay for patients undergoing laparoscopic colectomy was 4 days and, more than 88 % of patients were discharged routinely [8].

## Complications

The reported complication rate after laparoscopic left colectomy ranges from 10 to 40 %. A recent review of the American College of Surgeons National Surgical Quality Improvement Program database from the years 2005–2008 found that right colectomies were performed laparoscopically more often when compared to left colectomies. Perioperative mortality after a left colectomy was 1.2 %, and 17 % of cases had at least one complication. The most common surgical complications were superficial surgical site infection (8 %), sepsis (4 %), urinary tract infection (3 %), and respiratory complications (2 %). Almost 4 % of patients required reoperation during the same hospitalization [14].

## Conclusion

The potential benefits of the laparoscopic approach are particularly relevant in patients undergoing a left hemicolectomy, as the open approach requires a long incision to provide access from the splenic flexure to the pelvis. There is now conclusive evidence that laparoscopy provides an effective and safe approach to left colon cancer resection, without compromising oncologic principles. Thorough knowledge of the patient's anatomy, and appropriate laparoscopic experience and skill, are important to ensure safe and efficient performance. Exposure, adequate traction, countertraction, use of gravity for exposure, and defining the role of the assistant all contribute to a successful laparoscopic procedure.

## References

1. Lacy AM, Garcia-Valdecasas JC, Delgado S, Castells A, Taura P, Pique JM, et al. Laparoscopy-assisted colectomy versus open colectomy for treatment of non-metastatic colon cancer: a randomised trial. Lancet. 2002;359(9325):2224–9. doi:10.1016/s0140-6736(02)09290-5.
2. Laparoscopically assisted colectomy is as safe and effective as open colectomy in people with colon cancer Abstracted from: Nelson H, Sargent D, Wieand HS, et al; for the Clinical Outcomes of Surgical Therapy Study Group. A comparison of laparoscopically assisted and open colectomy for colon cancer. N Engl J Med 2004; 350: 2050-2059. Cancer Treat Rev. 2004;30(8):707–9. doi:10.1016/j.ctrv.2004.09.001.
3. Guillou PJ, Quirke P, Thorpe H, Walker J, Jayne DG, Smith AM, et al. Short-term endpoints of conventional versus laparoscopic-assisted surgery in patients with colorectal cancer (MRC CLASICC trial): multicentre, randomised controlled trial. Lancet. 2005;365(9472):1718–26. doi:10.1016/s0140-6736(05)66545-2.
4. Cirocco WC, Schwartzman A, Golub RW. Abdominal wall recurrence after laparoscopic colectomy for colon cancer. Surgery. 1994;116(5):842–6.
5. Fleshman J, Sargent DJ, Green E, Anvari M, Stryker SJ, Beart Jr RW, et al. Laparoscopic colectomy for cancer is not inferior to open surgery based on 5-year data from the COST Study Group trial. Ann Surg. 2007;246(4):655–62. doi:10.1097/SLA.0b013e318155a762; discussion 62–4.
6. Colon Cancer Laparoscopic or Open Resection Study Group, Buunen M, Veldkamp R, Hop WC, Kuhry E, Jeekel J, et al. Survival after laparoscopic surgery versus open surgery for colon cancer: long-term outcome of a randomised clinical trial. Lancet Oncol. 2009;10(1):44–52. doi:10.1016/s1470-2045(08)70310-3.
7. Green BL, Marshall HC, Collinson F, Quirke P, Guillou P, Jayne DG, et al. Long-term follow-up of

the Medical Research Council CLASICC trial of conventional versus laparoscopically assisted resection in colorectal cancer. Br J Surg. 2013;100(1): 75–82. doi:10.1002/bjs.8945.
8. Juo YY, Hyder O, Haider AH, Camp M, Lidor A, Ahuja N. Is minimally invasive colon resection better than traditional approaches?: first comprehensive national examination with propensity score matching. JAMA Surg. 2014;149(2):177–84. doi:10.1001/jamasurg.2013.3660.
9. Fowler DL, White SA. Laparoscopy-assisted sigmoid resection. Surg Laparosc Endosc. 1991;1(3):183–8.
10. Jacobs M, Verdeja JC, Goldstein HS. Minimally invasive colon resection (laparoscopic colectomy). Surg Laparosc Endosc. 1991;1(3):144–50.
11. Monson JR, Darzi A, Carey PD, Guillou PJ. Prospective evaluation of laparoscopic-assisted colectomy in an unselected group of patients. Lancet. 1992;340(8823):831–3.
12. Rouffet F, Hay JM, Vacher B, Fingerhut A, Elhadad A, Flamant Y, et al. Curative resection for left colonic carcinoma: hemicolectomy vs. segmental colectomy. A prospective, controlled, multicenter trial. French Association for Surgical Research. Dis Colon Rectum. 1994;37(7):651–9.
13. Vlug MS, Wind J, Hollmann MW, Ubbink DT, Cense HA, Engel AF, et al. Laparoscopy in combination with fast track multimodal management is the best perioperative strategy in patients undergoing colonic surgery: a randomized clinical trial (LAFA-study). Ann Surg. 2011;254(6):868–75. doi:10.1097/SLA.0b013e31821fd1ce.
14. Kwaan MR, Al-Refaie WB, Parsons HM, Chow CJ, Rothenberger DA, Habermann EB. Are right-sided colectomy outcomes different from left-sided colectomy outcomes?: study of patients with colon cancer in the ACS NSQIP database. JAMA Surg. 2013;148(6): 504–10. doi:10.1001/jamasurg.2013.1205.

## Key Operative Steps

1. Place the patient in modified lithotomy position.
2. Create pneumoperitoneum using a Veress needle.
3. Use medial-to-lateral dissection approach.
4. Identify, isolate, and divide the inferior mesenteric vein.
5. Identify, isolate, and divide the inferior mesenteric artery after identifying and preserving the left ureter.
6. Dissect the mesocolon from the retroperitoneal structures.
7. Mobilize the descending and sigmoid colon from the lateral abdominal wall. Mobilize the greater omentum and splenic flexure
8. Transect the rectosigmoid colon.
9. Use a Pfannenstiel or periumbilical incision for specimen extraction using a wound protector.
10. Perform extracorporeal placement of an anvil after proximal division of the left colon.
11. Perform laparoscopic intracorporeal end-to-end anastomosis using a circular stapler.
12. Perform an air leak test.

# 20 Open Technique for Low Anterior Resection

Erin Teeple and Ronald Bleday

## Incidence

Although the impact of colorectal cancer has been decreasing over the last 20 years due to increased screening and improved radiation and chemotherapeutic regimens, rectal cancer still poses significant morbidity and mortality. In the US in 2013, 40,340 cases for colorectal cancer were diagnosed with a mortality rate of approximately 8,500 [1, 2]. Rectal cancer alone comprises nearly 35 % of all colorectal cancers.

## Historical Perspective

The history of modern rectal cancer surgery, much like many other oncologic operations, mirrors the evolution of understanding its underlying pathophysiology. In 1884, Vincenz Cerny was the first to describe a combined abdominal and perineal approach for a rectal tumor [3]. Charles Mayo reported his technique for an abdominoperineal resection (APR) in 1904, emphasizing resection of lymphatics [4, 5]. However, it was in 1908 that Sir Ernest Miles highlighted "the zone of upward spread" that he had found in a series of postmortem analysis of recurrent rectal tumors [6]. He stressed the importance of removal of "the whole pelvic colon" so as to eliminate this zone of upward spread. Because Miles' initial paper of 12 patients had a prohibitively high mortality rate of 42 %, the technique was not adopted until improved 5-year survival was robustly demonstrated in his follow-up paper published in 1914 [7].

## Anatomic Highlights

The rectum typically measures 15 cm in length and extends from the distal sigmoid to the anal canal. The rectosigmoid junction is signified by the coalescence of the longitudinal muscles of the colon wall called taeniae coli. The proximal portion of the rectum is intraperitoneal while the distal 6–8 cm are extraperitoneal. Posteriorly, the rectum is connected to the sacrum at the level of S4 by the rectosacral fascia called Waldeyer's fascia (Fig. 20.1). In a male, the anterior rectum is separated from the prostate and seminal vesicles by Denonvillier's fascia, a double layer of peritoneum. In a female, the anterior peritoneal reflection forms the pouch of Douglas, which extends to the cervix anteriorly and the mid-rectum posteriorly. The endopelvic fascia forms the fascia propria, a layer which encloses the

E. Teeple, M.D.
Department of Surgery, Thomas Jefferson University/ AI DuPont Hospital for Children, 1600 Rockland Rd., Wilmington, DE 19803, USA

R. Bleday, M.D. (✉)
Division of Colorectal Surgery, Department of Surgery, Brigham and Women's Hospital, Harvard Medical School, 75 Francis Street, Boston, MA 02115, USA
e-mail: rbleday@partners.org

J. Kim and J. Garcia-Aguilar (eds.), *Surgery for Cancers of the Gastrointestinal Tract: A Step-by-Step Approach*, DOI 10.1007/978-1-4939-1893-5_20, © Springer Science+Business Media New York 2015

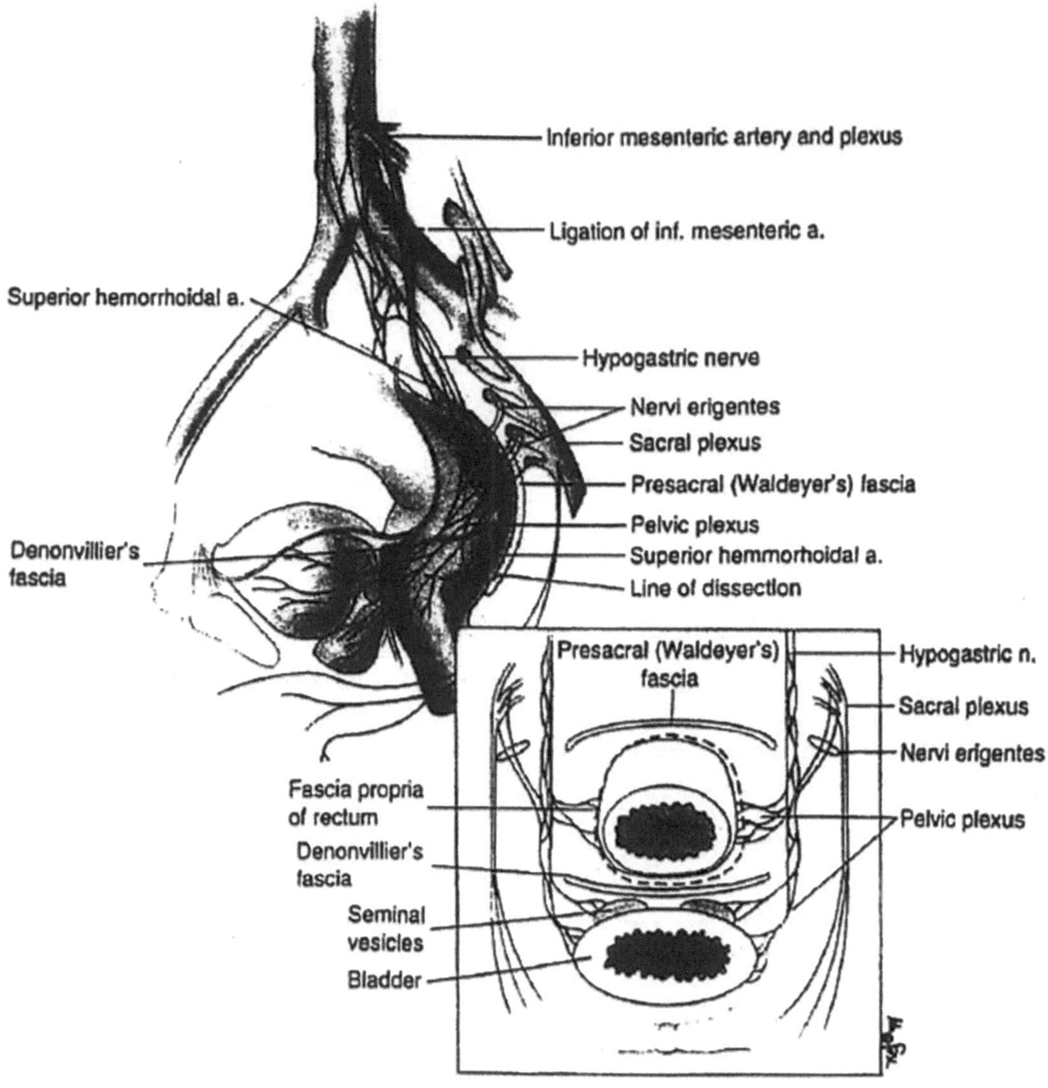


**Fig. 20.1** Diagram illustrating the fascial planes. The rectum is connected to the sacrum at the level of S4 by the rectosacral fascia called Waldeyer's fascia

rectum along with the mesorectal fat, lymphatics, and vascular supply. This fascia propria becomes an important plane of distinction during a total mesorectal excision (TME).

The dentate line signifies the anorectal junction. The top of the anal canal can be identified on palpation of a muscular complex consisting of the internal and external sphincters as well as the puborectalis sling. Distance of the tumor from this important landmark determines the ability to preserve the sphincters during resection. The tumor must be proximal enough from the anorectal ring to ensure a 1–2 cm distal margin. If this margin cannot be achieved, or if sphincter function would be compromised, then an APR should be performed.

The vascular supply of the upper and middle rectum is provided by the superior rectal artery as it branches off the inferior mesenteric artery. The inferior rectal artery branches off the internal pudendal arteries originating posterolaterally and supply the anal sphincters and anal epithelium. Although the lateral rectal stalks are thought to contain the middle rectal arteries, this is true only 22 % of the time [8]. These stalks predominantly contain nerves. The superior rectal vein drains

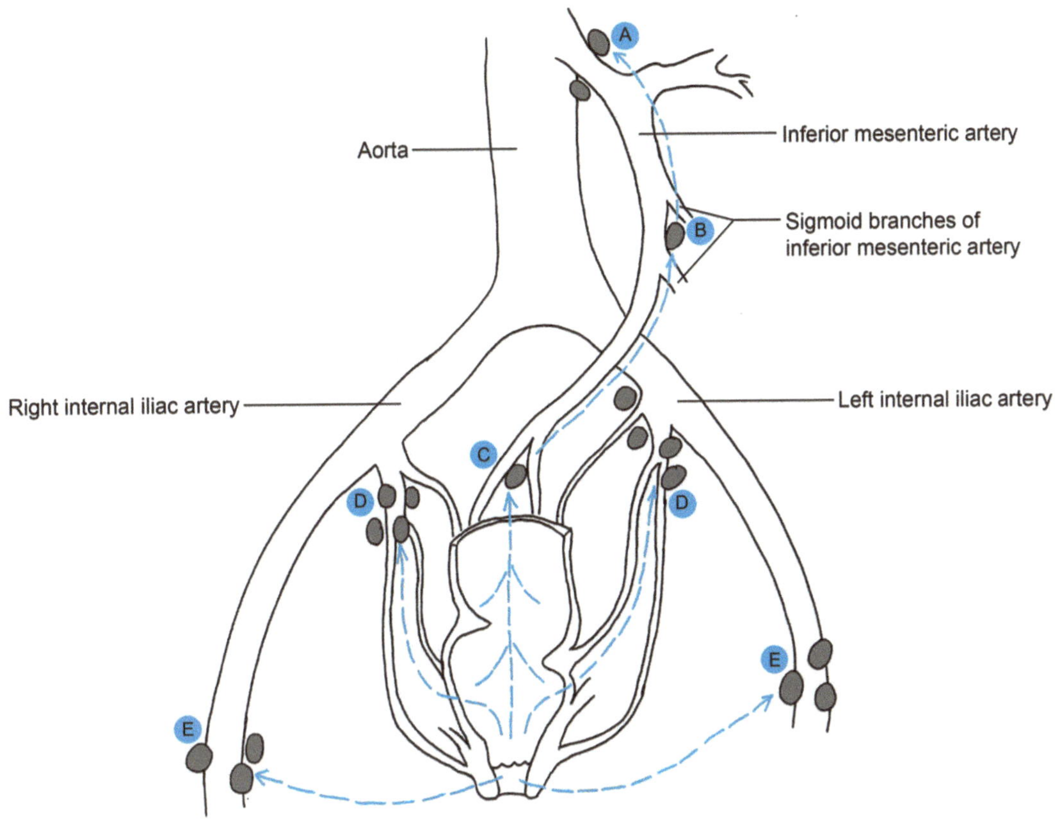


**Fig. 20.2** Lymphatic drainage of the rectum and anus. The nodes at the origin of (**a**) inferior mesenteric artery and (**b**) the sigmoid branches. The (**c**) sacral, (**d**) internal iliac, and (**e**) inguinal nodes are represented

the superior and middle rectum, emptying into the inferior mesenteric vein. The middle rectal vein drains the distal rectum and proximal anal canal via the internal iliac veins. Lastly, the inferior rectal veins drain the distal anal canal via the pudendal veins.

Lymphatic drainage is achieved within the mesorectum and follows the vascular supply (Fig. 20.2). Tumor cells can spread cranially along the superior rectal vessels necessitating a high ligation of the vascular supply at its origin for adequate staging and local control. The hypothesized amount of distal spread has influenced the recommended distal margin. Recently, distal spread has been shown to rarely extend beyond 1 cm allowing decreased distal margins for adequate control of disease [9–16] and improved sphincter preservation. Lymph traveling from the lower rectum can drain along any of the rectal arteries, emptying into the iliac vessels and ultimately the periaortic nodes.

Innervation within the pelvis consists of paired sympathetic (hypogastric) nerves, sacral parasympathetic nerves, and inferior hypogastric nerves. The sympathetic nerves originate from L1 to L3 and descend as the hypogastric nerves along the sacrum. The parasympathetic innervation (*nervi erigentes*) originate from S2 to S4, joining the hypogastric nerves anterior and lateral to the rectum. These nerves form the pelvic plexus as well as the periprostatic plexus. Fibers from these sympathetic and parasympathetic plexi innervate bladder, ureter, prostate, seminal vesicles, membranous urethra, and corpora cavernosa. Injury to these nerves during dissection can lead to side effects such as impotence, retrograde ejaculation, bladder dysfuction, urinary retention, and loss of normal defecatory mechanisms.

## Indications for Operation

Low anterior resection (LAR) is defined as resection of the rectum with extraperitoneal rectal anastomosis [17]. The most common indication for an LAR is rectal cancer. As with any oncologic procedure, proper patient selection is important. The primary goal is complete extirpation of the tumor and any involved lymphatics. Reestablishment of bowel continuity is a secondary goal. Preoperative staging with an endorectal ultrasound (ERUS) or magnetic resonance imaging (MRI) as well as distance from the anorectal ring dictate the ability to adequately resect using a transanal approach, LAR, or APR. Preoperative evaluation of patient comorbidity, fecal continence, and preoperative radiation are important influencing factors in the decision to reanastomose as well as the decision to create a diverting stoma proximal to the anastomosis.

Other indications for an LAR include inherited polyposis syndromes such as familial adenomatous polyposis (FAP) and proctitis refractory to medical management. Proctectomy for FAP is typically combined with total abdominal colectomy (TAC) for control of oncologic risk. LAR for medically refractory ulcerative colitis can be performed in combination with a TAC or may be part of a staged operation for ultimate control of disease.

## Preoperative Workup

Although patients usually present to the surgeon with a confirmed endoscopic diagnosis of cancer, they may present with an initial complaint of rectal bleeding, pain, tenesmus, fullness, change in bowel habit, obstruction or obstipation, and/or weight loss. Many tumors are found incidentally either on screening colonoscopy or other imaging. Important features of the review of systems include weight loss, indicating a more urgent obstructive process; back pain or pain with defecation, indicating tumor eroding into the sacrum or sphincters; fecal or flatal incontinence; and baseline sexual and urinary function. The remaining portion of the history and physical should be focused on identifying other medical comorbidities, which may require further evaluation and risk stratification prior to surgical intervention. A thorough family history should be obtained to help identify those patients with a strong family history who may be at risk for a familial syndrome or inflammatory bowel disease.

The physical examination should include both a rectal exam and, if appropriate, a rigid proctoscopy. The rectal exam should specifically note size, mobility, fixation, and anatomic location of tumor including laterality as well as distance from the anorectal ring and anal verge. Rigid proctoscopy can be used to delineate the distance from the anal verge, length of tumor, and its relation to critical structures such as sphincters, peritoneal reflection, vagina, and prostate. If not done so prior, a full colonoscopy should be performed to identify the possibility of synchronous cancers, which occur 2–8 % of the time [18–21].

Preoperative staging is important in rectal cancer to assess the need for neoadjuvant therapy as well as determining the appropriate approach to surgical eradication of the tumor and the presence of regional lymph nodes the depth of invasion can be assessed by type out all ERU & MRI. A computed tomography (CT) of the chest, abdomen and pelvis should be obtained to evaluate the possibility of distant metastasis. Laboratory studies are obtained preoperatively based on other medical comorbidities. A carcinoembryonic antigen (CEA) should be checked before removal of the tumor to risk stratify the patient, since a higher CEA signifies a worse prognosis than those patients with the same stage and a normal CEA [22–25]. Also, an elevated preoperative CEA, which does not normalize postoperatively, warrants a workup for persistent disease.

## Perioperative Preparation

Prior to the standard use of mechanical and preoperative antibiotics, the postoperative rate of infection was noted to be as high as 60 % [26]. Currently, a standard bowel preparation includes

1–3 days of clear liquids as well as some combination of hyperosmolar colonic irrigant such as polyethylene glycol or magnesium citrate and laxatives and/or enemas. Oral antibiotics are also used to decrease the bacteria count of the colon. Common choices are neomycin 1 g and erythromycin 1 g given at 5 p.m. and 10 p.m. the day before surgery. Metronidazole can be substituted to control a greater spectrum of anaerobes. Intravenous antibiotics are given per current Center for Medicare and Medicaid Services (CMS) recommendations [27]. According to the American Heart Association guidelines, the choice of perioperative intravenous antibiotic is broadened in those patients with cardiac prosthesis to include ampicillin [28]. The patient is also given a preoperative dose of 5,000 units of subcutaneous heparin. The abdomen is clipped as appropriate and cleaned using an antiseptic agent.

## Surgical Technique

### Operative Positioning and Exploration

The patient is brought to the operating room and general anesthesia is administered with the placement of an endotracheal tube. A foley catheter is sterilely placed within the bladder. The patient is then moved to the lithotomy position with the weight of the leg resting on the heel and appropriate support provided to alleviate pressure from both the low back and the lateral peroneal nerve of the lower leg. The arms are placed on arm boards bilaterally so as not to cause undue stretch on the brachial plexus (Fig. 20.3). Preoperative placement of urinary stents can aid in identification of bilateral ureters during dissection. A rectal exam is performed to reassess the tumor, its location, and possible fixation. The abdomen is prepped and draped in a sterile fashion, allowing appropriate access to the anus. A midline vertical subumbilical incision is made. If cephalad extension is required for mobilization of the splenic flexure, the incision should be continued on the contralateral side of any potential stoma. Once access to the abdomen is gained, the abdomen is explored for signs of metastatic disease including visualization and palpation of the peritoneal surfaces and the liver. The tumor is palpated within the pelvis to assess fixation and likelihood of invasion to surrounding structures. The abdominal self-retractor is used for adequate exposure. The patient is placed in slight Trendelenburg position and the small bowel is packed into the upper abdomen.

### Mobilization and Resection

Mobilization of the colon is begun laterally along the white line of Toldt (Fig. 20.4). The ureter is identified at the bifurcation of the common iliac artery. After mobilization of the colon is begun, the length of colon to be resected can be grossly estimated and, subsequently, the need to mobilize the splenic flexure assessed. During mobilization of the splenic flexure, tension on the left and transverse colon should be firm but not excessive and blunt dissection should be avoided to avoid inadvertent splenic injury. The omentum is freed from the transverse colon via sharp dissection in the avascular plane between the two structures.

The sigmoid colon is manually elevated in the air and the mesentery is scored on both sides to the level of the sacral promontory. The inferior mesenteric artery (IMA) pedicle is isolated and the left colic is identified and spared, if appropriate. The superior hemorrhoidal artery is ligated at its takeoff from the IMA. Two large Kelly clamps are placed proximally and one is placed distally. The pedicle is then transected and doubly ligated. The bowel is subsequently transected at a level ensuring adequate blood supply to the remaining colon (Fig. 20.5). The method of transection depends on the type of anastomosis planned, i.e., stapled or hand-sewn. A TME is undertaken and crucial for adequate oncologic resection. After identifying the sympathetic nerves traveling over the pelvic brim, electrocautery is used to dissect in the posterior avascular, alveolar plane between the fascia propria of the rectum and the parietal fascia of the pelvic floor structures while the rectum is being retracted anteriorly. This, when undertaken accurately, allows for sparing of the

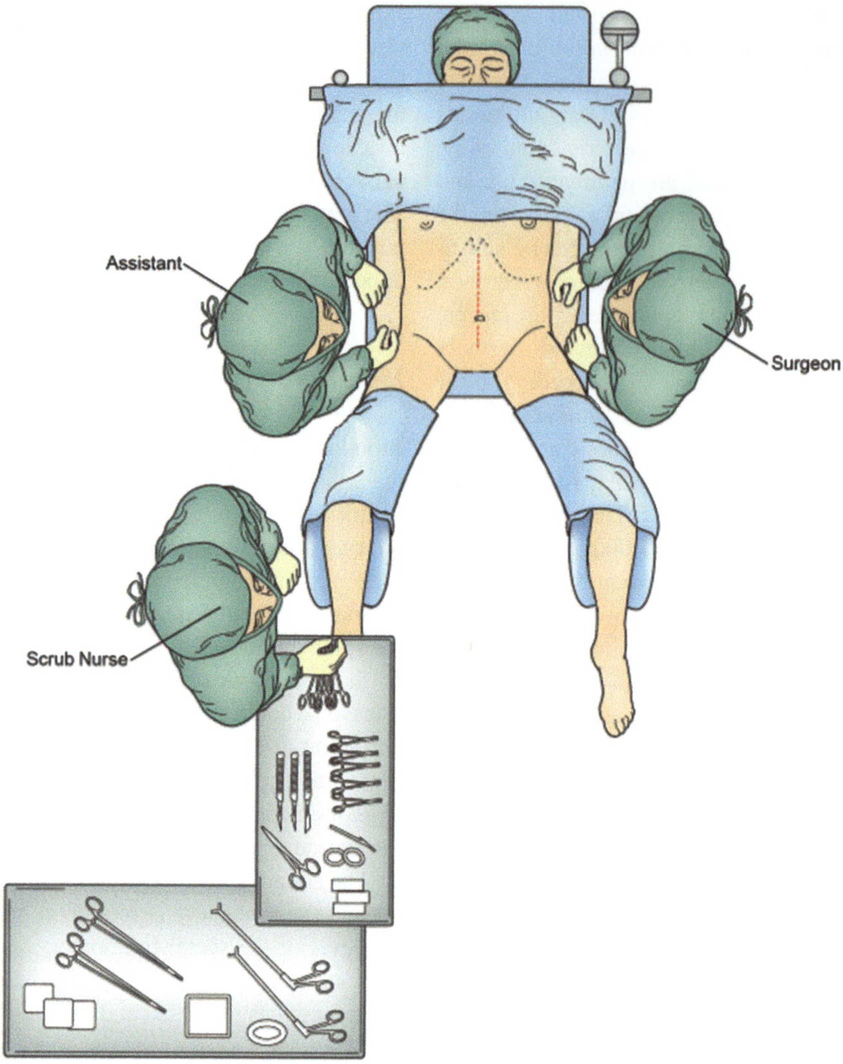


**Fig. 20.3** Operating room setup with the patient in lithotomy position with the upper extremities placed on arm boards

autonomic nerves as well as the surrounding pelvic structures and results in a smooth, bilobed mesorectal specimen.

The posterior dissection is carried inferiorly through Waldeyer's fascia to the level of the coccyx. A St. Mark's abdominal retractor facilitates retraction of the rectum in the deep pelvis. The lateral and anterior dissection is undertaken using electrocautery. The anterior peritoneum is incised at the groove between the rectum and the anterior structures, either the cervix/vagina in women or the seminal vesicles in men. As stated, the lateral stalks contain the middle rectal vessels in 22 % of patients [8]. As these are divided, care should be taken to preserve the hypogastric plexus that lies on the pelvic sidewall, lateral to the seminal vesicles in men and the cardinal ligaments in women. In Japan, dissection of these lateral lymph nodes are purposefully pursued and has been routinely practiced since 1940 [29]. However, there is minimal, if any, oncologic benefit to lymphadenectomy in these lateral spaces [30–37]. Avoiding this dissection helps prevent significant postoperative problems with sexual potency and

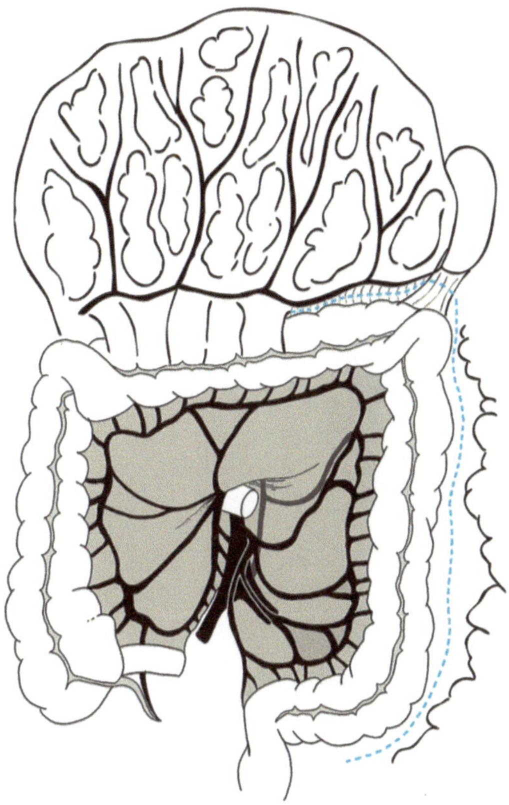

**Fig. 20.4** Mobilization of the colon is begun laterally along the white line of Toldt

urination [34, 38–41]. During the anterior dissection, the planes are less distinct and the fat on the anterior mesorectum is thin. The anterior pelvic structures are elevated off the anterior rectal wall using a lipped St. Mark's retractor. This dissection is carried through Denonvillier's fascia. This fascia is taken off the anterior structures and kept with the specimen in an oncologic operation.

The distal point of bowel transection depends on the level of the tumor. Middle and distal rectal tumors require removal of the entire mesorectum. An upper rectal tumor requires transection of the rectum and mesorectum 5–6 cm below the level of the tumor. Tumor spread within the mesorectum rarely extends beyond 3–4 cm distally [42, 43]. In addition, multiple studies have shown that a 2 cm margin of the mucosa is likely more than adequate [11–16]. A rigid sigmoidoscopy may be helpful in identifying the tumor when it is not palpable, particularly after neoadjuvant therapy. Mobilization of the rectum can increase the distance of the tumor from the dentate line allowing an adequate distal margin with preservation of the sphincters, which may not have been perceived before mobilization of the rectum. Once the level of transection has been established, the mesorectum should be divided with bipolar thermal energy or direct suture ligation. The rectal wall can then be transected using a stapling device, either a thoraco-abdominal (TA) linear stapler or a curved contour stapler dependent on the width of the pelvis. The length of the proximal colon is then evaluated for construction of a tension-free anastomosis. If more length is needed, a variety of maneuvers can be employed. The splenic flexure can be further mobilized, the inferior mesenteric vein can be identified and transected, and the mesentery can be further ligated (at the risk of necessitating further colon resection).

## Anastomosis

The size of end-to-end anastomosis (EEA) stapler is decided by the caliber of the colon. Dependent on the type of reconstruction planned (i.e., end-to-end or side-to-end), the anvil is either placed within the end of the colon after the staple line is amputated or a colotomy is made on the antimesenteric surface approximately 3 cm from the staple line and the anvil is placed within the colotomy. The anvil is secured with a purse-string using 3-0 prolene suture. The serosa of the colon is then cleaned of fat and small vessels within 1 cm of the shaft of the anvil to facilitate the bowel-to-bowel contact within the anastomosis.

Once the anvil is secured, the pelvis is then irrigated and excellent hemostasis is achieved prior to formation of the anastomosis, which will limit access to the deep pelvis. One member of the surgical team then gently dilates and places the lubricated circular stapler in the anus. The surgeon then guides the assistant to follow the curve of the sacrum and advance the stapler to the rectal staple line. Once in adequate position, the spike is deployed slowly ensuring proper positioning. We prefer to deploy the spike 2–3 mm posterior to the

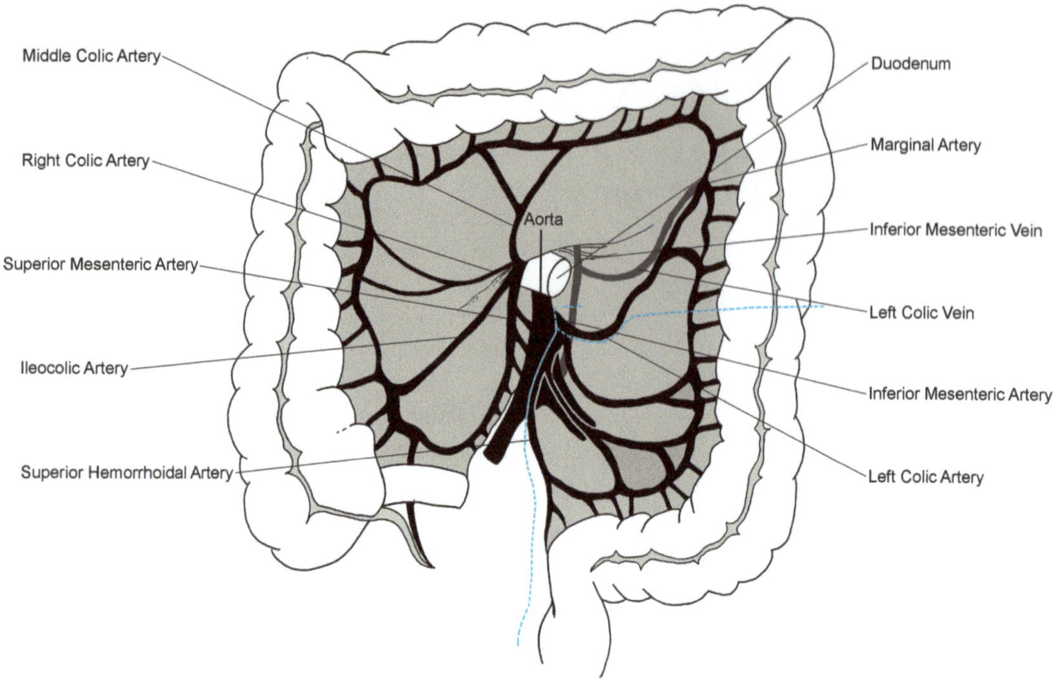


**Fig. 20.5** Transection of mesentery vessels and colon. The superior hemorrhoidal artery is divided and the left colon and mesentery are divided at the junction of the descending and sigmoid colon

staple line to discourage the capture of any anterior structures in the EEA anastomosis. Once the spike is completely deployed, the anvil is brought to the pelvis and secured onto the spike making sure the mesentery and colon are properly oriented (Fig. 20.6). The stapling device is slowly closed, ensuring all extraneous tissue is removed from the anastomosis. The stapler is then fired, opened partially, and gently removed from the anus. The anastomotic "donuts" are examined to ensure identification of complete rings of tissue. If incomplete rings are found, the anastomosis should be scrutinized for any compromise. An air test of the anastomosis is then performed. The surgeon fills the pelvis with irrigant and clamps the colon proximal to the anastomosis while the assistant insufflates the rectum with air via rigid proctoscopy. If bubbling is identified, the anastomosis is reinforced or refashioned.

## Ileostomy and Closure

A diverting loop ileostomy should be considered for any low anastomosis (<5 cm from the dentate line) where anastomotic leak rates are as high as 20 % [44, 45]. Other factors which increase the risk of anastomotic leak are malnutrition, previous radiation, immunosuppression, and a positive air leak test. Loop ileostomies can be closed after 8 weeks but are usually left in place until completion of any adjuvant therapy. Prior to ileostomy closure, a water-soluble contrast enema is performed to evaluate the colorectal anastomosis. Most surgeons advocate the use of drains for extraperitoneal anastomoses despite the lack of evidence to support them. We evaluate the need for drainage on a patient-by-patient basis but strongly advocate drainage in extraperitoneal anastomoses and APRs.

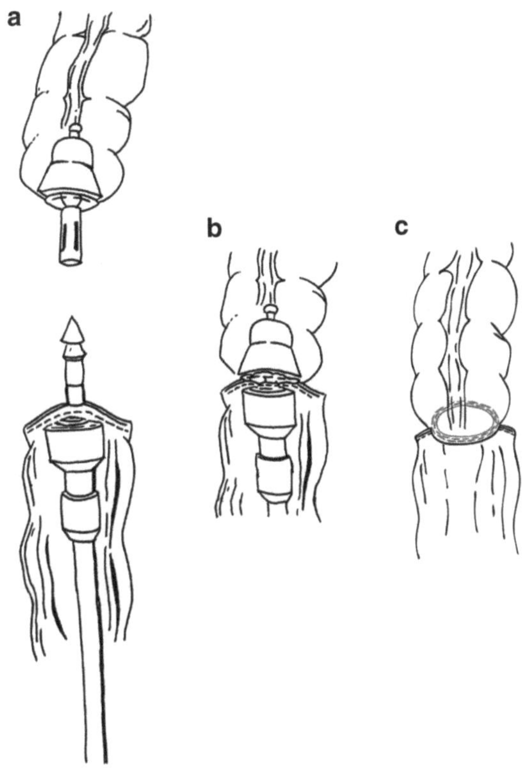


**Fig. 20.6** Double-staple colorectal anastomosis. (**a**) Insertion of circular stapler into the anus. (**b**) The anvil is secured to the spike and the stapling device is closed. (**c**) Firing and removal of the stapler leaves an anastomotic "donut"

## Postoperative Management

The patient does not leave the operating room with a nasogastric tube and can have liquids on postoperative day (POD) zero. Isotonic intravenous fluids are run at a maintenance rate on POD #0 then decreased to three-quarters maintenance and changed to a dextrose-containing formula on POD #1. The foley catheter is removed on POD #3 to allow for any sympathetic and parasympathetic neuropraxia to resolve as well as to allow time away from the general anesthetic. An epidural is used for pain control with the addition of parenteral narcotics when needed. The epidural is typically left in place for 3 days as long as it is functional. Subcutaneous heparin venothrombotic prophylaxis is continued postoperatively. Sequential compression devices are also placed on the lower extremities. The diet is advanced on POD #3 unless the patient is distended or nauseated.

## Complications

Complications of an LAR can include those associated with any major intraabdominal operation including bleeding, deep and superficial infections, wound dehiscence, venothrombotic or embolic complications, cardiac or respiratory compromise, and renal failure. Those germane to proctectomy include impotence, retrograde ejaculation, urinary retention, anastomotic leak, and intraoperative hemorrhage during pelvic dissection.

Impotence can occur in up to 50 % of men postoperatively, making it imperative to discuss sexual function with the patient preoperatively [46–48]. The majority of these patients will respond to phosphodiesterase inhibitors (i.e., sildenafil) postoperatively. Women may also experience a change in sexual function, including increased dryness or even dyspareunia, particularly if the vagina was distorted during the rectal resection.

As previously stated, the leak rate in a low pelvic anastomosis can be as high as 20 % [44, 45]. Patients will typically present with fever, tachycardia, and leukocytosis on POD #5–#7. Other presenting symptoms can include tachypnea, arrhythmia, enterocutaneous fistula, and frank peritonitis. If the patient is clinically stable without signs of peritonitis, the leak may be managed conservatively with *nil per os* (NPO), intravenous fluid, and intravenous antibiotics. A percutaneous drain can be placed in a perianastomotic pelvic abscess to facilitate resolution. If clinical compromise or peritonitis is present then return to the operating room for exploration and diverting ileostomy or colostomy is needed. An anastomosis is rarely deconstructed and should not be reconstructed in the presence of sepsis.

Urinary retention can occur in both men and women. Men with benign prostatic hypertrophy may be predisposed to urinary retention as well as those women whose tumor necessitated dissection of the anterior vagina where neural control of urination resides. Urinary retention typically resolves spontaneously after days to weeks. It can be treated with an indwelling foley and void trials, or follow-up with a urologist as needed.

Massive arterial and venous bleeding can occur when the presacral plane is disrupted during posterior dissection of the rectum or dissection in the lateral plane encroaches on the iliac vessels. Presacral venous bleeding is typically lateral to midline and can be controlled with either a sterile thumbtack or electrocauterization of autologous tissue onto the bleeding vessel (i.e., rectus muscle). Iliac bleeding must be controlled and closely evaluated as nonspecific ligation is discouraged and can be hazardous.

## Conclusion

The evolution of LAR for rectal cancer will continue as understanding of the oncologic process grows. Excellent surgical technique to achieve adequate margins and ensure a true TME is imperative to achieving a favorable oncologic result.

## References

1. American Cancer Society. Cancer Facts & Figures, 2013. 2013. http://www.cancer.org/Research/CancerFactsFigures/index. Accessed 9 Jan 2014.
2. Bleday R, Brindzei N. Surgical treatment of rectal cancer. In: Beck D, Roberts P, Saclarides T, Senagore A, Stamos M, Wexner S, editors. The ASCRS textbook of colon and rectal surgery. 2nd ed. New York: Springer; 2011.
3. Rankin FW. How surgery of the colon and rectum developed. Surg Gynecol Obstet. 1937;64:705–10.
4. Mayo CH. Cancer of the large bowel. Med Sentinel. 1904;12:466–73.
5. Mayo CH. Cancer of the sigmoid and rectum. Surg Gynecol Obstet. 1906;3:236–41.
6. Miles WE. A method of performing abdomino-perineal excision for carcinoma of the rectum and of the terminal portion of the pelvic colon (1908). CA Cancer J Clin. 1971;21(6):361–4.
7. Shleton A, Goldberg S. Evolution of the surgical management of rectal cancer. In: Audisio R, Geraghty J, Longo W, editors. Modern management of cancer of the rectum. London: Springer; 2001. p. 3.
8. Sato K, Sato T. The vascular and neuronal composition of the lateral ligament of the rectum and the rectosacral fascia. Surg Radiol Anat. 1991;13(1):17–22.
9. Rutkowski A, Bujko K, Nowacki MP, Chmielik E, Nasierowska-Guttmejer A, Wojnar A. Distal bowel surgical margin shorter than 1 cm after preoperative radiation for rectal cancer: is it safe? Ann Surg Oncol. 2008;15(11):3124–31. doi:10.1245/s10434-008-0125-6.
10. Moore HG, Riedel E, Minsky BD, Saltz L, Paty P, Wong D, et al. Adequacy of 1-cm distal margin after restorative rectal cancer resection with sharp mesorectal excision and preoperative combined-modality therapy. Ann Surg Oncol. 2003;10(1):80–5.
11. Shirouzu K, Isomoto H, Kakegawa T. Distal spread of rectal cancer and optimal distal margin of resection for sphincter-preserving surgery. Cancer. 1995;76(3):388–92.
12. Andreola S, Leo E, Belli F, Lavarino C, Bufalino R, Tomasic G, et al. Distal intramural spread in adenocarcinoma of the lower third of the rectum treated with total rectal resection and coloanal anastomosis. Dis Colon Rectum. 1997;40(1):25–9.
13. Ueno H, Mochizuki H, Hashiguchi Y, Ishikawa K, Fujimoto H, Shinto E, et al. Preoperative parameters expanding the indication of sphincter preserving surgery in patients with advanced low rectal cancer. Ann Surg. 2004;239(1):34–42. doi:10.1097/01.sla.0000103070.13030.eb.
14. Williams NS, Dixon MF, Johnston D. Reappraisal of the 5 centimetre rule of distal excision for carcinoma of the rectum: a study of distal intramural spread and of patients' survival. Br J Surg. 1983;70(3):150–4.
15. Lazorthes F, Voigt JJ, Roques J, Chiotasso P, Chevreau P. Distal intramural spread of carcinoma of the rectum correlated with lymph nodal involvement. Surg Gynecol Obstet. 1990;170(1):45–8.
16. Madsen PM, Christiansen J. Distal intramural spread of rectal carcinomas. Dis Colon Rectum. 1986;29(4):279–82.
17. Lowry AC, Simmang CL, Boulos P, Farmer KC, Finan PJ, Hyman N, et al. Consensus statement of definitions for anorectal physiology and rectal cancer. Colorectal Dis. 2001;3(4):272–5.
18. Travieso Jr CR, Knoepp Jr LF, Hanley PH. Multiple adenocarcinomas of the colon and rectum. Dis Colon Rectum. 1972;15(1):1–6.
19. Heald RJ, Bussey HJ. Clinical experiences at St. Mark's Hospital with multiple synchronous cancers of the colon and rectum. Dis Colon Rectum. 1975;18(1):6–10.
20. Reilly JC, Rusin LC, Theuerkauf Jr FJ. Colonoscopy: its role in cancer of the colon and rectum. Dis Colon Rectum. 1982;25(6):532–8.
21. Langevin JM, Nivatvongs S. The true incidence of synchronous cancer of the large bowel. A prospective study. Am J Surg. 1984;147(3):330–3.

22. Tarantino I, Warschkow R, Worni M, Merati-Kashani K, Koberle D, Schmied BM, et al. Elevated preoperative CEA is associated with worse survival in stage I-III rectal cancer patients. Br J Cancer. 2012;107(2):266–74. doi:10.1038/bjc.2012.267.
23. Wallin U, Rothenberger D, Lowry A, Luepker R, Mellgren A. CEA - a predictor for pathologic complete response after neoadjuvant therapy for rectal cancer. Dis Colon Rectum. 2013;56(7):859–68. doi:10.1097/DCR.0b013e31828e5a72.
24. Wang L, Zhong XG, Peng YF, Li ZW, Gu J. Prognostic value of pretreatment level of carcinoembryonic antigen on tumour downstaging and early occurring metastasis in locally advanced rectal cancer following neoadjuvant radiotherapy (30 Gy in 10 fractions). Colorectal Dis. 2014;16(1):33–9. doi:10.1111/codi.12354.
25. Huang CS, Lin JK, Wang LW, Liang WY, Lin CC, Lan YT, et al. Assessment of the value of carcinoembryonic antigen reduction ratio as a prognosis factor in rectal cancer. Am J Surg. 2014;208(1):99–105. doi:10.1016/j.amjsurg.2013.08.054.
26. Clarke JS, Condon RE, Bartlett JG, Gorbach SL, Nichols RL, Ochi S. Preoperative oral antibiotics reduce septic complications of colon operations: results of prospective, randomized, double-blind clinical study. Ann Surg. 1977;186(3):251–9.
27. Centers for Medicare and Medicaid Services. Surgical Care Improvement Project Measures. 2014. https://www.cms.gov/Medicare/Demonstration-Projects/DemoProjectsEvalRpts/downloads/ACEQualityMeasures.pdf. Accessed 11 Feb 2014.
28. Wilson W, Taubert KA, Gewitz M, Lockhart PB, Baddour LM, Levison M, et al. Prevention of infective endocarditis: guidelines from the American Heart Association: a guideline from the American Heart Association Rheumatic Fever, Endocarditis, and Kawasaki Disease Committee, Council on Cardiovascular Disease in the Young, and the Council on Clinical Cardiology, Council on Cardiovascular Surgery and Anesthesia, and the Quality of Care and Outcomes Research Interdisciplinary Working Group. Circulation. 2007;116(15):1736–54. doi:10.1161/circulationaha.106.183095.
29. Kuru M. Cancer of the rectum. J Jpn Surg Soc. 1940;41:832–77.
30. Bacon HE. Cancer of the colon, rectum and anal canal. Philadelphia: JB Lippincott; 1964.
31. Stearns Jr MW, Deddish MR. Five-year results of abdominopelvic lymph node dissection for carcinoma of the rectum. Dis Colon Rectum. 1959;2(2):169–72.
32. Glass RE, Ritchie JK, Thompson HR, Mann CV. The results of surgical treatment of cancer of the rectum by radical resection and extended abdomino-iliac lymphadenectomy. Br J Surg. 1985;72(8):599–601.
33. Kusters M, Beets GL, van de Velde CJ, Beets-Tan RG, Marijnen CA, Rutten HJ, et al. A comparison between the treatment of low rectal cancer in Japan and the Netherlands, focusing on the patterns of local recurrence. Ann Surg. 2009;249(2):229–35. doi:10.1097/SLA.0b013e318190a664.
34. Nagawa H, Muto T, Sunouchi K, Higuchi Y, Tsurita G, Watanabe T, et al. Randomized, controlled trial of lateral node dissection vs. nerve-preserving resection in patients with rectal cancer after preoperative radiotherapy. Dis Colon Rectum. 2001;44(9):1274–80.
35. Fujita S, Yamamoto S, Akasu T, Moriya Y. Lateral pelvic lymph node dissection for advanced lower rectal cancer. Br J Surg. 2003;90(12):1580–5. doi:10.1002/bjs.4350.
36. Watanabe T, Tsurita G, Muto T, Sawada T, Sunouchi K, Higuchi Y, et al. Extended lymphadenectomy and preoperative radiotherapy for lower rectal cancers. Surgery. 2002;132(1):27–33.
37. Moreira LF, Hizuta A, Iwagaki H, Tanaka N, Orita K. Lateral lymph node dissection for rectal carcinoma below the peritoneal reflection. Br J Surg. 1994; 81(2):293–6.
38. Enker WE, Havenga K, Polyak T, Thaler H, Cranor M. Abdominoperineal resection via total mesorectal excision and autonomic nerve preservation for low rectal cancer. World J Surg. 1997;21(7):715–20.
39. Enker WE. Potency, cure, and local control in the operative treatment of rectal cancer. Arch Surg. 1992;127(12):1396–401; discussion 402.
40. Hojo K, Sawada T, Moriya Y. An analysis of survival and voiding, sexual function after wide iliopelvic lymphadenectomy in patients with carcinoma of the rectum, compared with conventional lymphadenectomy. Dis Colon Rectum. 1989;32(2):128–33.
41. Koch M, Kienle P, Antolovic D, Buchler MW, Weitz J. Is the lateral lymph node compartment relevant? Recent Results Cancer Res. 2005;165:40–5.
42. Haggitt RC, Glotzbach RE, Soffer EE, Wruble LD. Prognostic factors in colorectal carcinomas arising in adenomas: implications for lesions removed by endoscopic polypectomy. Gastroenterology. 1985;89(2):328–36.
43. Hida J, Yasutomi M, Maruyama T, Fujimoto K, Uchida T, Okuno K. Lymph node metastases detected in the mesorectum distal to carcinoma of the rectum by the clearing method: justification of total mesorectal excision. J Am Coll Surg. 1997;184(6):584–8.
44. Vignali A, Fazio VW, Lavery IC, Milsom JW, Church JM, Hull TL, et al. Factors associated with the occurrence of leaks in stapled rectal anastomoses: a review of 1,014 patients. J Am Coll Surg. 1997;185(2):105–13.
45. Dietz D. Postoperative complications. In: Beck D, Roberts P, Saclarides T, Senagore A, Stamos M, Wexner S, editors. The ASCRS textbook of colon and rectal surgery. 2nd ed. New York: Springer; 2011.
46. Pocard M, Zinzindohoue F, Haab F, Caplin S, Parc R, Tiret E. A prospective study of sexual and urinary function before and after total mesorectal excision with autonomic nerve preservation for rectal cancer. Surgery. 2002;131(4):368–72.

47. Kim NK, Aahn TW, Park JK, Lee KY, Lee WH, Sohn SK, et al. Assessment of sexual and voiding function after total mesorectal excision with pelvic autonomic nerve preservation in males with rectal cancer. Dis Colon Rectum. 2002;45(9):1178–85. doi:10.1097/01.dcr.0000027125.03278.26.
48. Junginger T, Kneist W, Heintz A. Influence of identification and preservation of pelvic autonomic nerves in rectal cancer surgery on bladder dysfunction after total mesorectal excision. Dis Colon Rectum. 2003;46(5):621–8. doi:10.1097/01.dcr.0000059327.55102.96.

## Key Operative Steps

1. Place the patient in lithotomy position.
2. Perform complete abdominal exploration to rule out metastatic disease
3. Mobilize the colon along the white line of Toldt.
4. Identify the ureter at the bifurcation of the common iliac artery.
5. If necessary, mobilize the splenic flexure.
6. Elevate the sigmoid colon and isolate the inferior mesenteric artery and left colic artery, which should be spared if appropriate. Ligate the superior hemorrhoidal artery at its takeoff from the inferior mesenteric artery.
7. Transect the colon to ensure adequate blood supply.
8. Start total mesorectal excision. Dissect posterior to the rectum between the fascia propria of the rectum and the parietal fascia of the pelvic floor.
9. Carry the dissection through Waldeyer's fascia to the level of the coccyx.
10. Use electrocautery for anterior and lateral dissection.
11. Transect the rectum once an adequate distal margin has been reached.
12. Assure a tension-free colorectal anastomosis.
13. Create the anastomosis using a circular stapling device.
14. Perform a "leak test" on the anastomosis.
15. Create a diverting ileostomy when indicated.

# Laparoscopic Technique for Low Anterior Resection

# 21

Marta Jiménez Toscano and Antonio M. Lacy

## Historical Perspective

Rectal resection for cancer has evolved over the last century from the radical abdominoperineal resection proposed by Miles in 1908, to the sphincter sparing surgery introduced by Abel in 1931, to the total mesorectal excision (TME) by Heald in 1979. Since then, TME has become the standard surgical treatment for rectal cancer [1]. Recent advances in laparoscopic equipment and techniques have facilitated the application of minimally invasive approaches to rectal cancer surgery. It is now clear that laparoscopic TME can reduce length of stay and expedite recovery without compromising oncologic outcomes. Furthermore, the laparoscopic approach may allow for easier mobilization of the splenic flexure, easier dissection of critical vessels, and easier identification of important structures such as the ureters and pelvic nerves [2–4]. Reducing the size of the abdominal incision results in lower wound infection rates and lower risk of incisional hernia formation [5]. In some series, the laparoscopic approach to rectal cancer surgery has also been associated with improvements in local recurrence, functional results, and quality of life [6].

## Indications

The laparoscopic approach was initially limited to low rectal cancers that were candidates for abdominoperineal excision of the rectum. With the advances in laparoscopic stapling devices, the laparoscopic approach can be used to treat malignant tumors of the rectum as low as 3–4 cm from the anal verge. Lower tumors can be resected using a partial internal sphincter resection and transanal hand-sewn anastomosis [6]. Because of enhanced visualization, laparoscopy can be particularly useful in patients with a narrow pelvis.

## Contraindications

Laparoscopic TME can be particularly challenging in morbidly obese patients. Paradoxically, these are the patients more likely to benefit from

Electronic supplementary material: Supplementary material is available in the online version of this chapter at 10.1007/978-1-4939-1893-5_21. Videos can also be accessed at http://www.springerimages.com/videos/978-1-4939-1892-8.

M.J. Toscano, M.D.
Department of Gastrointestinal Surgery, University of Barcelona School of Medicine, Clinic Hospital, Quiron Hospital, Barcelona, Spain

A.M. Lacy, M.D., Ph.D. (✉)
Department of Gastrointestinal Surgery, University of Barcelona School of Medicine, Clinic Hospital, Quiron Hospital, Barcelona, Spain

Centro Esther Koplowitz, University of Barcelona, Villarroel, 170, 08036 Barcelona, Spain
e-mail: lacy@clinic.ub.es

J. Kim and J. Garcia-Aguilar (eds.), *Surgery for Cancers of the Gastrointestinal Tract: A Step-by-Step Approach*,
DOI 10.1007/978-1-4939-1893-5_21, © Springer Science+Business Media New York 2015

a minimally invasive approach. Laparoscopy may also be challenging in some patients with T4 tumors or recurrent cancers particularly when complex multiorgan resections and reconstruction may be contemplated. An early decision to convert may be wise if tumor involvement of adjacent structures is unexpectedly encountered during laparoscopic TME for cancer.

## Anatomic Considerations

Because of the lack of tactile sensation, a clear understanding of the arterial supply to the rectum and its relationship to the hypogastric plexus and the left ureter is particularly important during laparoscopy to avoid intraoperative complications and long-term functional sequelae. The pneumoperitoneum tends to open the areolar space that separates the mesorectal fascia from the surrounding structures facilitating dissection. Finally, it is important to be aware of the curvature of the sacrum to avoid bleeding from the presacral plexus at the insertion of Waldeyer's fascia, where the distal sacrum curves anteriorly.

## Preoperative Considerations

Our preoperative studies do not differ from ones that are used for approaches to rectal cancer with other techniques. The complete workup includes:

- Clinical evaluation including family history, bowel function, sexual and urinary function, weight loss, rectal bleeding, and abdominal and rectal examination
- Laboratory analysis including hemoglobin and carcinoembryonic antigen level
- Complete colonoscopy and tumor biopsy
- Computed tomographic scan of the chest, abdomen, and pelvis
- Endorectal ultrasound or rectal magnetic resonance imaging
- Preoperative marking by an enterostomal nurse

## Preoperative Considerations

Although perioperative preparation of the patient begins days before surgery, the 24 h before surgery is the most important period. The preparation consists of:

- Clear liquid diet for at least 24 h
- Mechanical bowel preparation the day before surgery with or without oral antibiotics
- Intravenous prophylactic antibiotics
- Thoracic epidural catheter for pain control
- Central venous catheter
- Intermittent lower extremity compression stockings and adjustable leg stirrups
- Irrigation of the rectal stump (1 % diluted iodine solution)

## Surgical Technique

The patient is placed in Lloyd Davis position with the legs in stirrups for lithotomy position (Fig. 21.1). Occasionally a supine position with open legs in a split table is sufficient to perform a stapled anastomosis comfortably. The arms are tucked at the patient's side. A bandage is placed around the thorax to secure the patient to the OR table to prevent patient movement with steep Trendelenburg position. The abdomen is prepared with antiseptic solution and draped sterilely.

The surgeon works from the patient's right with an assistant to the left of the surgeon and on the left side of the patient. We prefer to use two monitors on the left side of the patient; one is placed at hip level for optimal surgeon's view and a second one opposite to the first assistant. A third monitor in the right side of the patient may be useful to the second assistant. The operating nurse and instrument table should be on the right side, close to the foot of the patient.

The pneumoperitoneum is made by a Veress needle inserted in a periumbilical location or in the left upper quadrant (Palmer's point). The abdomen is insufflated with $CO_2$ gas. When a 12 mmHg pressure is obtained, a 10/12-mm port

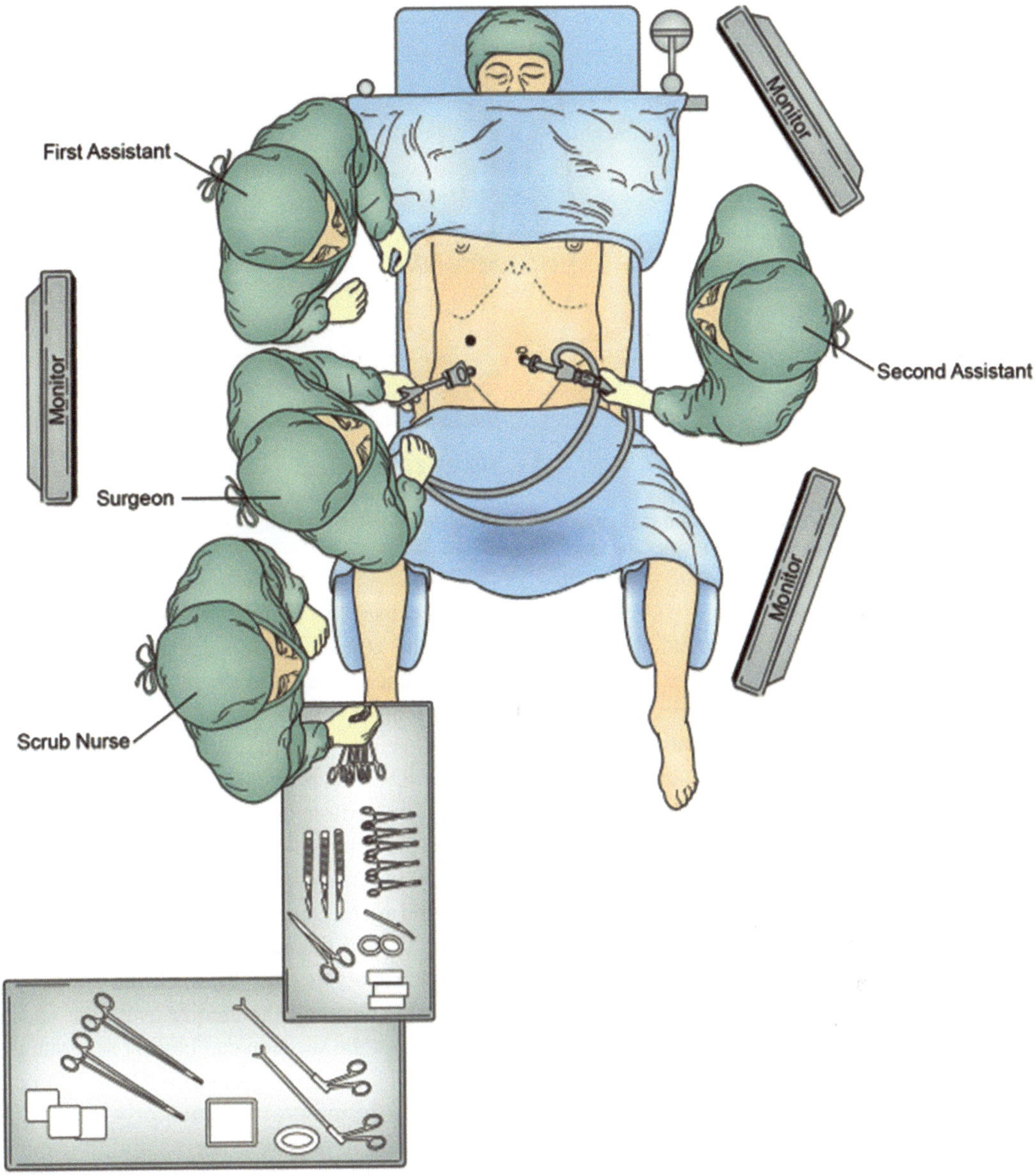


**Fig. 21.1** Theater organization for laparoscopic low anterior resection

is inserted at the level of the umbilicus and a 30° camera is introduced. Two 5-mm trocars are introduced in the right side of the abdomen and in the left lower quadrant. Finally, a 5/12-mm trocar is introduced in right lower abdominal region (Fig. 21.2). Additional trocars can be introduced as needed. Care is needed during trocar placement to avoid injury to the inferior epigastric vessels.

First, the surgeon should explore the abdominal cavity laparoscopically looking for tumor implants or liver metastasis. A steep Trendelenburg and right side down position of the table is adopted and the small bowel is moved to the right upper quadrant. We favor a medial-to-lateral approach to the superior rectal vessels, however there are some situations in which early mobilization of the lateral attachments of the

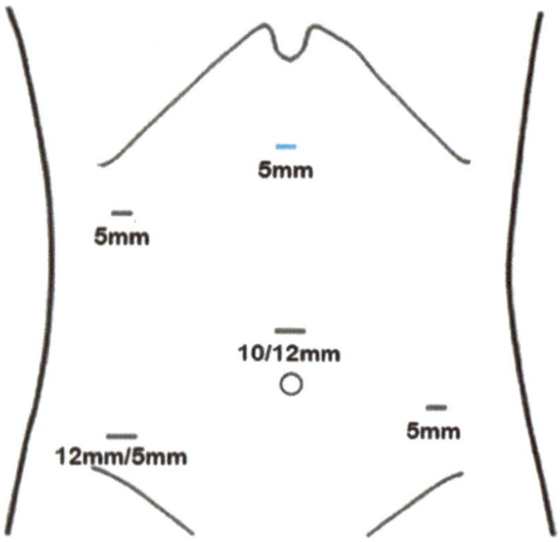


**Fig. 21.2** Trocar positions for the abdominal approach. The blue 5-mm trocar is used if a splenic flexure approach is necessary

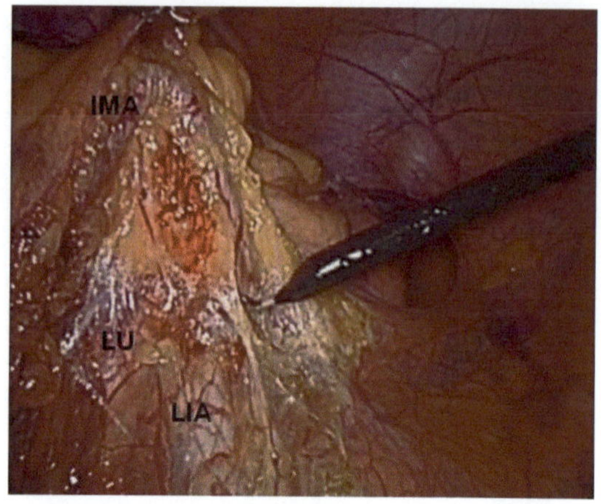


**Fig. 21.3** Laparoscopic view of the pelvis. Traction of the inferior mesenteric artery (IMA) allows the correct visualization of the left ureter (LU) and left iliac artery (LIA)

sigmoid colon and a lateral to medial approach may be advantageous.

We use the 5-mm LigaSure device (Covidien) as a hemostatic device and a monopolar energy device (e.g., hook) to perform the surgery. A gentle skyward traction of the sigmoid colon is made by the assistant with a grasping forceps so the inferior mesenteric vessels are retracted. In general, grasping the colon should be avoided to prevent bowel injury. The surgeon incises the peritoneum at the base of the sigmoid mesentery over the right iliac vessels and the space between the superior rectal vessels and the retroperitoneum is bluntly dissected. The inferior mesenteric artery and vein are dissected separately and the left ureter is localized over the left common iliac artery (Fig. 21.3). The gonadal vessels should also be identified lateral to the ureter before ligating the mesenteric vessels. The inferior mesenteric artery is divided 1 cm from its origin using clips, a laparoscopic linear stapler, or simply with the LigaSure device (Fig. 21.4). The inferior mesenteric vein is found next to the pancreas and similarly divided. The mesentery of the descending and sigmoid colon is released from medial to lateral all the way to the line of Toldt (Fig. 21.5). Care should be taken to avoid injuries to the mesenteric arcades to guarantee a correct blood supply to the descending colon. Gauze is used for hemostasis and to protect the ureter and gonadal vessels and is left as a marking reference to assist in the takedown of the lateral attachments from the left side. The assistant surgeon gently pulls the sigmoid colon medially to expose the peritoneal attachment in the left gutter. The peritoneum is incised from the pelvic brim to the splenic flexure.

Now, the attention is turned to the pelvis to begin the rectal surgery. By pulling the rectum upward toward the anterior abdominal wall, the surgeon separates the mesorectum from the promontory opening the areolar avascular space. At this point the surgeon can bluntly separate the mesorectal fascia from the presacral fascia propia by pushing the mesorectum anteriorly (Fig. 21.6). As such, the hypogastric nerves and, more distally, the pelvic nerve plexus are exposed and protected from potential injury. The dissection should be meticulous to avoid injuring the sacral venous plexus.

The dissection is then continued laterally, opening the peritoneum all the way to the anterior peritoneal reflection in the cul-de-sac and dividing the lateral ligaments. The position of both ureters and hypogastric nerves should be checked at this point and preserved. Finally, the surgeon incises the peritoneum of the rectovesical pouch in men or the rectovaginal pouch in women, exposing Denonvilliers' fascia. The dissection is

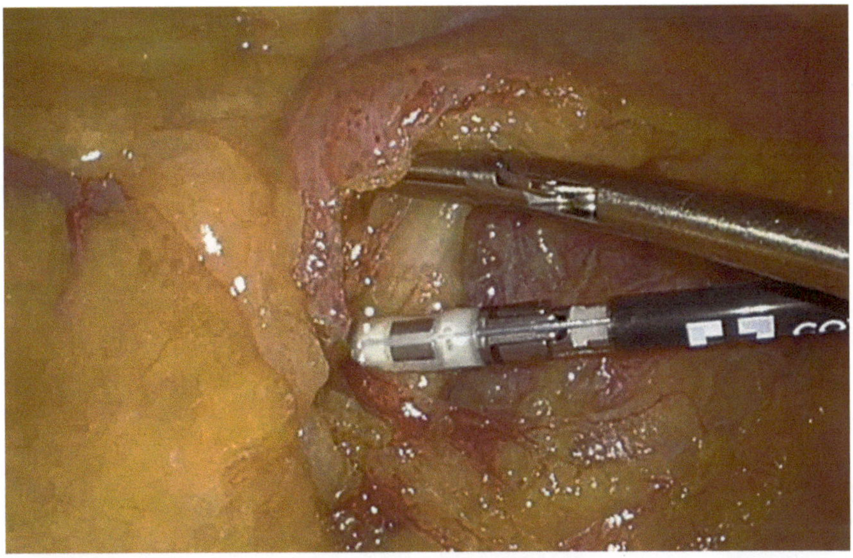

**Fig. 21.4** Division of the inferior mesenteric artery with the LigaSure device

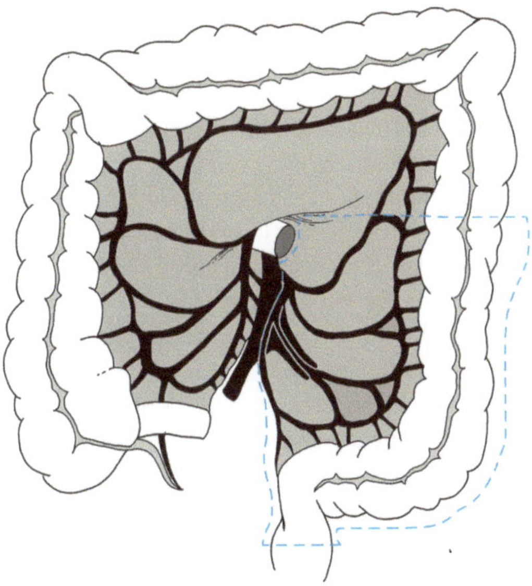

**Fig. 21.5** Schematic of the resection

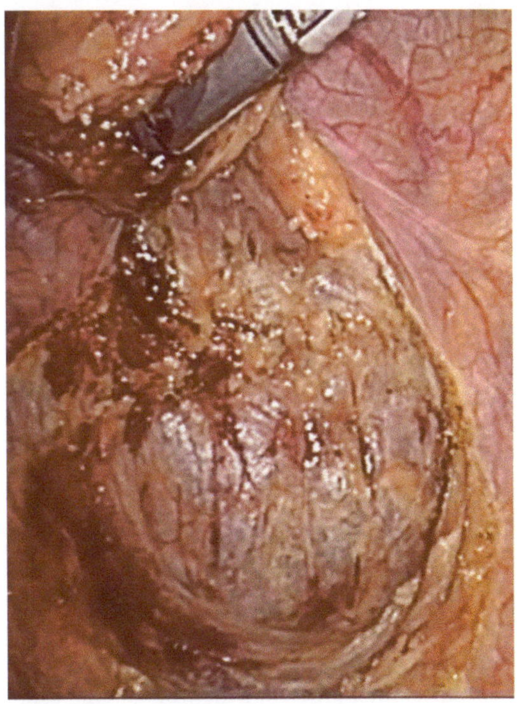

**Fig. 21.6** Dissection of the mesorectum in an avascular presacral plane. The instrument is holding the rectum up against the anterior abdominal wall

continued, alternating right and left side, until the distal rectum is completely freed taking care to preserve the neurovascular bundles. Once the rectosacral ligament is incised at the level of the fourth sacral vertebra, the dissection meets the levator ani muscle and the pelvic floor. When a TME is performed, the rectum is divided at the level of the pelvic floor, ideally leaving a margin of at least 2 cm distal to the tumor. An articulating linear stapler is commonly used to divide the rectum (Fig. 21.7). In very low rectal tumors, an intersphincteric resection is necessary using a perineal transanal approach.

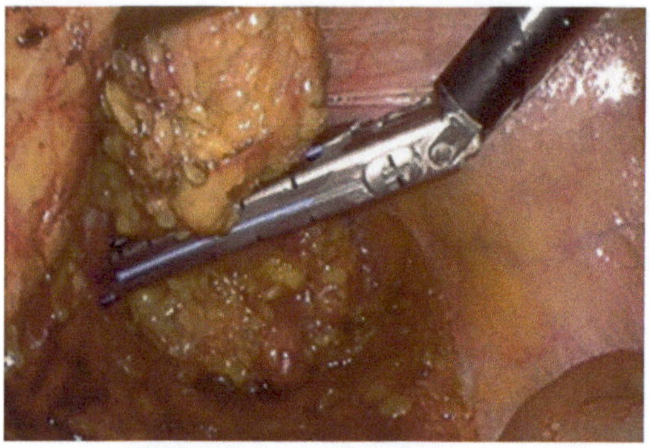

**Fig. 21.7** Distal resection of the low rectum with an articulating laparoscopic linear stapler

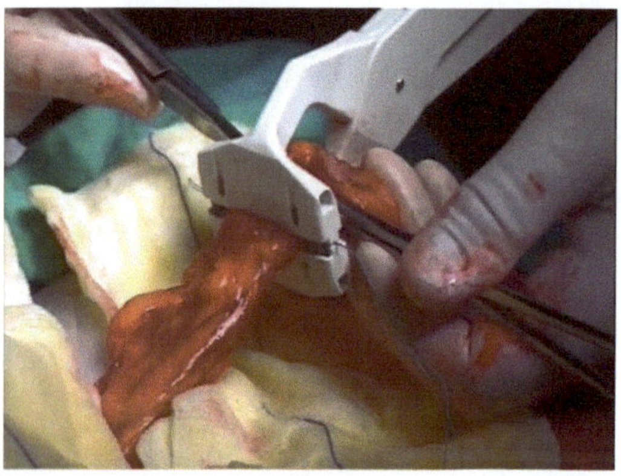

**Fig. 21.8** Proximal resection of the rectum with a purse-string device. B Introduction of the circular stapler anvil

## Anastomotic Technique

Depending on the patient and the location of the tumor, the anastomosis can be performed mechanically or hand-sewn.

### Mechanical Anastomosis

For middle or high rectal tumors we exteriorize the rectum and sigmoid colon with a Pfannenstiel incision. The specimen is drawn out of the peritoneal cavity after protecting the wound (e.g., using a plastic ring drape) and divided proximally with scissors to verify the blood supply. A 2-0 polypropylene purse-string suture is then applied to the open end of the proximal colon (Fig. 21.8). The anvil of a circular stapler is inserted and secured with the purse-string suture (Fig. 21.9). The mesenteric fat is cleared from the end of the bowel close to the anvil and the bowel is returned to the abdomen closing the fascia behind. The pneumoperitoneum is established again to finish the anastomosis.

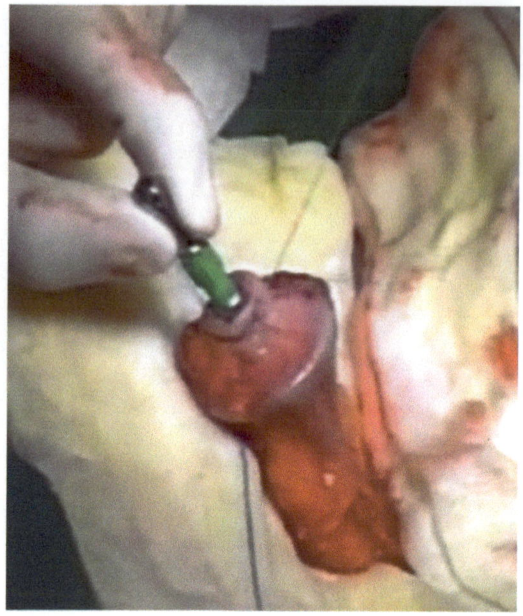

**Fig. 21.9** The purse-string is tied around the anvil

It is important to verify that the length of the colon will be sufficient to perform a tension-free anastomosis. If the anvil and colon are positioned correctly in the pelvis, then anastomotic tension is not expected. If there is tension, we mobilize the splenic flexure from its attachments to the spleen and to the left kidney over Gerota's fascia. We can approach the flexure by elevating the omentum and dissecting it off the transverse colon. This way we can enter the lesser sac to expose the stomach, pancreas, and retroperitoneum and finish the dissection of the splenic flexure comfortably. Sometimes, long instruments, another 5-mm trocar, and the surgeon positioned between the legs are needed to completely mobilize the splenic flexure.

The circular stapler is introduced carefully through the anus and advanced until the cartridge is seen pushing against the rectal stump. The spike is advanced and pushed though the rectal wall close to the transverse staple line (Fig. 21.10). The anvil is then connected to the spike. Before closing and firing the stapler, we confirm the

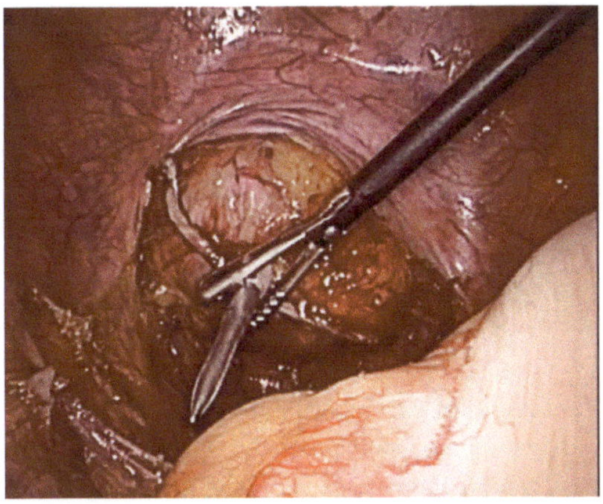

**Fig. 21.10** The circular stapler is introduced into the rectal stump and the spike is opened close to the transverse staple line

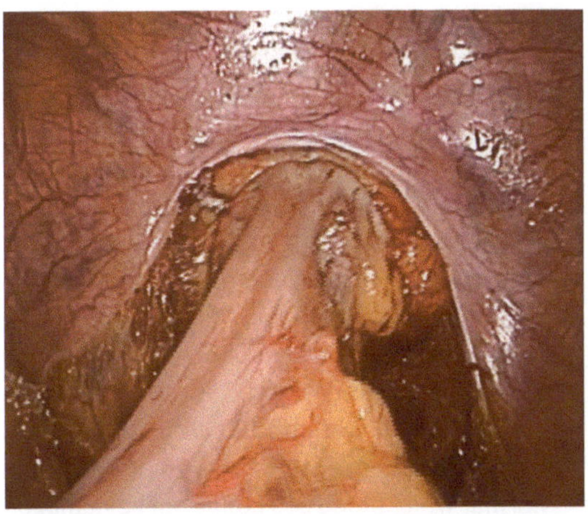

**Fig. 21.11** Intra-abdominal view of the completed anastomosis showing proper orientation of the bowel and mesentery

correct position of the colon by following the colonic taeniae and the cut edge of the mesentery (Fig. 21.11). The stapler device is slowly closed without tension or torsion with visual control from the abdominal side, ensuring that the surrounding tissues (vagina and lateral pelvic tissues) are not caught in the anastomosis. Once the stapler has been fired and removed, the tissue rings are inspected for completeness. In low rectal cancer, we prefer to use the circular stapler that is used for stapled hemorroidectomy, because it provides larger tissue rings and possibly a longer distal margin (Fig. 21.12).

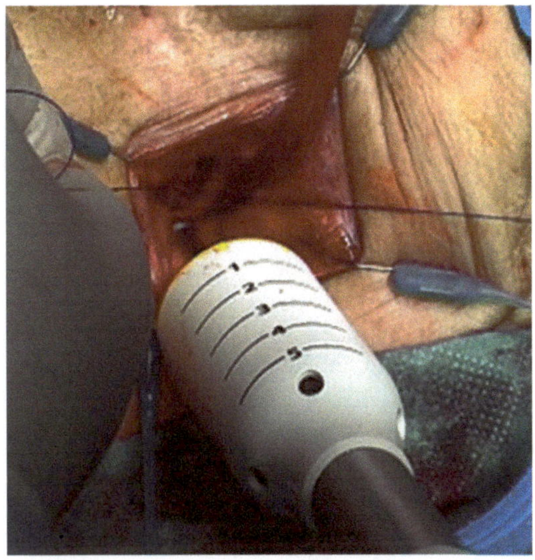

**Fig. 21.12** For low rectal tumors, a circular stapler for stapled hemorrhoidectomy (Covidien) is used

## Hand-Sewn Anastomosis

For very low tumors, an intersphinteric resection is performed, the specimen is removed transanally, and a hand-sewn end-to-end colo-anal anastomosis is fashioned. Our hand-sewn colo-anal anastomosis starts with four quadrant sutures of 2-0 reabsorbable sutures placed through the distal anal canal and muscle. After these four quadrant sutures are tied, we complete the anastomosis with interrupted 3-0 reabsorbable sutures. A Lone Star Retractor (CooperSurgical) is very useful to expose the anal canal and distal rectum and complete the anastomosis.

Before closing, hemostasis is insured and the abdominal cavity is irrigated with 1 % povidone iodine. A closed suction drain is introduced from the left port into the pelvis leaving the proximal end close to the rectal anastomosis. From the anus, a rectal drainage is placed across the anastomosis and secured to the perianal skin.

## Port Site Closure

Usually, we do not close the fascia of the 5-mm port sites. If one of them is bleeding or we have to increase the size for any reason we close the orifice with a Reverden needle with vicryl suture.

## Indication for Ileostomy

When a low anastomosis is performed, we prefer to add a defunctioning loop ileostomy. The distal small bowel is localized laparoscopically and the afferent and efferent limbs are identified. The 5-mm port on the right side is used to get the bowel out. A diverting loop ileostomy is performed with 3-0 reabsorbable sutures orienting the afferent limb superiorly. The ileostomy is closed in 8 weeks after checking the integrity of the anastomosis with a gastrografin enema.

## Postoperative Management

- The nasogastric tube is removed in the operating room
- Oral liquid intake is started the first day after surgery
- Antibiotics are not routinely used after surgery
- The Foley catheter is removed on postoperative day #1 if urine output is adequate
- The abdominal drain is removed on postoperative day #3 if output is <50 mL.
- The epidural catheter is usually removed on postoperative day #2 at which point pain is controlled using oral analgesics
- The patient is discharged home when a soft diet is tolerated and the stoma is functioning properly

## Complications

### Perioperative Complications

Management of complications begins with the anticipation of potential anastomotic and technical challenges. Some of the more common intraoperative complications include:

- Presacral hemorrhage and prostatic bleeding. Usually we can stop the hemorrhage with local pressure with gauze. Occasionally hemostatic agents may be necessary. Placements of stitches or thumbtacks are rarely necessary.
- Anastomotic bleeding. We can control bleeding using a transanal approach to obtain hemostasis with bipolar cautery or reabsorbable sutures.
- Injury of the rectal stump during distal posterior dissection is best avoided by minimizing direct traction and grasping of the rectal wall. When perforation occurs, it can be repaired with sutures, incorporated in the surgical specimen or incorporated in the anastomosis.
- Ureteral damage is repaired primarily when possible or, if not possible, the ureter is reimplanted into the bladder. If diagnosed after surgery, an ureteral injury may require stenting and/or reoperation.
- Iliac vessel damage requires conversion to open surgery and repair with 4-0 or 5-0 prolene sutures.

### Postoperative Complications

- One of the most common early complications is anastomotic dehiscence and pelvic sepsis. Depending on the magnitude of the defect and the clinical presentation, anastomotic leaks are treated in different ways. Patients with small leaks, minimal clinical symptoms, and a normal white blood cell count can be managed conservatively with bowel rest, antibiotics, and percutaneous drainage if an abscess is present. If the patient has peritonitis, a reoperation with washout, drainage, and a diverting ileostomy or colostomy is performed in addition to antibiotic therapy and resuscitation maneuvers.
- We use the transanal minimally invasive surgery (TAMIS) approach to evaluate and repair anastomotic dehiscence when possible.
- Bladder dysfunction often requires urinary catheter for several weeks.
- Long-term complications include sexual and urinary dysfunction, as well as defecatory problems known as the low anterior resection syndrome.

## Conclusion

Laparoscopic TME can now be safely performed for most rectal cancer patients. However, due to the limitations of current laparoscopic instrumentation, the dissection of the distal rectum is still challenging. Recently, we have developed the transanal Natural Orifice Transluminal Endoscopic Surgery with Total Mesorectal Excision (NOTES-TME) that allows the entire rectal and mesorectal dissection using a transanal approach [7]. Using this combined abdominal/transanal approach to TME, improved visualization and precise resection is possible even in difficult scenarios such as patients with narrow pelvis, visceral obesity, and low rectal tumors. Studies are currently underway to determine if using this TAMIS/NOTES-TME approach is oncologically acceptable compared to current open, laparoscopic, and robotic techniques.

## References


1. Heald RJ, Moran BJ, Ryall RD, Sexton R, MacFarlane JK. Rectal cancer: the Basingstoke experience of total mesorectal excision, 1978–1997. Arch Surg. 1998;133(8):894–9.
2. Tytherleigh MG, Mc CMNJ. Options for sphincter preservation in surgery for low rectal cancer. Br J Surg. 2003;90(8):922–33. doi:10.1002/bjs.4296.
3. Boutros M, Hippalgaonkar N, Silva E, Allende D, Wexner SD, Berho M. Laparoscopic resection of rectal cancer results in higher lymph node yield and better short-term outcomes than open surgery: a large single-center comparative study. Dis Colon Rectum. 2013;56(6):679–88. doi:10.1097/DCR.0b013e318287c594.
4. Agha A, Benseler V, Hornung M, Gerken M, Iesalnieks I, Furst A, et al. Long-term oncologic outcome after laparoscopic surgery for rectal cancer. Surg Endosc. 2013;28(4):1119–25. doi:10.1007/s00464-013-3286-8.
5. Ng SS, Lee JF, Yiu RY, Li JC, Hon SS, Mak TW, et al. Laparoscopic-assisted versus open total mesorectal excision with anal sphincter preservation for mid and low rectal cancer: a prospective, randomized trial. Surg Endosc. 2014;28(1):297–306. doi:10.1007/s00464-013-3187-x.
6. Rullier E, Denost Q, Vendrely V, Rullier A, Laurent C. Low rectal cancer: classification and standardization of surgery. Dis Colon Rectum. 2013;56(5):560–7. doi:10.1097/DCR.0b013e31827c4a8c.
7. Sylla P, Bordeianou LG, Berger D, Han KS, Lauwers GY, Sahani DV, et al. A pilot study of natural orifice transanal endoscopic total mesorectal excision with laparoscopic assistance for rectal cancer. Surg Endosc. 2013;27(9):3396–405. doi:10.1007/s00464-013-2922-7.


## Key Operative Steps

1. The abdominal cavity is accessed and the small bowel and omentum are moved toward the right upper quadrant.
2. The inferior mesenteric artery is divided near its origin after identifying the left ureter.
3. The descending colon and sigmoid colon are mobilized using a medial-to-lateral approach.
4. The inferior mesenteric vein is divided.
5. The splenic flexure is mobilized.
6. Start total mesorectal excision with dissection into the presacral plane.
7. Dissect the peritoneal attachments on the right and left sides of the rectum and on the anterior peritoneal reflection.
8. For middle and proximal rectal tumors, exteriorize the specimen with a Pfannenstiel incision, resect the proximal colon, and introduce the anvil of the circular stapler. For ultralow tumors, the specimen is exteriorized transanally, the proximal rectum is transected, and a hand-sewn anastomosis is performed.
9. Close ports that are 10–12 mm in size.
10. Create diverting ileostomy.

# 22 Totally Robotic Low Anterior Resection

J. Joshua Smith, Leandro Feo, and Julio Garcia-Aguilar

## Principles and Justification

Over the past two decades the popularity of laparoscopic-assisted surgery has risen dramatically. The short-term benefits of the minimally invasive approach, compared to open surgery, include less physiologic stress and blood loss, less postoperative pain, less use of analgesic medication, faster recovery, shorter length of stay, and smaller incisions with better cosmetic results [1, 2]. These advantages and appealing short-term outcomes often make minimally invasive surgery the procedure of choice. Although there was initial controversy and concern if the short-term and long-term outcomes were as oncologically sound as those of open surgery [3], several randomized trials in colon cancer have shown that the outcomes are equivalent [4–6].

However, rectal cancer surgery is more complex. This is largely because the surgical field is in the bony pelvis, a much more restrictive anatomical area. The major limitations are due to the need to perform a circumferential dissection in this confined pelvic space, making optimal retraction and visualization difficult [7, 8]. Thus, while laparoscopic low anterior resection (LAR) for rectal cancer offers short-term advantages compared with the open approach, this procedure has not gained widespread acceptance among rectal cancer surgeons because of the associated technical challenges.

As an effective alternative to traditional open surgery and conventional laparoscopy, minimally invasive procedures for rectal cancer can now be performed with the assistance of a robotic system: the da Vinci Surgical System (Intuitive). From the surgeon's point of view, the superior precision and dexterity of the four-arm DaVinci robotic system (Intuitive) give it a clear advantage over conventional laparoscopy in rectal cancer surgery [9–12]. The four arms provide superior retraction, making reliance on a highly skilled assistant unnecessary. The precise articulation of the robotic instruments

Electronic supplementary material: Supplementary material is available in the online version of this chapter at 10.1007/978-1-4939-1893-5_22. Videos can also be accessed at http://www.springerimages.com/videos/978-1-4939-1892-8.

J.J. Smith, M.D., Ph.D.
Department of Surgery,
Memorial Sloan Kettering Cancer Center,
1275 York Avenue, Room C-1067,
New York, NY, USA
e-mail: smithj5@mskcc.org

L. Feo, M.D.
Department of Surgery, Memorial Sloan Kettering Cancer Center, 1275 York Avenue, Room C-1067,
New York, NY, USA
e-mail: leandrofeo@gmail.com

J. Garcia-Aguilar, M.D., Ph.D. (✉)
Department of Surgery,
Benno C. Schmidt Chair in Surgical Oncology,
Memorial Sloan Kettering Cancer Center,
1275 York Avenue, Room C-1067,
New York, NY, USA
e-mail: garciaaj@mskcc.org

J. Kim and J. Garcia-Aguilar (eds.), *Surgery for Cancers of the Gastrointestinal Tract: A Step-by-Step Approach*, DOI 10.1007/978-1-4939-1893-5_22, © Springer Science+Business Media New York 2015

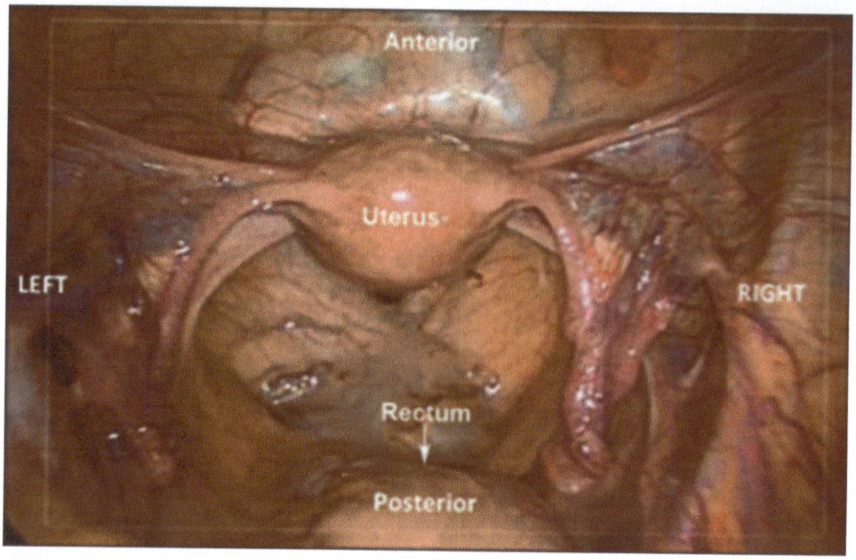


**Fig. 22.1** High-definition three-dimensional camera and visualization of pelvic structures. The female pelvic anatomy is demonstrated

enables the surgeon to follow the contours of the rectum and mesorectum with greater ease than is possible with conventional straight laparoscopic instruments [13]. In addition, the high-definition three-dimensional (3D) camera provides an ideal visualization of all pelvic structures (Fig. 22.1).

A number of trials comparing robotic TME (RTME) and laparoscopic TME with respect to feasibility and long-term oncologic outcomes are forthcoming [14–16]. Recent review of outcomes associated with robotic-assisted, laparoscopic, and open surgical approaches to colorectal cancer indicates that the robotic approach is safe and feasible, demonstrating comparable short-term outcomes [17]. In a comparison of robotic-assisted versus open surgery for rectal cancer, Pigazzi et al. reported reduced complications and a reduction in postoperative pain allowing many patients undergoing robotic-assisted procedures to begin adjuvant treatment sooner [18]. Pigazzi et al. also reported no operative mortality, 7.3 % rate of conversion, 8.6 % rate of anastomotic leak, 13.1 lymph nodes retrieved, and 97.6 % negative circumferential resection margin in another series of 82 rectal cancer patients treated with RTME [19]. These outcomes are similar to other reports showing favorable results in patients undergoing RTME [19, 20, 28].

RTME is associated with similar short-term quality of life outcomes, similar rates of post-operative complications, equivalent short-term surrogate outcomes such as circumferential resection margin, number of harvested lymph nodes, and rates of clear distal margin but lower intraoperative conversion rates, compared to conventional laparoscopic TME [15, 16, 19, 21–23].

It should be noted that, while RTME facilitates pelvic dissection, it requires a longer operative time than open or traditional laparoscopic surgery. This is true even after the learning curve is reached, although the amount of operative time has been shown to decrease with surgeon experience [24]. Additionally, there is a relatively high learning curve of at least 15–20 cases [24–26]. The robotic system comes at a high price. This includes not only the cost of the robotic system itself (approximately $1.65–$2.5 million USD), but its maintenance [11, 27], raising significantly the costs per patient hospitalization compared to conventional laparoscopy (average $84,000 vs. $63,000, respectively).

## Surgeon Requirements

As mentioned above, RTME requires a longer operative time. RTME technique is technically demanding, with a high associated learning curve [25, 26, 28]. Surgeons wishing to embrace RTME should meet the following criteria:

1. Experience and comfort performing laparoscopic segmental colon resection without hand assistance.
2. Robotic experience with inanimate models/simulators and animal and cadaveric models.
3. A thorough understanding of the principles of TME and an adequate yearly volume of rectal procedures.

## Patient Selection

We use robotic LAR for the patient who presents with nonsphincter-invading mid and low rectal cancer. However, surgeons who are just beginning to use the robotic system should offer this procedure more selectively. For a double-stapled anastomosis after LAR, the surgical distance between the lower edge of the tumor and the anorectal ring should be at least 1–2 cm. Thus, at the start of the learning curve, female patients with normal body mass index (BMI) and tumor located high above the anal verge are ideal patients.

## Preoperative Considerations

Preoperative imaging of all patients with rectal cancer should involve chest X-ray, computed tomography (CT) scan of the abdomen and pelvis, and endorectal ultrasound (ERUS) or pelvic magnetic resonance imaging (MRI). Neoadjuvant chemoradiation (CRT) treatment should be offered to patients with locally advanced cancer, according to the surgeon's preference and experience. A bowel preparation is recommended the day before surgery, as this makes intestinal manipulation easier.

## Patient Positioning

We routinely place a large foam mat under the patient to prevent sliding during changes in the position of the operating bed. The upper chest is secured with a velcro strap and tested. After induction of general anesthesia, the patient is moved into a modified lithotomy position. A digital rectal examination is performed to confirm the location of the tumor. Routine rectal irrigation with water or an iodine-based solution is done. A urinary catheter is inserted once the patient is prepped and draped. The perineum is prepped in sterile fashion only if a transanal extraction and hand-sewn coloanal anastomosis are anticipated.

## Totally Robotic Approach

Previously, we performed a hybrid/laparoscopic approach, but we now complete the procedure in a completely robotic manner. We complete the operation with one docking maneuver and minor patient repositioning. The entire intracorporeal procedure with transanal extraction and minimal incision will be described. It is important to note that this approach requires considerable expertise with robotic port placement and cart positioning, in order to avoid collisions with the robotic arm. This should become less problematic with the new generation robotic systems.

## Port Placement

A Veress needle is inserted in the left subcostal region (Palmer's point) and the abdomen is insufflated to 15 mmHg. A 12-mm camera (port C) is placed halfway between the pubis and xiphoid. As a general principle, robotic ports must be at least 8–10 cm apart to avoid collisions (Fig. 22.2). A 12-mm trocar (R1) is then placed roughly

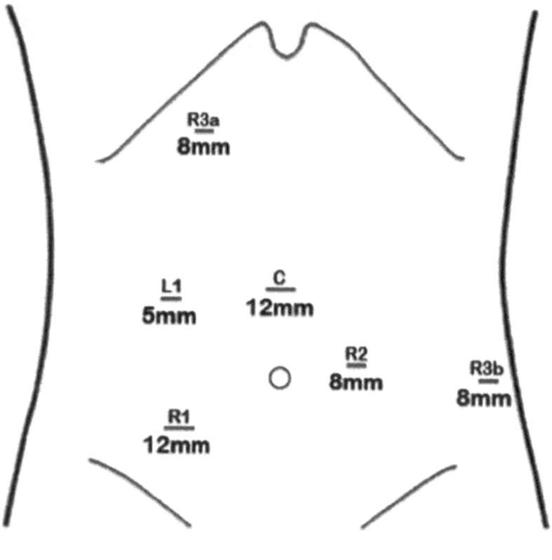


**Fig. 22.2** Trocar positioning for robotic total mesorectal excision. All robotic ports must be 8–10 cm apart to avoid collisions

halfway between C and the right anterior superior iliac spine (ASIS), which corresponds to the midclavicular line (MCL). Great care must be taken to avoid the inferior epigastric vessels in this area. R1 will be the main stapling/clipping port for vessels, mesentery, and bowel; this site may also serve for the protective ileostomy. R1 is used by the surgeon's right hand. A 5-mm laparoscopic port (L1) is placed 8–10 cm above R1 in the MCL. A robotic 8-mm trocar (R2) will be inserted in the same position on the left side. A third robotic port (R3a) is placed in the MCL, 8 cm above L1 (Fig. 22.2). The fourth robotic port (R3b) will be 8–10 cm more lateral to R2, usually just above the left ASIS. It is important to note that some variations in port set-up may be necessary depending on gender, body habitus, and tumor location. For example, in large male patients with low tumors, the four robotic ports will be shifted medially to prevent the robotic arms from hitting a narrow pelvic sidewall and to access the levator plane more easily.

## Mobilization of Splenic Flexure and Left Colon

For this portion of the procedure, the patient will be right side down and in moderate Trendelenburg position. The surgeon will control C, R1 and R3a, while the bedside assistant has L1. The surgeon can also utilize R2 to obtain better access to a high splenic flexure. A medial-to-lateral mobilization of the left and sigmoid colon is performed. The inferior mesenteric vein (IMV) is used as the initial anatomic landmark. To expose the IMV, the ligament of Treitz and attachments between the proximal jejunum and descending mesocolon may have to be divided, so the small bowel can be retracted towards the right upper quadrant (Fig. 22.3a).

Next, the peritoneum just under the IMV is incised, and medial-to-lateral dissection begins. Dissection proceeds, with care taken to identify and preserve the ureter and gonadal vessels. To avoid traction injuries, we recommend early division of the IMV near the pancreas, where the IMV is traveling alone without a paired artery (Fig. 22.3b). More distally, the IMV runs parallel to the left colic artery (LCA). Therefore, the IMV/LCA pedicle should be followed inferiorly and freed from its posterior attachments to the aorta up to the origin of the IMA. The peritoneum over the sacral promontory just medial to the right common iliac vessels is incised, entering the areolar plane posterior to the superior rectal artery. By extending this dissection plane to the cephalad, the origin of the IMA is identified; the vessels create a characteristic T-shaped structure.

After identification of the ureter and gonadal vessels in the retroperitoneal plane, the IMA can be divided. The medial-to-lateral dissection is taken laterally toward the abdominal wall. The colon is then retracted medially; the peritoneum along the white line of Toldt is opened, completely freeing the descending and sigmoid colon. Next, the splenic flexure is taken down by opening the gastrocolic omentum just below the gastroepiploic vessels or dividing the avascular colo-epiploic attachments next to the bowel wall. The splenocolic ligament is then divided. We recommend using an energy-based vessel-sealing device for these steps. Lastly, the attachments of the body and tail of the pancreas to the colonic mesentery are carefully divided to obtain a full splenic flexure release.

The mesentery of the descending colon is then divided from the stump of the IMA towards

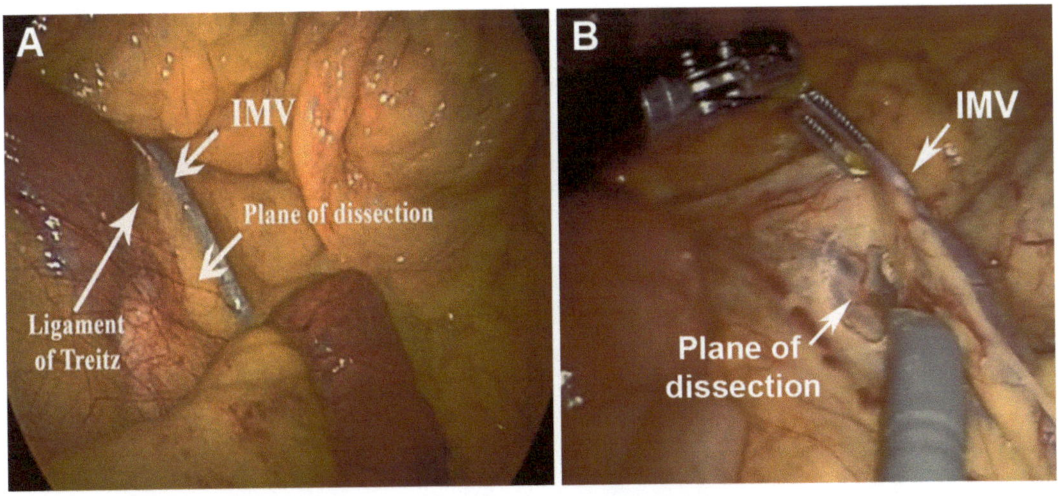


**Fig. 22.3** Exposure and division of the inferior mesenteric vein (IMV). (**a**) View of the IMV and ligament of Treitz, with the plane of dissection indicated. (**b**) A clip has been placed on the IMV, and the dashed line shows the IMV traveling with the left colic artery. The medial-to-lateral dissection plane can be seen beneath the vessels

the colon at the point of future division of the bowel, usually at the junction of the descending and sigmoid colon. The mesentery can be divided with an energy source or with several fires of a vascular stapler. We recommend dividing the marginal artery at this time to avoid tearing vessels during extraction, particularly if extraction of the specimen though the anus is anticipated.

## Total Mesorectal Excision

After completing colonic mobilization, pelvic dissection can begin. The robotic arms are detached from the trocar, the patient is levelled, and a significant degree of Trendelenburg positioning is necessary to maintain the small intestine out of the pelvis. The robotic system should be redocked over the patient's left hip, permitting access to the anus and perineum during the entire procedure (Fig. 22.4).

The camera arm with a zero degree telescope is placed in trocar C. Next, we attach a robotic trocar to arm 1 and "piggyback" this into the 12-mm R1 port. Arms 2 and 3 are docked to trocars R2 and R3b, respectively. With respect to instruments, we choose scissors for arm 1, a fenestrated bipolar grasper in arm 2, and a Prograsp grasper (Intuitive) in arm 3. The assistant remains on the right side, using ports L1 and R3a for suctioning and retraction of the rectum out of the pelvis.

With the assistant elevating the rectosigmoid junction, dissection begins posteriorly at the sacral promontory, entering the plane between the fascia propria of the rectum and the presacral fascia. Care must be taken to identify and preserve the hypogastric nerves bilaterally. The dissection is carried out almost exclusively with monopolar cautery, applied in short bursts with scissors to prevent excessive smoke accumulation and nerve injury. The TME proceeds along the areolar plane down to the rectococcygeal ligament. It is important to avoid grasping the mesorectum with robotic graspers because these instruments have considerable strength and can cause bleeding as well as injury to the fascia propria. We prefer to use the bipolar grasper in arm 2 as a retracting device.

Anteriorly, the peritoneal reflection is incised and the dissection is continued along the rectovaginal septum in women or the rectovesical/rectoprostatic fascia (Denonvillier's fascia) in men. Arm 3 is very useful for retracting the bladder and other anterior structures as dissection proceeds distally. The articulation of the robotic

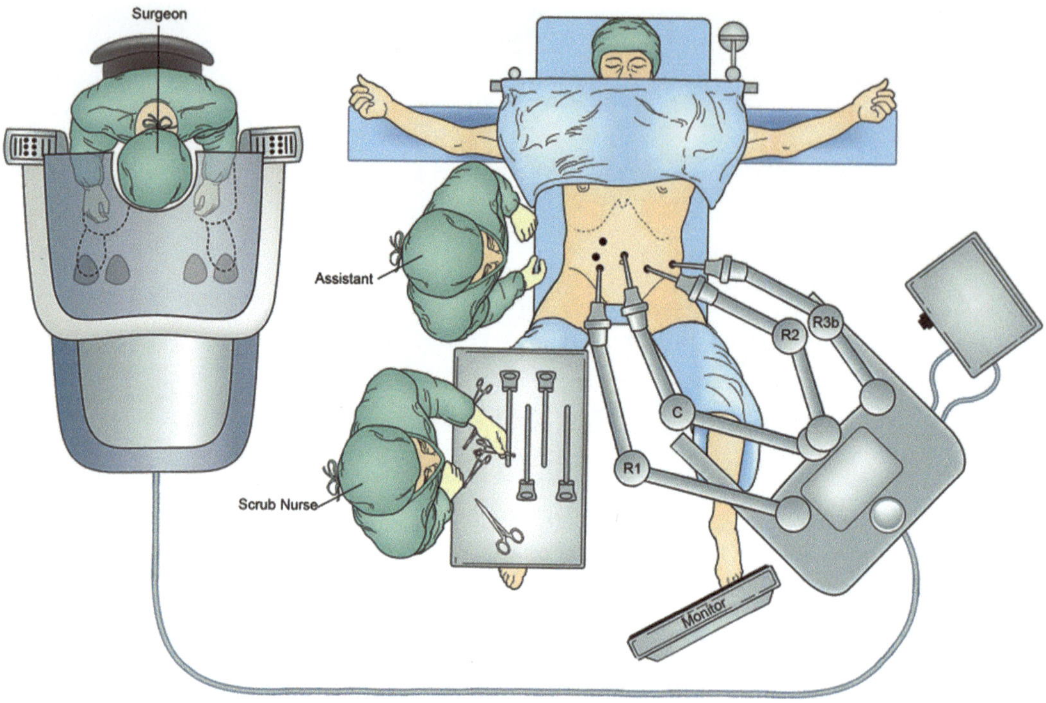


**Fig. 22.4** The patient is repositioned for the total mesorectal excision. The robot is docked using a left hip approach

scissor tips enables the surgeon to perform the dissection using ideal approach angles.

Laterally, dissection proceeds along the sidewalls medial to both ureters. Care must be taken to avoid injuring the autonomic pelvic plexus. The lateral stalks are controlled with bipolar cautery on arm 2 and are subsequently cut and divided.

Dissection continues down to the pelvic floor, separating the fatty mesorectum from the levators. In preparation for rectal division, digital rectal examinations and brief endoscopic exams are performed regularly to ascertain the level of the tumor. The rectum is lifted off the levator muscle and prepared circumferentially for division (Fig. 22.5).

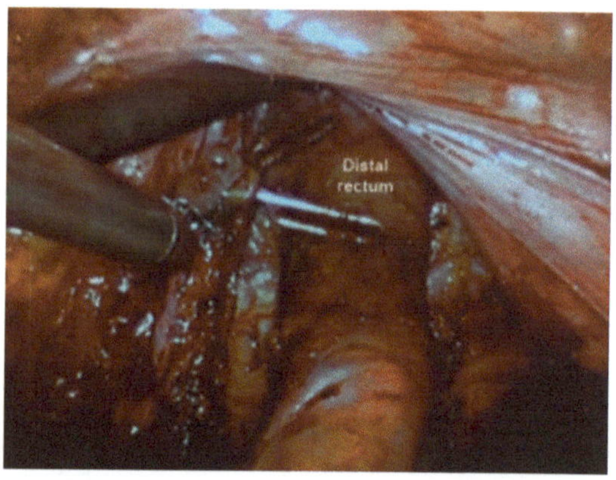


**Fig. 22.5** Robotic view of the distal dissection and preparation of the rectum. This image shows the completed dissection of the distal rectum to the level of the anal hiatus. Note the absence of mesorectum at this level

Before dividing the rectum, one member of the team performs a digital rectal exam and occasionally an endoscopic exam under direct visualization to fully assess the distal margin. In select cases we have tied a suture around the distal rectum to close off the rectal lumen and ensure application of the stapler below the level of the tumor. Because of the superb articulation of the robotic arms, this maneuver is not technically challenging.

The assistant can divide the rectum while the surgeon maintains proper exposure. Under ideal circumstances the 12-mm R1 trocar can be used after undocking the robotic arm, leaving the

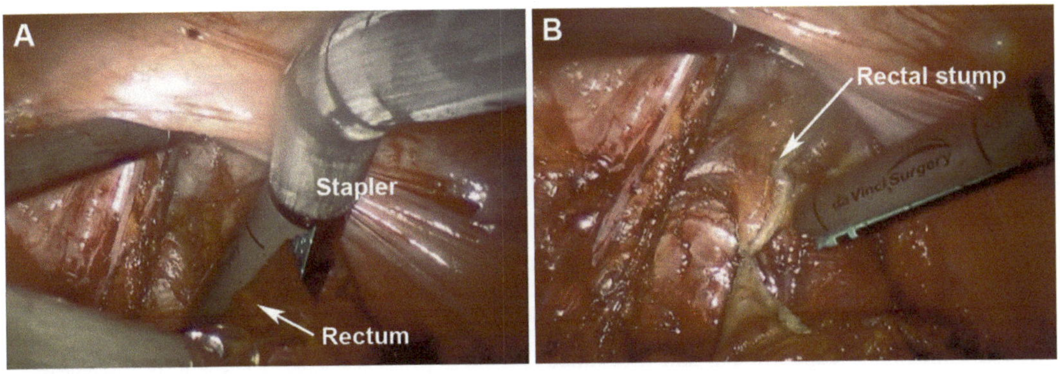


**Fig. 22.6** Division of the rectum. (**a**) The stapler is applied through a right lower quadrant port and the rectum is sequentially divided. (**b**) An intact stump can be seen just below the anorectal ring

surgeon with only R2 and R3. Stapler cartridge length should not exceed 45 mm; this permits easy application of the jaws across the rectum. Usually two to three fires are necessary, and it is important to maintain proper alignment in order to avoid crossing staple lines (Fig. 22.6). Given the thickness and pliability of the rectum, a green cartridge or the new purple cartridge (Covidien) may be indicated.

After division of the rectum, the robotic cart can be undocked. We routinely extract the specimen through a 3–4 cm suprapubic Pfannensteil mini-laparotomy covered with a plastic wound protector. The proximal bowel is divided and an anvil secured to the proximal colon with a hand-sewn purse-string suture. After closing the fascia of the Pfannensteil with interrupted absorbable sutures, the anastomosis is created with a circular stapler under direct laparoscopic visualization. In cases requiring a very low anastomosis a diverting loop ileostomy is indicated, especially after neoadjuvant CRT.

## Transanal Extraction Techniques

In lieu of an LAR with a traditional double-stapled anastomosis and transabdominal extraction, it is possible to extract the specimen transanally and perform the anastomosis manually. This technique is indicated when the tumor is very close to the anorectal ring, making safe application of the linear stapler difficult. The rectal wall is divided transanally at the beginning of the operation, with a clear view of the distal margin. The transanal dissection is then carried as far as possible outside of the rectum and mesorectum. The open lumen of rectum distal to the tumor is closed off with interrupted sutures, to avoid spillage during the pelvic dissection. The robotic dissection proceeds until the perineal dissection is approached and the bowel is passed through the rectal stump, covered with a wound protector, and delivered through the anus. The proximal bowel is divided outside the anus at the point where the mesentery and the marginal vessels have been previously divided. The anastomosis can then be accomplished manually with interrupted sutures.

These techniques obviate the need for an abdominal incision and the associated potential for wound complications and incisional pain. However, they require a higher degree of technical expertise and are, therefore, not recommended at the beginning of the surgeon's learning curve.

## Postoperative Regimen

Most patients experience only mild discomfort after RTME. Patient-controlled analgesia (PCA) is usually not necessary, and nasogastric suctioning is not indicated after robotic LAR. Patients can be started on clear liquids on postoperative day one and advanced as tolerated. If a protective ileostomy is placed, intravenous fluids are continued until the day of discharge. Proper education about fluid repletion is given to prevent dehydration while the patient recovers at home.

## Summary

The robotic surgical approach to rectal cancer offers the advantages of flexible instruments, wristed movement capabilities, self-assistance features via a third robotic arm, and high-definition, 3-D views from a mounted camera [13]. Optimized technical features enable more precise lateral dissection within the narrow, bony pelvis. No differences have been demonstrated in long-term oncologic outcomes, i.e., rectal cancer survival or recurrence rates [29], and the technique is not inferior to that of laparoscopic surgery [17]. Costs may be higher in the short term, but this gives us the opportunity to determine cost-saving measures going forward. After proper patient selection, sufficient learning experience, familiarity with intraoperative set-up, and prior mastery of TME skills, we believe that RTME is an effective tool in the hands of an experienced colorectal surgeon.

## References

1. McKay GD, Morgan MJ, Wong SK, Gatenby AH, Fulham SB, Ahmed KW, et al. Improved short-term outcomes of laparoscopic versus open resection for colon and rectal cancer in an area health service: a multicenter study. Dis Colon Rectum. 2012;55(1):42–50. doi:10.1097/DCR.0b013e318239341f.
2. Row D, Weiser MR. An update on laparoscopic resection for rectal cancer. Cancer Control. 2010; 17(1):16–24.
3. Milsom JW, de Oliveira Jr O, Trencheva KI, Pandey S, Lee SW, Sonoda T. Long-term outcomes of patients undergoing curative laparoscopic surgery for mid and low rectal cancer. Dis Colon Rectum. 2009;52((7)): 1215–22. doi:10.1007/DCR0b013e3181a73e81.
4. Guillou PJ, Quirke P, Thorpe H, Walker J, Jayne DG, Smith AM, et al. Short-term endpoints of conventional versus laparoscopic-assisted surgery in patients with colorectal cancer (MRC CLASICC trial): multicentre, randomised controlled trial. Lancet. 2005;365(9472):1718–26. doi:10.1016/s0140-6736(05)66545-2.
5. Jayne DG, Guillou PJ, Thorpe H, Quirke P, Copeland J, Smith AM, et al. Randomized trial of laparoscopic-assisted resection of colorectal carcinoma: 3-year results of the UK MRC CLASICC Trial Group. J Clin Oncol. 2007;25(21):3061–8. doi:10.1200/jco.2006.09.7758.
6. Buunen M, Veldkamp R, Hop WC, Kuhry E, Jeekel J, Haglind E, et al. Survival after laparoscopic surgery versus open surgery for colon cancer: long-term outcome of a randomised clinical trial. Lancet Oncol. 2009;10(1):44–52. doi:10.1016/S1470-2045(08)70310-3.
7. Kim JY, Kim YW, Kim NK, Hur H, Lee K, Min BS, et al. Pelvic anatomy as a factor in laparoscopic rectal surgery: a prospective study. Surg Laparosc Endosc Percutan Tech. 2011;21(5):334–9. doi:10.1097/SLE.0b013e31822b0dcb.
8. Kim YW, Lee HM, Kim NK, Min BS, Lee KY. The learning curve for robot-assisted total mesorectal excision for rectal cancer. Surg Laparosc Endosc Percutan Tech. 2012;22(5):400–5. doi:10.1097/SLE.0b013e3182622c2d.
9. Baek SK, Carmichael JC, Pigazzi A. Robotic surgery: colon and rectum. Cancer J. 2013;19(2):140–6. doi:10.1097/PPO.0b013e31828ba0fd.
10. Lin S, Jiang HG, Chen ZH, Zhou SY, Liu XS, Yu JR. Meta-analysis of robotic and laparoscopic surgery for treatment of rectal cancer. World J Gastroenterol. 2011;17(47):5214–20. doi:10.3748/wjg.v17.i47.5214.
11. Wexner SD, Bergamaschi R, Lacy A, Udo J, Brolmann H, Kennedy RH, et al. The current status of robotic pelvic surgery: results of a multinational interdisciplinary consensus conference. Surg Endosc. 2009;23(2):438–43. doi:10.1007/s00464-008-0202-8.
12. Trakarnsanga A, Weiser MR. Minimally invasive surgery of rectal cancer: current evidence and options. Am Soc Clin Oncol. 2012;32:214–8. doi:10.14694/EdBook_AM.2012.32.214.
13. Peterson CY, Weiser MR. Robotic colorectal surgery. J Gastrointest Surg. 2014;18(2):398–403. doi:10.1007/s11605-013-2313-3.
14. Hui VW, Guillem JG. Minimal access surgery for rectal cancer: an update. Nat Rev Gastroenterol Hepatol. 2014;11:158–65. doi:10.1038/nrgastro.2013.203.
15. Baik SH, Ko YT, Kang CM, Lee WJ, Kim NK, Sohn SK, et al. Robotic tumor-specific mesorectal excision of rectal cancer: short-term outcome of a pilot randomized trial. Surg Endosc. 2008;22(7):1601–8. doi:10.1007/s00464-008-9752-z.
16. Baik SH, Kwon HY, Kim JS, Hur H, Sohn SK, Cho CH, et al. Robotic versus laparoscopic low anterior resection of rectal cancer: short-term outcome of a prospective comparative study. Ann Surg Oncol. 2009;16(6):1480–7. doi:10.1245/s10434-009-0435-3.
17. Kim CW, Kim CH, Baik SH. Outcomes of robotic-assisted colorectal surgery compared with laparoscopic and open surgery: a systematic review. J Gastrointest Surg. 2014;18:816–30. doi:10.1007/s11605-014-2469-5.

18. Baek JH, McKenzie S, Garcia-Aguilar J, Pigazzi A. Oncologic outcomes of robotic-assisted total mesorectal excision for the treatment of rectal cancer. Ann Surg. 2010;251(5):882–6. doi:10.1097/SLA.0b013e3181c79114.
19. Baek JH, Pastor C, Pigazzi A. Robotic and laparoscopic total mesorectal excision for rectal cancer: a case-matched study. Surg Endosc. 2011;25(2):521–5. doi:10.1007/s00464-010-1204-x.
20. Pigazzi A, Luca F, Patriti A, Valvo M, Ceccarelli G, Casciola L, et al. Multicentric study on robotic tumor-specific mesorectal excision for the treatment of rectal cancer. Ann Surg Oncol. 2010;17(6):1614–20. doi:10.1245/s10434-010-0909-3.
21. Bianchi PP, Ceriani C, Locatelli A, Spinoglio G, Zampino MG, Sonzogni A, et al. Robotic versus laparoscopic total mesorectal excision for rectal cancer: a comparative analysis of oncological safety and short-term outcomes. Surg Endosc. 2010;24(11):2888–94. doi:10.1007/s00464-010-1134-7.
22. Kwak JM, Kim SH, Kim J, Son DN, Baek SJ, Cho JS. Robotic vs laparoscopic resection of rectal cancer: short-term outcomes of a case-control study. Dis Colon Rectum. 2011;54(2):151–6. doi:10.1007/DCR.0b013e3181fec4fd.
23. Patel CB, Ragupathi M, Ramos-Valadez DI, Haas EM. A three-arm (laparoscopic, hand-assisted, and robotic) matched-case analysis of intraoperaive and postoperative outcomes in minimally invasive colorectal surgery. Dis Colon Rectum. 2011;54(2):144–50. doi:10.1007/DCR.0b013e3181fec377.
24. Spinoglio G, Summa M, Priora F, Quarati R, Testa S. Robotic colorectal surgery: first 50 cases experience. Dis Colon Rectum. 2008;51(11):1627–32. doi:10.1007/s10350-008-9334-0.
25. Bokhari MB, Patel CB, Ramos-Valadez DI, Ragupathi M, Haas EM. Learning curve for robotic-assisted laparoscopic colorectal surgery. Surg Endosc. 2011;25(3):855–60. doi:10.1007/s00464-010-1281-x.
26. Akmal Y, Baek JH, McKenzie S, Garcia-Aguilar J, Pigazzi A. Robot-assisted total mesorectal excision: is there a learning curve? Surg Endosc. 2012;26(9):2471–6. doi:10.1007/s00464-012-2216-5.
27. Turchetti G, Palla I, Pierotti F, Cuschieri A. Economic evaluation of da Vinci-assisted robotic surgery: a systematic review. Surg Endosc. 2012;26(3):598–606. doi:10.1007/s00464-011-1936-2.
28. Jimenez-Rodriguez RM, Diaz-Pavon JM, de la Portilla de Juan F, Prendes-Sillero E, Dussort HC, Padillo J. Learning curve for robotic-assisted laparoscopic rectal cancer surgery. Int J Colorectal Dis. 2013;28(6):815–21. doi:10.1007/s00384-012-1620-6.
29. Park EJ, Cho MS, Baek SJ, Hur H, Min BS, Baik SH et al. Long-term oncologic outcomes of robotic low anterior resection for rectal cancer: a comparative study with laparoscopic surgery. Ann Surg. 2014. doi:10.1097/SLA.0000000000000613.

## Key Operative Steps

1. Place the patient in modified lithotomy position.
2. Place the robotic trocars 8–10 cm apart to avoid collisions.
3. Divide the IMV near its insertion and perform medial to lateral mobilization of the left and sigmoid colon.
4. After identifying the ureter and gonadal vessels, the inferior mesenteric artery can be divided.
5. Retract the colon medially and open the white line of Toldt.
6. Perform the splenic flexure takedown.
7. Divide the mesentery of the descending colon.
8. Elevate the rectosigmoid junction and begin posterior dissection at the sacral promontory. Proceed along the areolar plane down to the rectococcygeal ligament.
9. Incise the peritoneal reflection anteriorly and continue dissection along the rectovaginal septum in women or Denonvillier's fascia in men.
10. Laterally, dissection is medial to both ureters to the middle rectal vessels.
11. At the pelvic floor separate the rectum from the levator muscle.
12. Perform digital rectal exam to ensure location of tumor and then divide the rectum with a stapling device.
13. Once the rectum is divided, the robot is undocked and the specimen is extracted.
14. An anvil is placed in the proximal bowel and a laparoscopic anastomosis is created with a circular stapler.
15. A diverting loop ileostomy is created.

# Hybrid Laparoscopic-Robotic Low Anterior Resection

# 23

Raul M. Bosio and Alessio Pigazzi

## Introduction

Two main factors have slowed down the progress of minimally invasive techniques in rectal surgery: (a) the concern that oncologic outcomes may be worse with these techniques [1–3] and (b) the realization that minimally invasive rectal surgery is technically challenging [4, 5]. From an oncologic standpoint, 5-year follow-up after laparoscopic or open rectal cancer resection for patients included in the Conventional Versus Laparoscopic-Assisted Surgery in Colorectal Cancer (CLASICC) trial showed that despite a higher rate of positive circumferential resection margin in the laparoscopic arm, both local recurrence and survival were similar between groups [6]. More importantly, 5-year overall survival was 52.9 % and 60.3 % for patients in the open versus laparoscopic groups, respectively [7]. Recently published data from the COlon carcinoma Laparoscopic or Open Resection (COLOR) II trial that randomly assigned patients to laparoscopic or open rectal surgery revealed a 10 % rate of positive circumferential resection margins in both groups with similar mortality between the two groups [8]. Practice parameters from the American Society of Colon and Rectal Surgery now consider laparoscopic rectal resection equivalent to open resections from an oncologic standpoint when performed by experienced laparoscopic surgeons [9]. Although oncologic outcomes after robotic rectal resections appear comparable to open and laparoscopic procedures as evidenced by numerous published articles, large scale randomized controlled trials evaluating this technique are not yet available [10–19].

From a technical viewpoint, the pelvis makes rectal dissection complex since retraction is limited by its bony structure leading to frequent collision of instruments, loss of visibility, and inability to reach deep structures. Obesity, male gender, narrow pelvis, and large tumor size tend to further limit the ability to generate traction and counter-traction, which are vital for adequate tissue exposure and precise dissection. As a direct consequence, most rectal resections in the US are still performed open or with combined laparoscopic-open approaches [20, 21]. For cases started laparoscopically, the conversion rate is high (>10–15 %), underlying further the

Electronic supplementary material: Supplementary material is available in the online version of this chapter at 10.1007/978-1-4939-1893-5_23. Videos can also be accessed at http://www.springerimages.com/videos/978-1-4939-1892-8.

R.M. Bosio, M.D., M.S.B.S.,
A. Pigazzi, M.D., Ph.D. (✉)
Department of Surgery, University of California, Irvine School of Medicine, 333 City Blvd West Suite 850, Orange, CA 92868, USA
e-mail: apigazzi@uci.edu

J. Kim and J. Garcia-Aguilar (eds.), *Surgery for Cancers of the Gastrointestinal Tract: A Step-by-Step Approach*, DOI 10.1007/978-1-4939-1893-5_23, © Springer Science+Business Media New York 2015

technical challenges of these procedures [6, 22–24]. The use of a robotic platform for rectal resections may facilitate safe completion of this procedure as suggested by a lower conversion to open surgery when the robot is used. Improved three-dimensional (3-D) optics, a steady operating field with a surgeon-controlled camera, and instruments with wrist-like functions aid the surgeon with tissue retraction and facilitate visualization and dissection [4, 5]. As many of the laparoscopic skills transfer to the robotic platform, surgeons experienced in advanced laparoscopic techniques may find that using the robot may enhance their ability to complete rectal procedures, offering patients the benefits of a minimally invasive technique and enhanced recovery.

## Indications

Operations that involve dissecting deep in the pelvis (i.e., rectal prolapse) or that require dividing the middle or lower rectum (i.e., middle and distal third rectal lesions) are routinely performed in our practice using a hybrid laparoscopic-robotic approach as we will explain in this chapter. Robotic rectal resection should be performed following the same principles described for open partial or total mesorectal excision (TME). Obtaining adequate distal as well as circumferential radial margin is of paramount importance when treating rectal cancer. Intraoperative digital rectal examination or flexible endoscopy with carbon dioxide should be performed as needed, to ensure that the dissection has progresses beyond the tumor.

A number of technical principles are common to various rectal procedures. Entering the operating room with these concepts clear in mind is the key to prevent intraoperative complications and conversion. As we proceed to describe a hybrid laparoscopic-robotic low anterior resection in detail, technical principles that allow the surgeon to transition from step to step effortlessly and to achieve the goal of completing a minimally invasive procedure will also be reviewed [25–28].

## Anatomic Considerations

From the operating surgeon mindset, rectal resections can be divided in two major stages: (1) an abdominal stage that includes the mobilization of the left colon and splenic flexure and division of both the inferior mesenteric artery (IMA) and vein (IMV) and (2) a pelvic stage where rectal dissection is performed within a confined space.

The dissection during the abdominal stage can be accomplished in a number of ways: medial-to-lateral, lateral-to-medial, IMV-first approach, etc. Independent of the approach, it is our preference to perform this stage of the operation laparoscopically. Despite our expertise in robotic surgery, this part of the dissection can be performed faster than and with results similar to a robotic approach. Simple maneuvers such as changes in the patient's position that facilitate tissue exposure cannot be performed while the robot is docked. On the contrary, the use of the robotic platform facilitates the rectal dissection. Since the dissection is performed in a confined space, the endowrist function of the robotic arms, the 3-D optics, and the ability of the operating surgeon to control the camera make rectal resection technically less challenging.

High ligation of the IMA is necessary not only from an oncologic standpoint but also in order to obtain adequate colonic mobilization. The IMV is also routinely divided near the Ligament of Treitz. Failure to complete these steps usually limits the ability of the colon to reach the lower rectum or anal canal, increasing the risk of constructing an anastomosis under tension, a well-described factor that may lead to a higher anastomotic leak rate.

We usually start the dissection using a medial-to-lateral approach. However, changing approaches and dissection from lateral-to-medial may be required when structures such as the left ureter cannot be identified. It is important to emphasize that vascular division should not be performed until the left ureter is identified, as this structure travels lateral to but in very close proximity with the IMA, hidden from the surgeon's view when dissecting from medial-to-lateral.

We start the medial-to-lateral approach by dividing the peritoneum distal to the IMA as the classic first step. In our experience, the IMV-first approach offers an excellent alternative starting point for a medial-to-lateral technique and we have used this approach more often recently.

Preservation of autonomic nerves should also be considered one of the goals of these procedures. There are four anatomic areas where nerve injury is most likely to occur: (a) the superior hypogastric plexus during dissection of the IMA, (b) the hypogastric nerves at the sacral promontory as the surgeon gains access to the retrorectal space, (c) the pelvic plexus during lateral mobilization of the rectum, and (d) the anterior nervies erigenti during anterior dissection of the rectum below the peritoneal reflection.

Division of the rectum low in the pelvis can be challenging. The type of disease that is being treated and the individual patient's characteristics play a role during this part of the operation, however, the surgeon's experience remains key. A surgeon that has the knowledge and comfort in performing a hand-sewn coloanal anastomosis or an intersphincteric dissection may be all that is necessary from preventing a conversion to an abdominoperineal resection.

A Pfannenstiel incision, where both skin and fascia are opened transversely while the muscle is retracted laterally in the midline, is our preferred method for specimen extraction. A transanal extraction is feasible in select patients, which has the advantage of leaving the abdomen only with trocar-size incisions. Reconstruction can be performed by hand-sewn coloanal anastomosis or by double pursue-string stapled colorectal anastomosis. Opportunities to get adequate training with these techniques are limited outside specialty training and may contribute to a number of abdominoperineal resections being performed instead [29, 30]. Finally, the ileostomy site is also a possible extraction site as well.

Patients undergoing resection rectopexy may also benefit from transanal extraction. In these cases, intracorporeal proximal and distal division of the specimen is required prior to the transanal extraction. Subsequently, creation of both proximal and distal pursue-strings is needed to create a double purse-string stapled colorectal anastomosis. Purse-string constructions are facilitated by the hand-wrist capabilities of robotic instruments compared to standard laparoscopic ones.

## Hybrid Laparoscopic-Robotic Low Anterior Resection

### Room Setup and Positioning

Our preference is to place the patient on the operating room table in a modified lithotomy position (Fig. 23.1a). The patient's buttocks should be positioned by the edge of the table and the hips should be slightly flexed and abducted. It is important to avoid pressure on the lateral compartment of the lower extremities to avoid nerve injury. This is accomplished by loosely aligning the knee to the patient's opposite shoulder. The feet and legs should be ergonomically positioned and padded, ensuring that the patient's weight is transferred to the plantar aspects of the feet, which should be on foot rests.

Patient positioning should be completed in such a way that the operating room table can be placed in steep Trendelenburg or in extreme lateral positions without the patient sliding. Despite the numerous techniques described to prevent patient sliding, such as beanbags and different types of straps, patient injuries have been described and can be as devastating as brachial plexus injuries and lower extremity nerve injuries with and without associated compartment syndrome. Ensuring adequate positioning is key prior to starting the operation, since unintended changes in patient position may be difficult to assess once sterile drapes are in place.

Our preference is to position the patient directly on a large high-viscosity foam mat with Velcro straps that are then secured to the table. In theory, this mat provides a friction hold, decreasing in-line sliding that may occur either during Trendelenburg or reverse Trendelenburg position. A second Velcro strap is required to

a

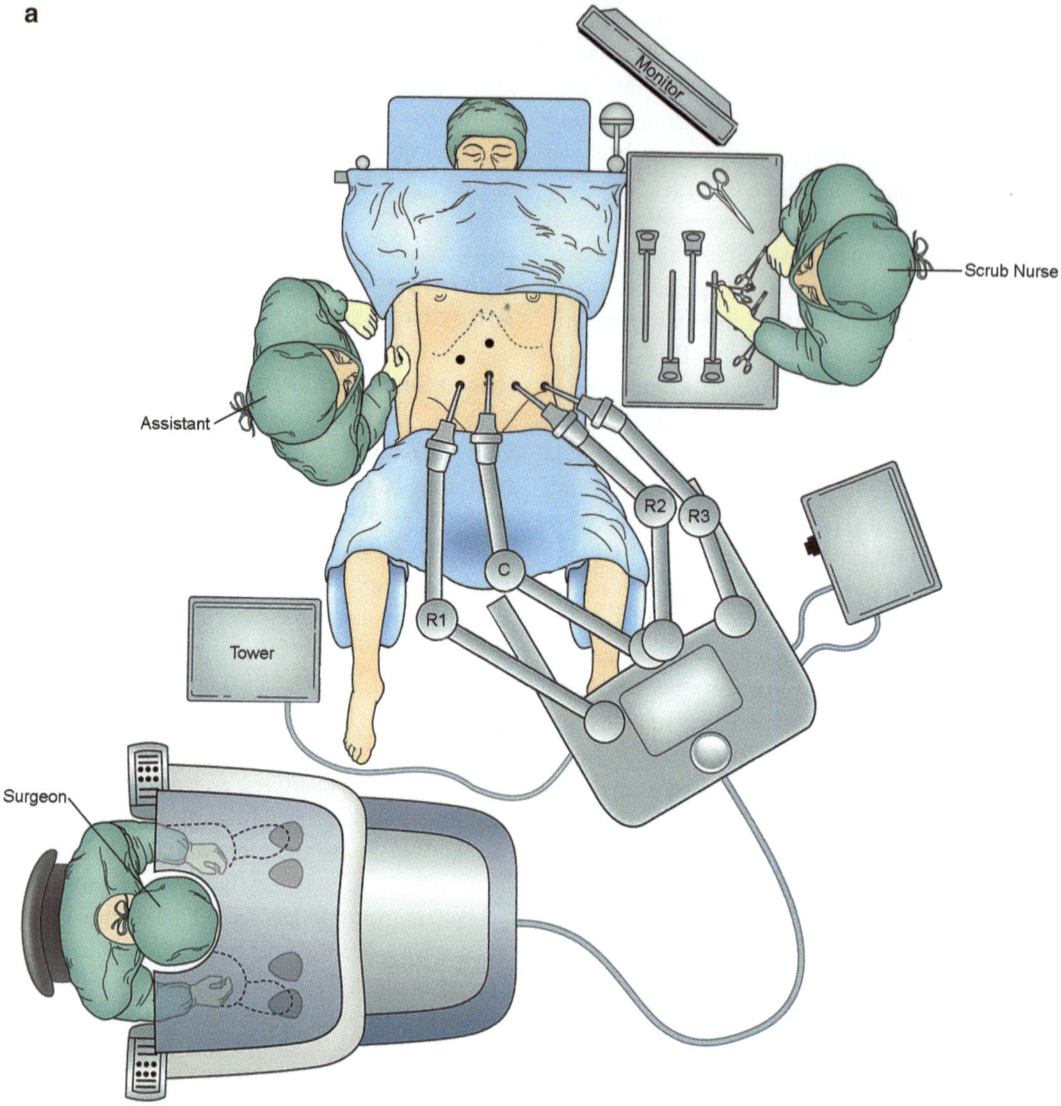


**Fig. 23.1** (**a**) Operative positioning of the patient, the surgical team, and the robot. (**b**) Trocar positioning of the robotic and assistant ports. A 12-mm camera port (**c**) is placed at the halfway point between the xiphoid process and the pubis symphysis. A line is drawn connecting the C port to the right and left anterior superior iliac spines. Three robotic ports (R) are then placed, four-finger breadths apart from each other. Two additional 5-mm laparoscopic ports (L) are also inserted. L1 is located along the right mid-clavicular line, four-finger breadths lateral to C and about four-finger breadths superior to R1. L2 is just lateral to the midline, four-finger breadths from L1

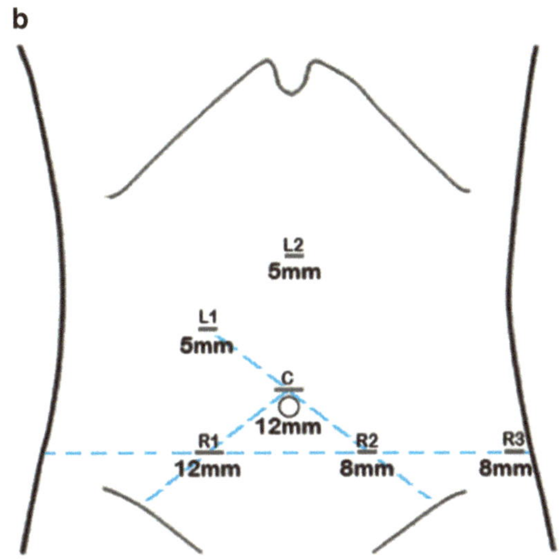


**Fig. 23.1** (continued)

prevent lateral sliding. It is placed across the chest and secured as well to the operating table at this level. It prevents sliding when the bed is tilted towards the right. It is our preference to tuck both arms, parallel to the patient on the operating table. However, it is not always necessary to tuck the left arm.

When treating rectal cancer or when transanal extraction is planned, we irrigate the rectum with water. A Foley catheter is utilized in all cases and intravenous preoperative antibiotics are administered. Ureteral stents are rarely used, except when a large inflammatory process is expected or in select reoperative cases. Digital rectal and/or vaginal exam is performed as necessary during the case and prior to dividing the rectum when treating distal tumors. Intraoperative flexible endoscopy with carbon dioxide is used in our practice routinely both for tumor location and anastomosis evaluation.

## Pneumoperitoneum and Port Placement

Pneumoperitoneum can be created in several ways. Entry into the abdominal cavity using either an open technique or by Veress needle has similar complication rates and both are valid starting options. It is our preference to create pneumoperitoneum by introducing a Veress needle at Palmer's point, right below the left costal margin at the left midclavicular line (MCL). Port location is decided after pneumoperitoneum has been created. This is of particular importance during the robotic part of the procedure, as we will describe later on this chapter.

It is standard in our practice to use a six-port technique during hybrid laparoscopic-robotic LAR, including one 12-mm umbilical port for the camera, two 8-mm left lower quadrant robotic ports, a 12/15-mm right lower quadrant (RLQ) port (an 8-mm robotic port is inserted in a trocar-in-trocar configuration at this location), and two 5-mm laparoscopic ports located in the right upper quadrant (RUQ) and epigastrium (Fig. 23.1b).

The keys to port location are as follows:

- A 12-mm camera port (C) is placed in the midline, at the halfway point between the xiphoid process and the pubis symphisis after pneumoperitoneum is completed. Placement could be at, below, or above the umbilicus. However, this trocar should be placed no further than 15 cm from the pubic symphisis. If this port is too high in the abdomen, the camera can hit the sacral promontory as dissection progresses into the pelvis, restricting close approach and visualization of the targets deep in the pelvis.

- Once the camera port is in place, a line connecting this port to the right and left anterior superior iliac spine should be drawn. This line will then serve as guidance for the three robotic ports (R) that will be inserted under direct visualization. Maintaining a distance of 8–12 cm between ports (four-finger breadths) is necessary to decrease the risk of arm collision during the robotic stage of the procedure.
- R1 is either a 12-mm laparoscopic trocar or 15-mm robotic trocar placed in the RLQ, four-finger breadths away from C. Another way to determine trocar position is by using the halfway point between C and the right anterior superior iliac spine (ASIS) or by selecting the point where the MCL intersects the line that connects C and the ASIS. An 8-mm robotic port needs to be introduced through this port (trocar-in-trocar) to allow for commonly used robotic instruments to be introduced and, therefore arm 1 to function.
- R2 is an 8-mm robotic trocar placed in the mirror image of R1 in the left lower quadrant (LLQ). R3 is also an 8-mm robotic trocar placed in the LLQ. It is inserted four-finger breadths apart (8–12 cm), lateral to R2. It is on the same transverse plane, directly above the left ASIS.
- Two 5-mm laparoscopic ports (L) are also routinely used in our practice. L1 is located in the RUQ, four-finger breadths lateral to C and about four-finger breadths (about 12 cm) from R1. L2 is inserted in the epigastric area, just lateral (either to the right or left) to the midline, four-finger breadths from L1.
- Instruments should always be introduced into the abdominal cavity under direct visualization. They should not be moving outside the field of vision. If an instrument moves outside the field of vision, it should be kept immobile until the camera is repositioned to find the instrument. Trying to blindly bring the instrument into the field of vision can lead to severe patient harm due to the lack of tactile feedback. Minimizing collision between arms is of paramount importance in robotic surgery as it could limit the range of motion of a particular instrument and the ability to reach the targeted structured.

## Initial Operative Steps

Once pneumoperitoneum has been created, both surgeon and assistant will stand on the right side of the patient, with the assistant towards the head. The abdominal cavity should be visualized entirely to rule out metastatic disease when treating rectal cancer. Subsequently, the patient is positioned in steep Trendelenburg and rotated to the right. This position facilitates retracting the small bowel and the cecum if necessary, out of the pelvis. If adhesions are present fixing either the small bowel or the cecum in the pelvis, it is of paramount importance to divide them prior to starting the robotic part of the procedure. Due to the lack of haptic feedback from the robotic platform, these structures are at risk of being inadvertently injured unless the surgeon is able to mobilize them out of the pelvis.

## Laparoscopic Medial-to-Lateral Dissection of the Left Colon

The RUQ and RLQ ports (L1 and R1 ports, respectively) are the operative ports during the abdominal portion of the operation. The C and L2 ports are controlled by the assistant and an atraumatic grasper in L2 usually aids with retraction. Dissection usually starts in a medial-to-lateral fashion. However, dissection may begin by dividing the peritoneum just distal to the IMA (classic approach) or at the level of the IMV (IMV-first approach).

Starting the dissection at the level of the IMV has the advantage that the avascular plane between the retroperitoneum and the mesocolon is very easy to identify and developed with blunt maneuvers. However, this approach requires excellent exposure of the fourth portion of the duodenum and the ligament of Treitz prior to dissecting. Placing the patient in slight reverse

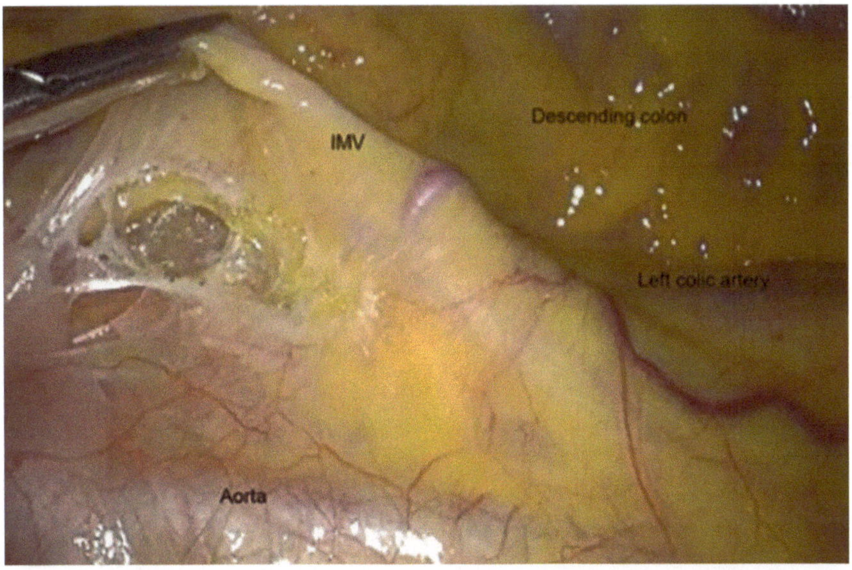


**Fig. 23.2** Dissection starting at the level of the inferior mesenteric vein. As the vein is gently grasped and lifted, the peritoneum is divided and the space between the mesocolon and the retroperitoneum is entered

Trendelenburg may help retract the small bowel out of this area. The IMV can usually be easily identified, traveling in a cranial to caudal direction in the mesocolon. This approach requires the small bowel to be displaced away from the LUQ, while the transverse colon should be positioned over the stomach high in the LUQ. Once the inferior mesenteric vein (IMV) is identified, we proceed to grasp the mesocolon (in many cases, the IMV itself is grasped) and gently retract it anteriorly towards the anterior abdominal wall. The peritoneum is then opened with monopolar cautery or hot-scissors just posterior to the IMV and following its course from the ligament of Treitz advancing caudally towards the IMA (Fig. 23.2). Visualization of areolar tissue usually indicates the surgeon is in the correct plane. Dissection progresses with blunt maneuvers since this is an avascular plane and allows the surgeon to mobilize the IMV and mesocolon off the retroperitoneum. Dissection advances laterally towards the lateral abdominal wall and towards the splenic flexure. Gerota's fascia is encountered and dissected down and away from the mesocolon. Caudally, the limit of the dissection is the IMA itself. The IMV can be divided at any point; although it is preferable to complete the dissection first, as this structure helps generate counter-traction (Fig. 23.3). Our preference is to clip it proximally and then divide it using a vessel sealer, preferable a bipolar device. Conversely, the IMV can be divided in between clips or using a vascular endostapler.

The lesser sac can be entered by continuing the dissection in the IMV plane. This maneuver may facilitate taking down the splenic flexure. However, this plane naturally continues under the pancreas. Therefore, carrying the dissection in this plane towards the LUQ will lead to lifting the pancreas along with the transverse mesocolon (Fig. 23.4). Unless clearly identified, our recommendation is not to continue towards the LUQ. Take-down of the splenic flexure and access to the lesser sac should be accomplished in a more traditional manner, after dividing the line of Toldt during the lateral to medial part of the procedure.

Dissection then continues, once the IMA has been identified, by gently lifting the superior hemorrhoidal pedicle towards the anterior abdominal wall. The parietal peritoneum below the superior hemorrhoidal artery is then divided advancing towards the sacral promontory. Blunt dissection allows entry into the same avascular

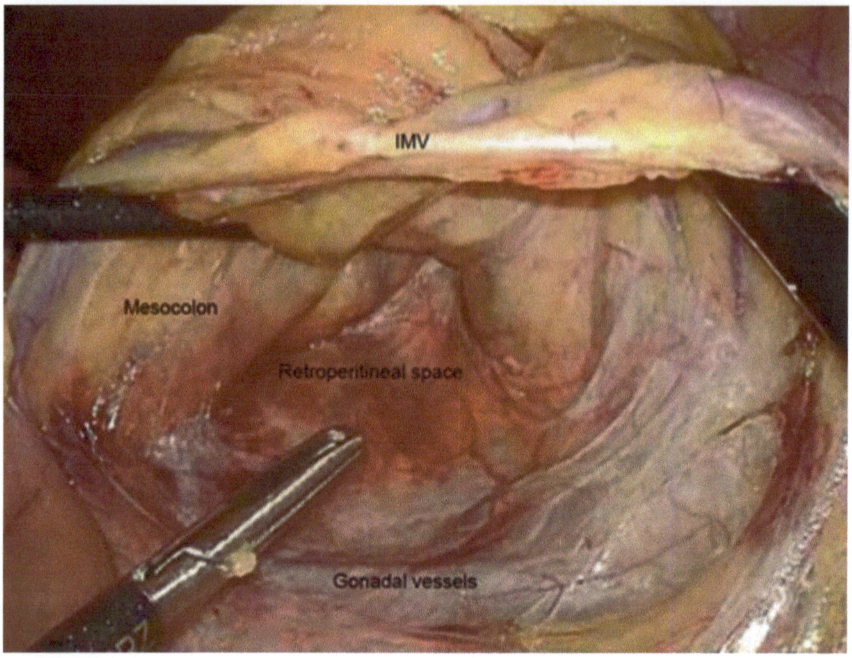


**Fig. 23.3** Development of the plane between the descending mesocolon and the retroperitoneum

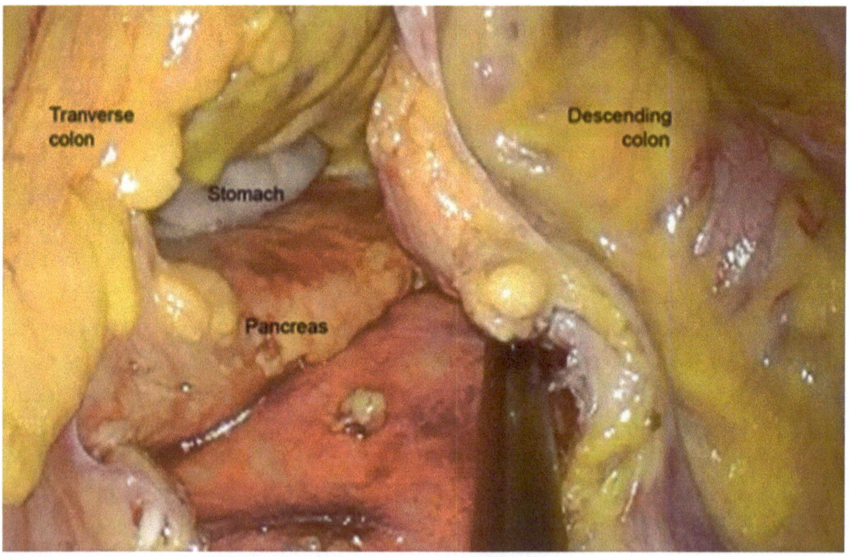


**Fig. 23.4** Dissection towards the left upper quadrant after dividing the IMV allows access to the lesser sac. The pancreas and the stomach are observed in this picture

plane that was developed before. From a practical standpoint, the surgeon should visualize the dissection area as a square where the floor is the retroperitoneum containing nerves and the iliac vessels and the roof is the superior hemorrhoidal artery. The left (cranial) "wall" demarcating this square is the IMA and the right (caudal) "wall" is the mesorectum (Fig. 23.5). Dissection is performed within this square in a medial to lateral fashion. As the gonadal vessels and the ureter are

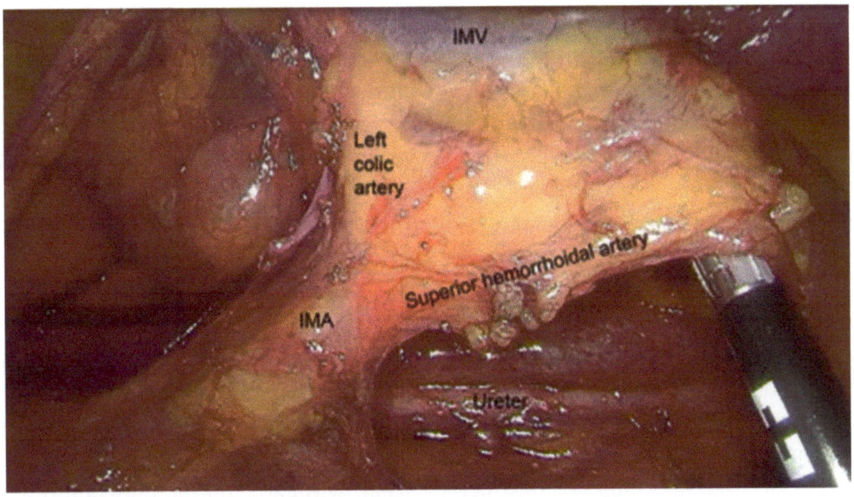


**Fig. 23.5** Medial-to-lateral dissection reveals the IMV and IMA

encountered, they should be dissected posteriorly towards the retroperitoneum. Visualization of the psoas muscle is usually indicative of a dissection that has proceeded in the wrong plane. The surgeon should reevaluate the plane of dissection; typically, both gonadal vessels and ureter have been inadvertently lifted with the mesocolon.

A common mistake that makes identification of the ureter difficult is starting the dissection through a small peritoneal opening. Starting the dissection by dividing the peritoneum from the IMA all the way to the rectum facilitates this part of the procedure. While keeping in mind the boundaries of the "square", creating a larger peritoneal opening allows for a larger area of blunt dissection and makes identification of the gonadal vessels and ureter easier. Care should be taken during this part of the procedure not to injure the hypogastric nerve plexus. Division of the IMA should not be performed prior to identification of these structures.

Once the peritoneum has been opened all the way from the IMV down to the mesorectum, a very characteristic "T" shaped configuration should be visualized as the mesocolon is retracted upwards towards the anterior abdominal wall. The IMA constitutes the vertical part of the "T", while its two branches, the left colic artery to the left and the superior hemorrhoidal artery to the right, form the horizontal parts (Fig. 23.5).

It is important to emphasize that the left ureter travels lateral just against the IMA and can be lifted and injured when attempting to divide the IMA if the dissection is not adequate. Therefore, the IMA should not be divided prior to visualization of the ureter. The IMA can then be divided in a number of ways, such as using a vessel sealing device, clips, or endostapler with a vascular load. We routinely clip the IMA prior to using an advanced bipolar device.

## Splenic Flexure Takedown

Once the medial-to-lateral dissection has been completed and both the IMA and IMV divided, the lateral attachments of the sigmoid and descending colon are taken down. The line of Toldt is divided with monopolar cautery, hot-scissors, or advanced bipolar device. Dissection usually starts at the LLQ and is facilitated by retracting the colon towards the midline. As the line of Toldt is divided, blunt maneuvers are also used as the initial medial dissection plane is easily encountered. As dissection progresses towards the LUQ, attachments from the omentum to the lateral abdominal wall and to the descending colon can be present. We usually divide the attachments to the colon, leaving those attachments between the omentum and the abdominal wall in place, unless they obstruct adequate visualization of our plane of dissection. Taking down the splenic flexure can be challenging from a technical standpoint. If progress stalls, approaching the splenic flexure from the transverse colon may make this part of the operation less cumbersome. In this case, the omentum is then divided off the distal transverse colon usually using a bipolar device. As dissection progresses, both the phrenocolic and splenocolic ligaments are encountered and divided. As the lesser sac is entered, mobilization of the colon is carried out at the base of the mesentery and allows for complete mobilization of the splenic flexure, a necessary step to be able to construct a tension-free anastomosis.

## Robotic Total Mesorectal Excision

It is our practice to perform the mesorectal dissection using a four-arm Da Vinci robot (Intuitive) docked at the patient's left hip. At the time of docking, the patient is in Trendelenburg and rotated to the right in such a way that the small bowel and right colon remain outside the pelvis. The central column of the Da Vinci cart is in-line with the patient's left ASIS and the right shoulder. Rectal procedures can also be completed by docking the robot in between the legs. However, intraoperative digital or endoscopic rectal examinations are difficult with this approach.

A 0-degree, 12-mm robotic camera is introduced in C. Although available, we rarely use a 30-degree camera. Arm 1 is docked to R1 and will be the access site later in the procedure for stapler devices. Laparoscopic staplers require a 12-mm port, while the robotic articulating stapler requires the use of a 15-mm robotic trocar in this location. An 8-mm robotic trocar using a trocar-in-trocar technique is required to use this port during dissection. A robotic hook or monopolar scissors is usually introduced through this port. A robotic bipolar fenestrated grasper is placed in Arm 2 and docked in R2, while Arm 3 is docked in R3 with a Prograsp (Intuitive). The assistant will remain on the right side of the patient generally using an extended-length suction irrigator in L1 and a locking grasper in L2. The suction-irrigator will play an important role generating counter-traction throughout the case.

Robotic TME (rTME) starts at the sacral promontory as the avascular plane between the endopelvic visceral fascia (EVF) that contains the mesorectum and the endopelvic parietal fascia (EPF) is entered (Fig. 23.6). Arms 2 and 3, controlled by the surgeon's left hand, will be key throughout the procedure as they provide retraction and expose the plane of dissection. In general, we prefer not to grasp the mesorectum with Arm 2, as the robotic arm may tear tissues easily. Arm 1, controlled by the surgeon's right hand, will carry on the dissection in this plane, using a combination of both monopolar cautery and blunt maneuvers (Fig. 23.7). As dissection starts, it is important to identify the hypogastric nerves in this area and gently push them away from the plane of dissection.

Dissection should be performed in the space delineated by the mesorectal fascia or EVF anteriorly and the EPF posteriorly, the so-called "holy plane" of rectal surgery described by Heald [31]. Dissecting posterior to the EPF places the surgeon in the presacral space, where the hypogastric nerves and presacral venous plexus are located and increases the risk of intraoperative complications and postoperative nerve dysfunction.

As dissection carries on distally, it is important to understand that the rectum curves upward and anteriorly as we approach the anorectal junction. Just above the levator ani muscle, the EPF fuses with the mesorectal fascia (commonly described as Waldeyer's fascia); as dissection continues beyond this point, a segment of rectum denuded of mesorectum is encountered. Continuing dissection further down may allow the surgeon to access the intersphincteric plane. Dissecting as far distal as possible in the posterior plane makes identification of the lateral stalks and dissection in the anterolateral areas easier. In most cases, however, surgery progresses with a combination of posterior and lateral dissection, as the surgeon alternates between these planes back and forth.

The surgeon and assistant work in conjunction using Arm 2 and the suction-irrigator, respectively,

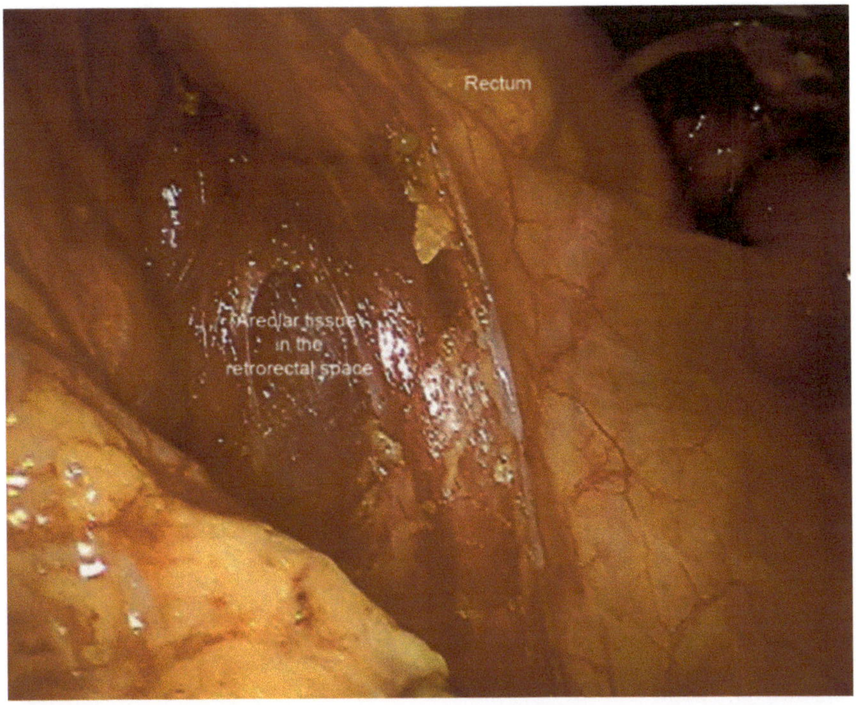


**Fig. 23.6** Starting the robotic rectal dissection at the level of the sacral promontory. As robotic arm 2 retracts the rectum towards the pubis, the areolar retrorectal tissue can be easily appreciated

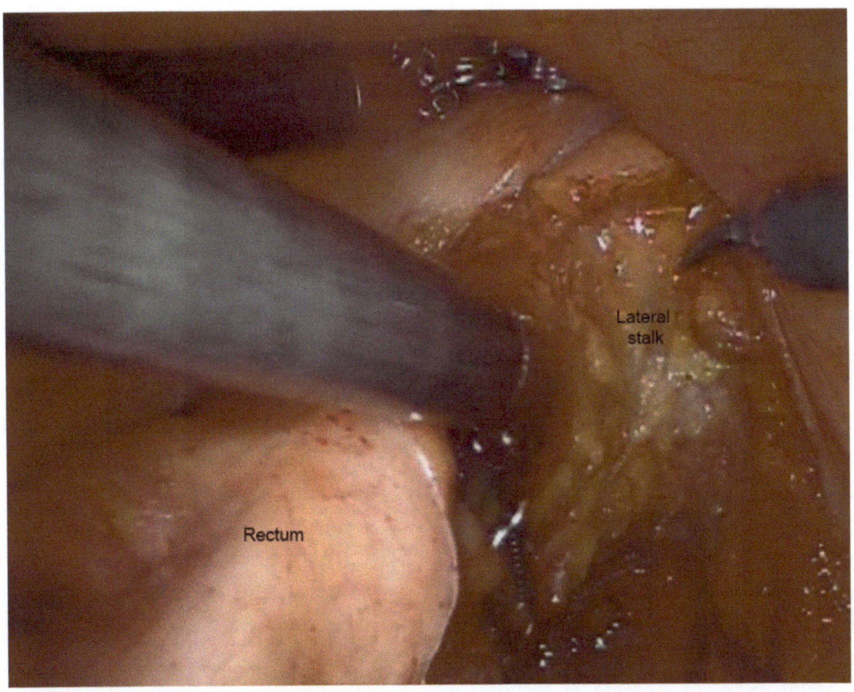


**Fig. 23.7** In this picture, robotic arm 3 is place anteriorly to retract the bladder. Arm 2 on the right side of the mesorectum retracts it to the left. Arm 1 with monopolar scissors carries on the dissection. Additional retraction with L1 and L2 is provided by the assistant holding the rectum out of the pelvis towards the abdomen

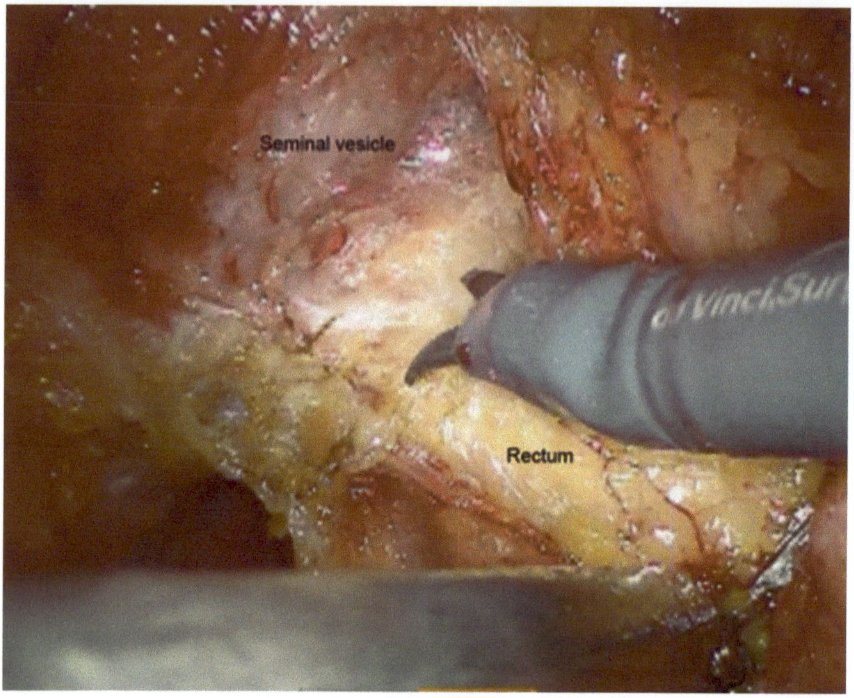


**Fig. 23.8** Dissecting anteriorly between the rectum and the prostate and seminal vesicles. Arm 3 retracts the bladder superiorly, while arm 2 retracts the rectum down and towards the sacrum

to create traction and counter-traction as the procedure progresses towards the right and left lateral stalks. As they are divided, dissection then moves anteriorly, towards the peritoneum between the rectum and seminal vesicles or upper vagina. As Arm 3 in an "L" configuration retracts these structures anteriorly towards the pubis, Arm 2 creates counter-traction by pushing the rectum down into the pelvis (Fig. 23.8). As the peritoneum is then divided, the plane between the vagina/seminal vesicles and rectum is exposed. As dissection advances distally (i.e., deeper) in this plane, access to the distal aspect of the lateral stalks is gained; terminal branches of the middle hemorrhoidal vessels can be found and may need to be divided with bipolar cautery by Arm 2 (Fig. 23.9). As the hypogastric nerves travel laterally in the mid-pelvis sidewall behind the EPF and beyond our plane of dissection, complete autonomic nerve preservation procedure is performed.

Digital rectal exam or flexible endoscopy is used as needed to confirm that the dissection has reached the desired level and that adequate margins can be obtained prior to dividing the rectum. Subsequently, the rectum is then divided using a laparoscopic or robotic stapler. The 8-mm robotic trocar is removed and either a 45-mm laparoscopic or robotic articulating stapler is introduced; either a green or black cartridge or a purple staple load is used. As the stapler is introduced, the rectum can be engaged from right to left, or in an anterior to posterior fashion (Fig. 23.10). More than one load is usually required to completely transect the rectum; care should be taken not to disrupt the staple line as upper traction is required to allow the stapler with subsequent loads to be positioned adequately. Once the rectum is divided, the robot is undocked.

## Specimen Extraction and Laparoscopically-Assisted Colorectal Anastomosis

A suprapubic Pfannenstiel incision is our preferred extraction site. A wound protector is routinely placed and the specimen is extracted. The colon is then divided taking care to include

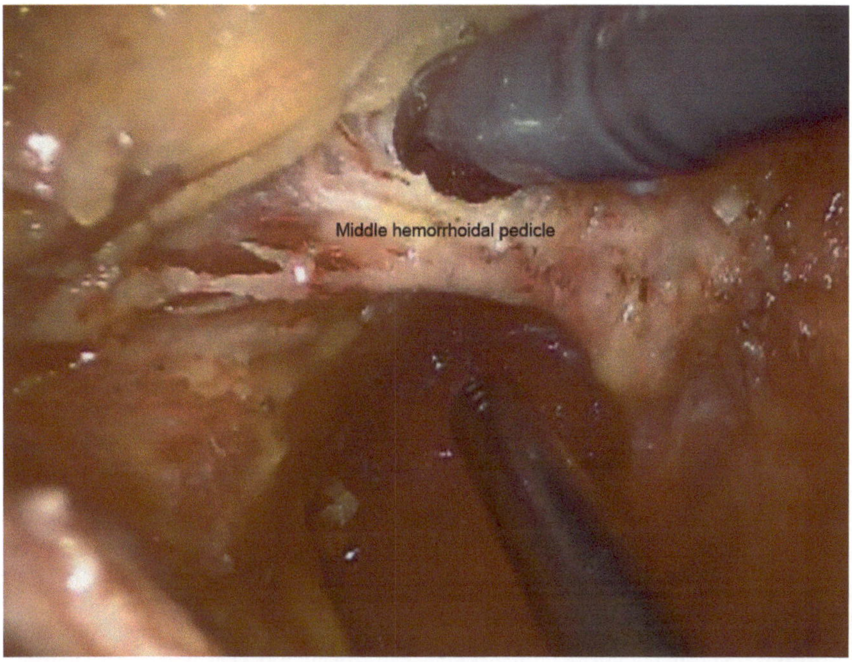


**Fig. 23.9** Dissecting the lateral stalks. The middle hemorrhoidal vessels are identified and subsequently divided with bipolar cautery (arm 2)

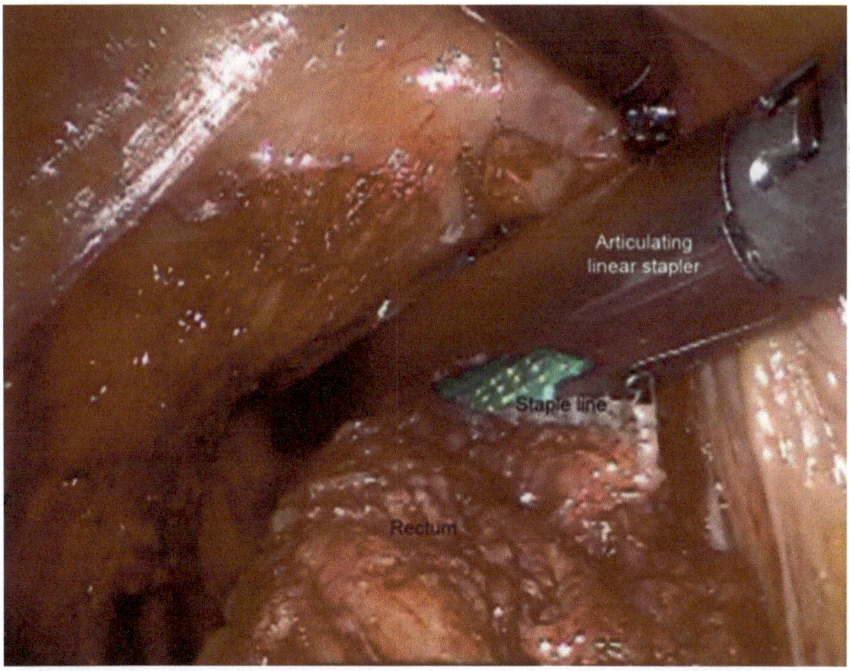


**Fig. 23.10** The rectum is divided with a laparoscopic or robotic stapler. It can be engaged in an anterior to posterior fashion as in this picture, or from right to left, as space allows

the IMA pedicle with the specimen. A pursue-string is then created tight around the anvil of a circular stapler. When a colonic J pouch is planned, the colon is divided using a linear stapler with a blue load. Subsequently, an enterotomy is created in the antimesenteric border and a 75-mm linear stapler with a blue load introduced to create a 5-cm pouch. The enterotomy site is then used to introduce the anvil of the circular stapler.

The incision is then closed and a circular colorectal anastomosis is created laparoscopically. The pelvis is then filled with water and an air-leak test is performed. Incomplete donuts are worrisome and may suggest a problem with the anastomosis. If there is an air leak, a decision must be made to reinforce versus redoing the anastomosis. A flexible endoscopy is routinely performed to evaluate the anastomosis in our practice; however, this reflects our personal preference and it is not a routine step. A loop ileostomy is usually created in high-risk patients or when the anastomosis is located within 7 cm of the anal verge.

## Conclusion

Training and cost are two main barriers that prevent widespread adoption of this platform. Personal experience suggests that the robot facilitates pelvic dissection and construction of ultralow-coloanal anastomoses. Furthermore, most of the skill set required in robotic surgery is quickly learned, as more and more surgeons adopting this technology are well versed in laparoscopic surgery. Although robotic surgery may contribute to lower conversion rates compared to open surgery, studies are needed to further determine the role of robotics in rectal surgery.

## References

1. Laparoscopically assisted colectomy is as safe and effective as open colectomy in people with colon cancer Abstracted from: Nelson H, Sargent D, Wieand HS, et al.; for the Clinical Outcomes of Surgical Therapy Study Group. A comparison of laparoscopically assisted and open colectomy for colon cancer. N Engl J Med 2004; 350: 2050–9. Cancer treatment reviews. 2004;30(8):707–9. doi:10.1016/j.ctrv.2004.09.001.
2. Colon Cancer Laparoscopic or Open Resection Study Group, Buunen M, Veldkamp R, Hop WC, Kuhry E, Jeekel J, et al. Survival after laparoscopic surgery versus open surgery for colon cancer: long-term outcome of a randomised clinical trial. Lancet Oncol. 2009;10(1):44–52. doi:10.1016/s1470-2045(08)70310-3.
3. Veldkamp R, Kuhry E, Hop WC, Jeekel J, Kazemier G, Bonjer HJ, et al. Laparoscopic surgery versus open surgery for colon cancer: short-term outcomes of a randomised trial. Lancet Oncol. 2005;6(7):477–84. doi:10.1016/s1470-2045(05)70221-7.
4. Baik SH. Robotic colorectal surgery. Yonsei Med J. 2008;49(6):891–6. doi:10.3349/ymj.2008.49.6.891.
5. Bianchi PP, Luca F, Petz W, Valvo M, Cenciarelli S, Zuccaro M, et al. The role of the robotic technique in minimally invasive surgery in rectal cancer. Ecancermedicalscience. 2013;7:357. doi:10.3332/ecancer.2013.357.
6. Jayne DG, Guillou PJ, Thorpe H, Quirke P, Copeland J, Smith AM, et al. Randomized trial of laparoscopic-assisted resection of colorectal carcinoma: 3-year results of the UK MRC CLASICC Trial Group. J Clin Oncol. 2007;25(21):3061–8. doi:10.1200/jco.2006.09.7758.
7. Jayne DG, Thorpe HC, Copeland J, Quirke P, Brown JM, Guillou PJ. Five-year follow-up of the Medical Research Council CLASICC trial of laparoscopically assisted versus open surgery for colorectal cancer. Br J Surg. 2010;97(11):1638–45. doi:10.1002/bjs.7160.
8. van der Pas MH, Haglind E, Cuesta MA, Furst A, Lacy AM, Hop WC, et al. Laparoscopic versus open surgery for rectal cancer (COLOR II): short-term outcomes of a randomised, phase 3 trial. Lancet Oncol. 2013;14(3):210–8. doi:10.1016/s1470-2045(13)70016-0.
9. Monson JR, Weiser MR, Buie WD, Chang GJ, Rafferty JF, Buie WD, et al. Practice parameters for the management of rectal cancer (revised). Dis Colon Rectum. 2013;56(5):535–50. doi:10.1097/DCR.0b013e31828cb66c.
10. McKay GD, Morgan MJ, Wong SK, Gatenby AH, Fulham SB, Ahmed KW, et al. Improved short-term outcomes of laparoscopic versus open resection for colon and rectal cancer in an area health service: a multicenter study. Dis Colon Rectum. 2012;55(1):42–50. doi:10.1097/DCR.0b013e318239341f.
11. Braga M, Frasson M, Vignali A, Zuliani W, Capretti G, Di Carlo V. Laparoscopic resection in rectal cancer patients: outcome and cost-benefit analysis. Dis Colon Rectum. 2007;50(4):464–71. doi:10.1007/s10350-006-0798-5.
12. Kang SB, Park JW, Jeong SY, Nam BH, Choi HS, Kim DW, et al. Open versus laparoscopic surgery for mid or low rectal cancer after neoadjuvant

chemoradiotherapy (COREAN trial): short-term outcomes of an open-label randomised controlled trial. Lancet Oncol. 2010;11(7):637–45. doi:10.1016/s1470-2045(10)70131-5.
13. Laurent C, Leblanc F, Wutrich P, Scheffler M, Rullier E. Laparoscopic versus open surgery for rectal cancer: long-term oncologic results. Ann Surg. 2009;250(1):54–61. doi:10.1097/SLA.0b013e3181ad6511.
14. Baek JH, Pastor C, Pigazzi A. Robotic and laparoscopic total mesorectal excision for rectal cancer: a case-matched study. Surg Endosc. 2011;25(2):521–5. doi:10.1007/s00464-010-1204-x.
15. Baek SJ, Al-Asari S, Jeong DH, Hur H, Min BS, Baik SH, et al. Robotic versus laparoscopic coloanal anastomosis with or without intersphincteric resection for rectal cancer. Surg Endosc. 2013;27(11):4157–63. doi:10.1007/s00464-013-3014-4.
16. Kwak JM, Kim SH, Kim J, Son DN, Baek SJ, Cho JS. Robotic vs laparoscopic resection of rectal cancer: short-term outcomes of a case-control study. Dis Colon Rectum. 2011;54(2):151–6. doi:10.1007/DCR.0b013e3181fec4fd.
17. Park JS, Choi GS, Lim KH, Jang YS, Jun SH. Robotic-assisted versus laparoscopic surgery for low rectal cancer: case-matched analysis of short-term outcomes. Ann Surg Oncol. 2010;17(12):3195–202. doi:10.1245/s10434-010-1162-5.
18. Scarpinata R, Aly EH. Does robotic rectal cancer surgery offer improved early postoperative outcomes? Dis Colon Rectum. 2013;56(2):253–62. doi:10.1097/DCR.0b013e3182694595.
19. Collinson FJ, Jayne DG, Pigazzi A, Tsang C, Barrie JM, Edlin R, et al. An international, multicentre, prospective, randomised, controlled, unblinded, parallel-group trial of robotic-assisted versus standard laparoscopic surgery for the curative treatment of rectal cancer. Int J Colorectal Dis. 2012;27(2):233–41. doi:10.1007/s00384-011-1313-6.
20. Ahmed K, Khan MS, Vats A, Nagpal K, Priest O, Patel V, et al. Current status of robotic assisted pelvic surgery and future developments. Int J Surg. 2009;7(5):431–40. doi:10.1016/j.ijsu.2009.08.008.
21. Halabi WJ, Kang CY, Jafari MD, Nguyen VQ, Carmichael JC, Mills S, et al. Robotic-assisted colorectal surgery in the United States: a nationwide analysis of trends and outcomes. World J Surg. 2013;37(12):2782–90. doi:10.1007/s00268-013-2024-7.
22. Lin S, Jiang HG, Chen ZH, Zhou SY, Liu XS, Yu JR. Meta-analysis of robotic and laparoscopic surgery for treatment of rectal cancer. World J Gastroenterol. 2011;17(47):5214–20. doi:10.3748/wjg.v17.i47.5214.
23. Memon S, Heriot AG, Murphy DG, Bressel M, Lynch AC. Robotic versus laparoscopic proctectomy for rectal cancer: a meta-analysis. Ann Surg Oncol. 2012;19(7):2095–101. doi:10.1245/s10434-012-2270-1.
24. Yang Y, Wang F, Zhang P, Shi C, Zou Y, Qin H, et al. Robot-assisted versus conventional laparoscopic surgery for colorectal disease, focusing on rectal cancer: a meta-analysis. Ann Surg Oncol. 2012;19(12):3727–36. doi:10.1245/s10434-012-2429-9.
25. Kang J, Hur H, Min BS, Lee KY, Kim NK. Robotic coloanal anastomosis with or without intersphincteric resection for low rectal cancer: starting with the perianal approach followed by robotic procedure. Ann Surg Oncol. 2012;19(1):154–5. doi:10.1245/s10434-011-1952-4.
26. Leong QM, Son DN, Cho JS, Baek SJ, Kwak JM, Amar AH, et al. Robot-assisted intersphincteric resection for low rectal cancer: technique and short-term outcome for 29 consecutive patients. Surg Endosc. 2011;25(9):2987–92. doi:10.1007/s00464-011-1657-6.
27. Peterson CY, McLemore EC, Horgan S, Talamini MA, Ramamoorthy SL. Technical aspects of robotic proctectomy. Surg Laparosc Endosc Percutan Tech. 2012;22(3):189–93. doi:10.1097/SLE.0b013e31824be924.
28. Rullier E, Denost Q, Vendrely V, Rullier A, Laurent C. Low rectal cancer: classification and standardization of surgery. Dis Colon Rectum. 2013;56(5):560–7. doi:10.1097/DCR.0b013e31827c4a8c.
29. Richardson DP, Porter GA, Johnson PM. Population-based use of sphincter-preserving surgery in patients with rectal cancer: is there room for improvement? Dis Colon Rectum. 2013;56(6):704–10. doi:10.1097/DCR.0b013e3182758c2b.
30. Tilney HS, Tekkis PP. Extending the horizons of restorative rectal surgery: intersphincteric resection for low rectal cancer. Colorectal Dis. 2008;10(1):3–15. doi:10.1111/j.1463-1318.2007.01226.x; discussion 6.
31. Heald RJ. The 'Holy Plane' of rectal surgery. J R Soc Med. 1988;81(9):503–8.

## Key Operative Steps

1. The patient is placed on the operating room table in modified lithotomy position and secured to prevent movement when the bed is changed to different positions.
2. The abdominal cavity is accessed and insufflated. Ports are placed after insufflation is complete.
3. The abdomen is thoroughly explored to rule out metastatic disease.
4. The inferior mesenteric vessels are identified then divided and the mesocolon is dissected away from retroperitoneal structures in a medial-to-lateral fashion. Care is taken to identify and protect the ureter.
5. The lateral attachments along the line of Toldt are divided and the splenic flexure is then mobilized.
6. Once the colon has been mobilized, the ureter identified, and the inferior mesenteric vessels divided, the robotic portion of the procedure begins.
7. rTME starts at the sacral promontory as the avascular plane between the EVF that contains the mesorectum

and the endopelvic parietal fascia is entered. As dissection starts, it is important to identify the hypogastric nerves in this area and gently dissected them away from the operating field.

8. Dissecting as far distal as possible in the posterior plane makes identification of the lateral stalks and dissection in the anterolateral areas easier.
9. As the peritoneal reflection is opened anteriorly, precise sharp dissection helps prevent injury to the seminal vesicles and prostate in men and the vaginal wall in women. As dissection progresses, the lateral stalks are divided.
10. The distal rectum is then transected at the desired level with a stapler. The robot is then undocked.
11. A Pfannenstiel incision is then made and the specimen delivered into the operative field. The proximal margin of resection is then divided with a stapler.
12. A circular stapler is used to create the colorectal anastomosis. Anastomotic integrity is checked and then the trocars are removed and all incisions are closed.

# Open Abdominoperineal Resection

# 24

Lin Wang, Jin Gu, and Philip Paty

## Indications for Abdominoperineal Resection

Abdominoperineal resection (APR) is the procedure of choice for treatment of rectal adenocarcinoma arising in the distal rectum or anal canal. APR involves removal of the entire rectum, mesorectum, anal canal, levator muscle, and portions of the ischiorectal fat and perineal skin. A permanent end-colostomy is constructed in the abdominal wall [1]. It is also the optimal surgical treatment for patients with anal squamous cell carcinoma that persists or recurs after chemotherapy and radiation, because these tumors usually involve the anal canal and levator muscle [2].

Occasionally, APR is required for less common tumors of the anorectal region such as anal melanoma, sarcoma, or gastrointestinal stromal tumors. An extended APR is sometimes performed for vulvar, vaginal, or prostate cancers involving the distal rectum or anal sphincter complex. In addition, APR is part of total proctocolectomy performed for patients with familial adenomatous polyposis or other hereditary polyposis syndromes. Finally, APR is commonly performed in patients with inflammatory bowel disease, either as part of a proctocolectomy for ulcerative or granulomatous colitis, or as a separate procedure in the setting of isolated anorectal Crohn's disease.

The aim of APR is to obtain negative distal and circumferential resection margins [3]. For locally advanced adenocarcinoma of the distal rectum, neoadjuvant chemoradiation is recommended, and tumors are typically assessed for resection approximately 6 weeks after chemoradiation. Sphincter-preserving resection may be considered if a macroscopic distal margin of at least 1 cm can be achieved while preserving the levator and anal sphincter muscles [4]. In general, APR is indicated when tumor penetrates beyond the muscularis propria and infiltrates the levator or anal sphincter muscles [5].

Before making the decision for APR, a digital examination should be performed. This provides valuable information about the relationship of the tumor to the anal canal. The top of the anal canal (the anorectal ring), where the muscular wall of the rectum turns into the anal canal around the sling formed by the puborectalis muscles, can be palpated dynamically as the patient voluntarily tightens his or her anal canal. High-resolution magnetic resonance imaging (MRI) can provide

Electronic supplementary material Supplementary material is available in the online version of this chapter at 10.1007/978-1-4939-1893-5_24. Videos can also be accessed at http://www.springerimages.com/videos/978-1-4939-1892-8.

L. Wang, M.D. • J. Gu, M.D., F.A.C.S.
Department of Colorectal Surgery, Peking University Cancer Hospital, Beijing, People's Republic of China

P. Paty, M.D. (✉)
Division of Colon & Rectal Surgery, Department of Surgery, Memorial Sloan Kettering Cancer Center, 1275 York Avenue, New York, NY 10065, USA
e-mail: patyp@mskcc.org

J. Kim and J. Garcia-Aguilar (eds.), *Surgery for Cancers of the Gastrointestinal Tract: A Step-by-Step Approach*,
DOI 10.1007/978-1-4939-1893-5_24, © Springer Science+Business Media New York 2015

axial, sagittal, and coronal views, demonstrating the relationship of tumor to the levator muscle and the external anal sphincter [6]. MRI is superior to computed tomography (CT) because it provides better discrimination of soft tissue planes. MRI can also measure the distance between the distal edge of the tumor to the anorectal ring, predicting the achievable distal margin in sphincter-preserving resection [7].

Although the mortality associated with APR has decreased dramatically in the last century, it is still a formidable operation associated with significant morbidity. Patients must be informed about the potential risks and complications of the procedure. They should also be counseled about prognosis and functional outcomes; in particular, the risk of sexual and urinary dysfunction. Before surgery, patients must be marked at the colostomy site. Finally, they should be educated by an enterostomal therapist regarding the practicalities of living with a permanent stoma.

The need for full mechanical bowel cleansing preoperatively is controversial, with recent evidence from randomized trials suggesting that it reduces the incidence of postoperative infection [8]. Patients should receive perioperative antibiotics and deep venous thrombosis prophylaxis.

## Surgical Approaches to Abdominoperineal Resection

Recent publications have emphasized the importance of resecting the levator muscles in continuity with the distal rectum [9]. This revisitation of the surgical planes, as described in the original Miles procedure, is now often referred to as "cylindrical APR" or "extralevator APR," as opposed to conventional APR [5, 10]. After dividing the lateral ligaments and releasing the mid-rectum from the pelvic sidewalls, the abdominal dissection ends at the top of the levator muscles. The levator muscles are then transected near their origin via the perineal approach, which can be accomplished in either the lithotomy or prone position [11, 12]. Some authors favor the prone position, arguing that it provides superior exposure, lighting, and assistance [13].

The open APR procedure performed from start to finish in lithotomy position has several advantages. First, it is time- and cost-effective. Second, multivisceral resection for bulky tumor via the open approach is easier and safer because access to sites of bleeding from the pelvic sidewall, vagina, prostate, and base of the penis is available from both the abdominal and pelvic perspectives. Third, the perineal dissection is made precise and efficient by the simultaneous approach of the abdominal and perineal surgeons, who can guide each other by using a finger or instrument to identify correct surgical planes. This helps prevent injury to adjacent organs, as well as inadvertent "coning-in" during division of the levator muscles. Fourth, additional procedures, such as intraoperative radiotherapy, urinary diversion, or rectus myocutaneous flap reconstructions, can be accomplished when the surgical specimen is extracted from the pelvis, providing continued access from both the abdominal and perineal perspective.

APR in lithotomy position provides adequate exposure during the perineal dissection, a key element to a successful operation. A high lithotomy position is required for visualizing and dividing the levator muscles at their origin, and performing an accurate anterior dissection (Fig. 24.1). High lithotomy is particularly helpful in male patients if the rectum and anal sphincters adhere tightly to the prostate and deep perineal structures. Two perineal surgeons are required. Ideally, an assistant will also be present to provide guidance from the abdominal approach and anterior retraction in the perineum.

## Securing the Radial Margin in Low Rectal Cancer

Although total mesorectal excision (TME) and improved anastomotic methods have enhanced the indications for and success of sphincter-preserving surgery (SPS), many low rectal cancers are better treated by APR. In the setting of T2/T3 tumors that invade the anal sphincters, APR is required in order to obtain negative radial and distal margins. In the setting of bulky T3 and

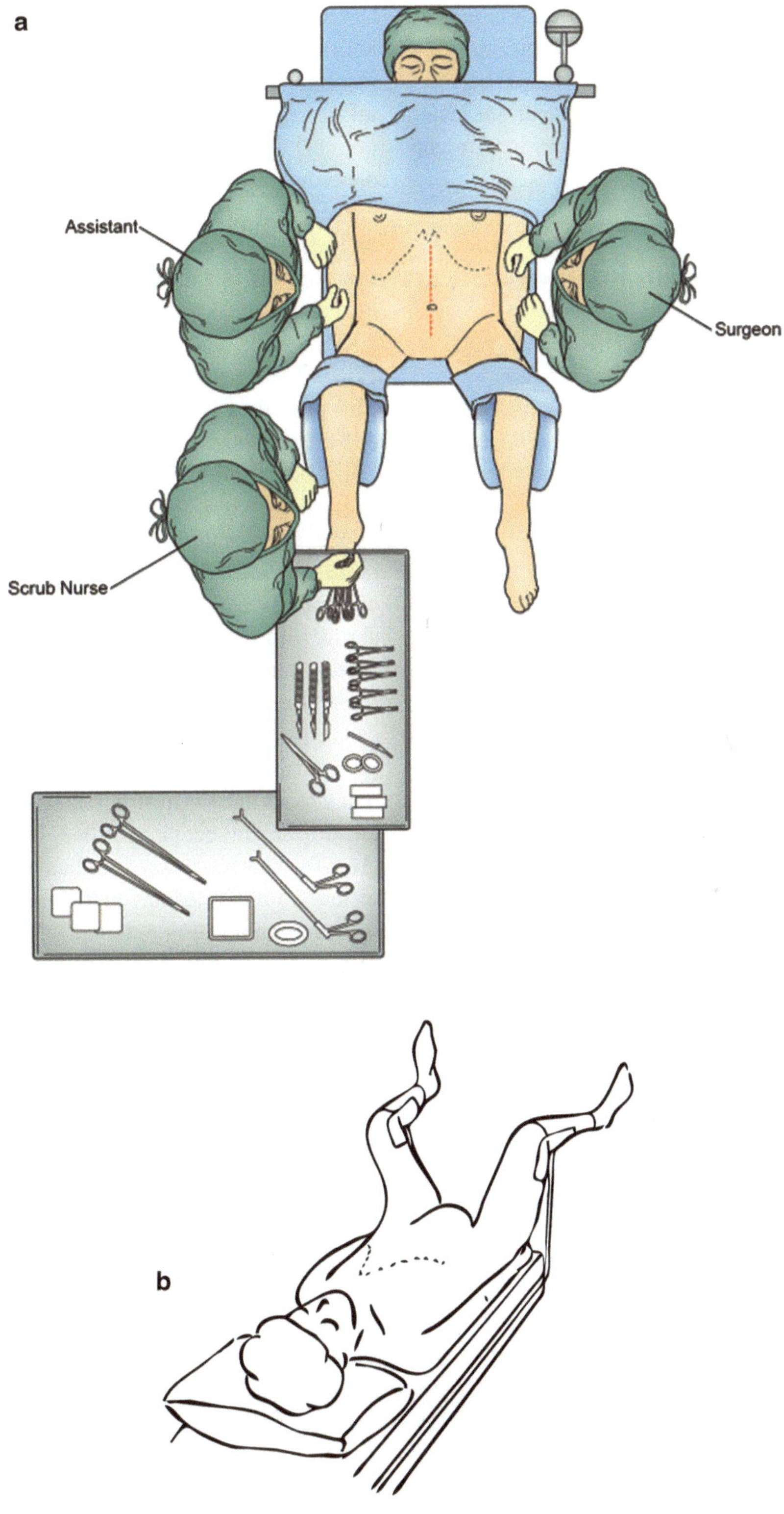


**Fig. 24.1** (**a**) Operative positioning of patient for APR in lithotomy position. (**b**) High lithotomy position used for this technique

T4 tumors that penetrate the muscularis propria and abut or invade the levator muscle, ultralow SPS requires opening of the hiatus between tumor and levator down to the anal sphincter. This can lead to tumor spillage and local recurrence [14].

## Variations in the Surgical Plane

### Standard Abdominoperineal Resection

Three variations of standard APR can be described based on the plane of dissection in the perineal phase.

#### Intralevator

This procedure is equivalent to the conventional APR described in the last decade [5, 10, 15, 16]. Dissection of the mesorectum is taken down close to the anorectal ring, opening the space between the rectum and the levator ani muscles (pubococcygeus, iliococcygeus, and ischiococcygeus) (Fig. 24.2a). The levator muscles are transected medially, near the anal canal. Most of the levator muscle and adipose tissue in the ischiorectal fossa is preserved. This procedure minimizes removal of tissue from the deep perineal space, but compromises radicality around the low rectum and anal canal. It may be successful for treatment of benign disease and low T1/T2 cancers without extrarectal spread, but it is not advisable in the setting of more advanced tumors [17].

#### Extralevator

This procedure is equivalent to the cylindrical or extralevator APR, as described in the last decade [5, 10, 16]. Abdominal dissection of the mesorectum stops at the origin of the levator muscles (tendinous arch of the obturator internus muscle). The perineal surgeon makes a conservative incision around the anus, dissects along the outer border of the anal sphincters and levator muscles, enters the pelvis anterior to the coccyx, and resects the levator ani muscles from below. The lower rectum, the entire funnel-shaped levator ani musculature, and the anal canal are resected in continuity. The adipose tissue in the ischiorectal fossa is preserved, limiting dead space in the perineal closure (Fig. 24.2b). Indications for this procedure are radical resection for low T2/T3/T4 cancers that threaten to invade the anal sphincters or levator ani, but show no evidence of infiltration into the ischiorectal adipose tissue or perineal skin.

#### Wide Perineal Resection

This procedure is equivalent to the original Miles APR described in the early twentieth century [18, 19]. Abdominal mobilization of the mesorectum stops at the top of the levator muscles, as is done in the extralevator APR. The perineal surgeon makes a wide skin incision around the anus. The adipose tissue of the ischiorectal fossa is resected, along with the anal sphincters, by outward dissection toward the ischial tuberosities. The rectum, the entire funnel of levator ani muscles, anal canal, ischiorectal fat, and a portion of perineal skin are completely resected (Fig. 24.2c). In many cases there is insufficient tissue for perineal closure, and myocutaneous flap repair is required [16, 20]. This procedure is indicated in the setting of low T3 or T4 lesions that invade or penetrate the levator ani and/or external sphincter muscles. Tumors that invade the perineal skin also require wide perineal resection. For posterior tumors that penetrate the rectal wall and abut or invade the coccyx, a complete resection of the ischiococcygeus muscle and coccyx is required (Fig. 24.3) [21]. Removal of these posterior structures is not routinely required in the setting of small or anteriorly located tumors.

The types of procedures and associated extent of resection are shown in Table 24.1. In tailored decision-making, these three variations of standard APR can be combined according to the quadrant of tumor location, to avoid unnecessary resection of normal tissue and delayed perineal healing. Precise preoperative examination and imaging are critical in optimizing the surgical dissection.

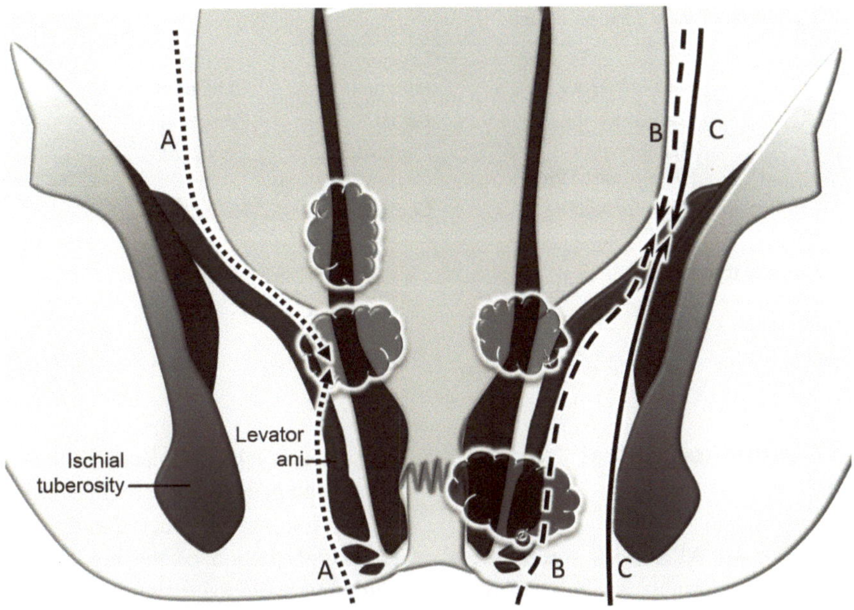


**Fig. 24.2** Comparison of the three surgical planes for APR. (**a**) Intra-levator APR for mid-low T2-3 rectal cancer without levator invasion but wide radial margin inside the levator (*dotted lines*). (**b**) Extra-levator APR for T3-4 rectal cancer with levator invasion (*dashed lines*). (**c**) Wide perineal resection for T4 rectal cancer at low rectum or anal canal, penetrating the levator or the external sphincter to the ischiorectal fat (*solid line*)

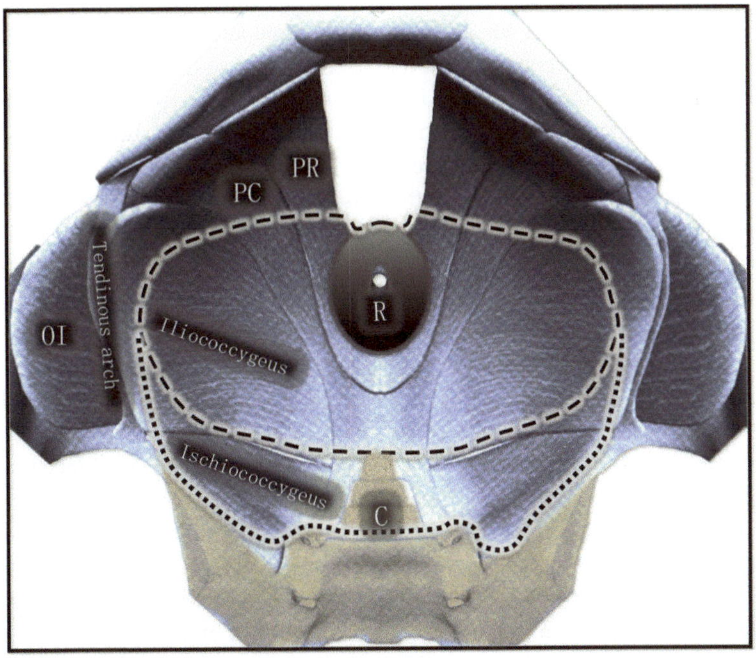


**Fig. 24.3** Surgical planes for APR with normal levator resection or extended posterior levator resection plus coccygectomy. *C* coccyx, *OI* obturator internus, *PC* pubococcygeus, *PR* puborectalis, *R* rectum

**Table 24.1** Comparison of three APR procedures

| Procedure | Also known as | Levator resection | Tissue in ischiorectal fossa | Perineal skin defect |
|---|---|---|---|---|
| Intralevator APR | Conventional APR | Partial | Preserved | Minor[a] |
| Extralevator APR | Cylindrical or Extralevator APR | Complete | Preserved | Minor[a] |
| APR with wide perineal resection | Miles' procedure | Complete | Resected | Large[b] |

*APR* abdominoperineal resection
[a]Primary suture repair
[b]Requires reconstruction with flaps

## Extended Abdominoperineal Resection

In selected cases an APR with multivisceral resection such as seminal vesiculectomy or prostatectomy in male patients, or partial vaginectomy in female patients can preserve urinary function without compromising the principles of en bloc R0 resection. Extended perineal dissections that include portions of the penis, scrotum, vulva, and pubic rami are sometimes required in the setting of bulky perineal tumors.

In summary, surgical dissection for an APR candidate should be planned preoperatively by high-quality imaging and thorough physical examination. It must be accomplished with strict attention to tumor size and location, circumferential margin, distal margin, and invasion of the levator muscle and adjacent organs.

## Positioning of the Patient

Patients are anesthetized in the supine position and then moved downward until the iliac spine reaches the lower edge of the operating table. A gel pad can be placed beneath the upper/mid-sacrum to elevate the buttocks and facilitate skin preparation. The buttocks should protrude from the end of the operating table, providing adequate exposure of the perineum [22].

The stirrups should be placed as low as possible on the rail of the operating table, so that they do not interfere with the position of the surgeon or assistants during the abdominal part of the procedure. The patient's legs are placed in the stirrups and aligned and padded properly to avoid pressure on the common peroneal nerve and popliteal artery [22]. Hyperflexion of the hip joints should be avoided to avoid excessive traction impinging on the sciatic nerve. Appropriate fitting of the leg in the stirrup is particularly important in obese patients, because excessive compression can lead to compartment syndrome [23]. When positioning is completed, the surgeon should reconfirm tumor location by digital exam and/or endoscopy. An irrigation-suction system is used to lavage the anal canal and rectal lumen, mitigating contamination in case of intraoperative bowel perforation. Following irrigation, the surgeon performs a double purse-string suture to close the anus.

## Abdominal Phase of Abdominoperineal Resection

### Abdominal Incision

A midline incision below the umbilicus is optimal in APR and can be used in most cases. A transverse or Pfannenstiel incision, which causes less pain and is cosmetically more appealing, may be used in selected patients. When a rectus muscle flap is required to close the perineal wound, it is necessary to make a midline incision. Exposure of the pelvis is achieved with self-retaining retractors. After entering the abdomen, exploratory examination is necessary to rule out extrapelvic metastases, particularly peritoneal dissemination.

## Sigmoid Mobilization

The small bowel is packed into the upper abdomen. Retracting the sigmoid colon medially exposes the lateral peritoneal reflection (the white line of Toldt). Mobilization begins along the left pelvic brim, using sharp dissection with electrocautery or scissors. Upon entering the retrosigmoid space, the left ureter and gonadal vessels should be identified and pushed lateral to the mesocolon. Dissection in this space reaches the brim of pelvis. Dissection beyond the lower descending colon is rarely necessary, as the proximal sigmoid colon is generally sufficient for constructing a colostomy. Next, the right lateral peritoneum is incised over the sacral promontory, and extended cephalad toward the origin of the inferior mesenteric artery. In general, the right ureter is well lateral to the incision and does not require exposure. Incisions on both sides are extended caudally, beyond the sacral promontory to the upper rectum.

## Low Ligation of the Inferior Mesenteric Artery

A typical ligation includes superior rectal artery/vein and the first trunk of sigmoid vessels. Additional ligation of vessels depends on the redundancy of the sigmoid colon [24]. The root of the inferior mesenteric artery (IMA) should be mobilized and palpated to discern any suspicious lymph nodes. Clinically positive lymph nodes should be removed [25]. The surgeon must be cautious when mobilizing the IMA to avoid injuring the sympathetic nerves of the hypogastric plexus and/or the left ureter.

## Transection of the Sigmoid Colon

Following ligation of the major vessels, the sigmoid mesocolon is divided at the level chosen to create the end-sigmoid colostomy. The proximal end of the divided sigmoid or descending colon should be sufficiently mobilized to ensure a tension-free, well-vascularized colostomy. The sigmoid colon is then transected using a linear stapler. Anterior retraction of the lower sigmoid colon exposes the retrorectal space and facilitates identification of the preaortic/hypogastric sympathetic nerves and the origin of the hypogastric nerves.

## Mobilization of the Upper Rectum

By retracting the lower sigmoid and rectum anteriorly away from the sacral promontory with tension, the plane between the visceral and pleural layer of the pelvic fascia can be sharply divided with minimal hemorrhage. The surgical plane should be developed anterior to the hypogastric nerve trunks. Tight adhesion between the hypogastric nerves and mesorectum requires meticulous dissection [26]. If the tumor invades unilateral or bilateral nerve trunks posteriorly, an en bloc resection is required. Injury to the hypogastric nerve trunks can lead to ejaculatory dysfunction in male patients.

Mobilization of the middle and low rectum comprises anterior dissection, posterior dissection, and management of the lateral ligaments. Some surgeons completely mobilize posteriorly in the presacral plane before starting the lateral or anterior dissection. However, release of the anterolateral peritoneal attachments as an initial maneuver provides mobility and better exposure of the retrorectal space. This also prevents tearing of the anterior rectum and tumor cell spillage, and provides better definition of the lateral ligaments. Suture retraction of the bladder in men or the uterus in women improves exposure of the pelvic cul-de-sac. Anterior dissection of the mid-rectum begins by incising the peritoneal reflection at the level of the seminal vesicles or vagina. Denonvillier's fascia is identified and dissection continues in front of it, reaching the level of the upper prostate or mid-vagina [27].

Following the anterior dissection, the rectum can be more ventrally retracted. Two layers of pelvic fascia converge to form the recto-sacral fascia (Waldeyer's fascia), which presents as firm fibrous ligaments at the S3/4 level. This fascia should be cut close to the mesorectum with electrocautery and followed to the tip of the coccyx. Accurate dissection of the lateral ligaments requires firm retraction of the rectum to the contralateral side. The middle rectal vessels, if present, must be ligated at their attachment at the visceral pelvic fascia. This prevents injury to the inferior hypogastric plexus and the urogenital nerve bundle, which crosses the middle rectal vessels and fans out behind the seminal vesicles or posterior vaginal wall.

## Levator Resection in the Abdominal Phase

Following lateral dissection carried to the origin of the levator muscle, the lateral attachment of the iliococcygeal muscle to the tendinous arch of the obturator internus can be exposed, and partially or completely incised by electrocautery to establish the plane of extralevator resection (Fig. 24.3) [28]. When possible, release of the iliococcygeal muscle should begin on the tumor-free side, exposing the adipose tissue in the ischiorectal fossa. If the exposure is adequate, this initial release of the levator muscle can be extended anteriorly and medially to include the pubococcygeus. The levator dissection can then continue posteriorly through the ischiococcygeus muscle toward the coccyx. It should be noted that the posterior attachments of the levator muscles cover much of the anterior surface of the coccyx. Therefore, the ischiococcygeus muscle may be resected with the coccyx (for a posterior tumor) or divided and separated from the coccyx (for an anterior tumor), as required for a clear posterior surgical margin. Having established these anatomic landmarks in the pelvic floor, the surgeon may then complete the levator dissection near the tumor with added confidence.

## Perineal Phase of Abdominoperineal Resection

A perineal tray with a separate set of instruments is prepared, including self-retaining retractors such as a Beckman-Adson and a pair of Gelpi retractors. A narrow Deaver is also useful for anterior retraction of the perineal skin to expose the perineal body and levator muscles. The use of a headlight is strongly recommended, as it affords sufficient illumination during resection in the deep pelvis and perineum.

An elliptical incision is made around the anus. The subcutaneous dissection is performed around the anal sphincter muscles. Anteriorly, dissection continues to the perineal body. Laterally and posteriorly, the extent of skin and fat resection in the ischiorectal fossa depends upon tumor infiltration. The incision is carried though the ischiorectal fossa until the anococcygeal ligament and the posterior/lateral levator muscles are exposed. Wide retraction of the perineal skin is secured with fixed retractors.

If the coccyx is to be preserved, the anococcygeal ligament is transected at the tip of the coccyx. With the abdominal surgeon lifting the rectum anteriorly and providing guidance with the tip of the fingers, the perineal surgeon can use electrocautery to divide the levator muscle at its attachment to the coccyx. Dissection is continued laterally and superiorly in the extralevator plane until the obturator fascia is reached. This creates a semicircular opening of the posterior and lateral pelvic diaphragm.

The anterior resection of the deep perineal space starts between the transverse superficial perineal muscle and perineal body [29]. Anterior retraction of the perineal skin is provided by the abdominal surgeon. Release of the levator muscles is continued from the existing dissection through the remaining pubococcygeus muscle. Bilateral stalks of the puborectalis muscles are divided from lateral to medial.

In male patients, the adhesions between the prostate, membranous urethra, bulbar urethra, and the anterior rectal wall can be dense and difficult to dissect from the perineal approach. Reversion of the rectal specimen to facilitate dissection is often difficult and may produce tearing of tissue, tumor exposure, or even bowel perforation. An alternative technique is to dissect from lateral to medial and proximal to distal along the posterior capsule of the prostate. This begins by transecting one stalk of the puborectalis muscle at the tumor-free side. The surgeon passes an index finger between the prostate and the anterior wall of the rectum, dissecting across the midline following the prostate capsule, and finally dividing the other stalk of the puborectalis muscle [14]. In female patients, dissection of the posterior vaginal wall away from the rectum can be guided by intermittent digital palpation of the posterior vaginal wall.

Once the rectal specimen has been removed, the surgical field is extensively irrigated. Drainage of the distal pelvis and deep perineal space is essential, and can be accomplished by drains brought through the abdominal wall or perineum [30]. The perineal defect is closed by approximating the deep layer of subcutaneous tissue with interrupted, absorbable sutures. The skin is closed by vertical mattress nylon sutures to assure watertight closure.

## Extended Abdominoperineal Resection

### Seminal Vesicle/Prostate Capsule Resection in Men

In selected male patients with anterior T3/T4 rectal cancer that abuts or focally invades anteriorly, APR combined with seminal vesiculectomy and partial prostatectomy may achieve clear surgical anterior margins, thus avoiding total pelvic exenteration and urinary diversion (Fig. 24.4) [31]. Preoperative high-quality MRI is essential for patient selection, and placing bilateral double J ureteral catheters is also recommended to identify the ureters intraoperatively [32].

### Vaginectomy in Women

In female patients the rectum and/or tumor may adhere tightly to the vagina. Wide excision of the vagina at any point of tumor adherence should be considered (Fig. 24.5) [33]. Small vaginal defects can be closed primarily, but may lead to vaginal stricture. Larger defects require flap reconstruction.

## Postoperative Management

Routine care following bowel resection includes bowel rest, intravenous fluids, pain management, deep venous thrombosis prophylaxis, and early ambulation. The lower limbs should be checked for skin integrity, arterial pulses, sensation, femoral and sciatic nerve function, and absence of compartment syndrome. Urinary catheters are maintained until the patient is fully ambulatory; this is typically 5 days in men with history of obstructive voiding symptoms. Pelvic drains protect the perineal wound from ascitic leak and are removed prior to discharge. The patient should avoid excessive pressure on the perineal closure, and is instructed to use a pillow to distribute pressure when sitting upright. The colostomy is monitored for vascularity and integrity and an enterostomal therapist instructs the patient in the use of stoma appliance and routine skin and stoma care.

## Complications

Intraoperative complications can be minimized by good planning, careful positioning, and accurate dissection. Ureteral catheters, placed by cystoscopy to protect the ureters, are sometimes helpful in the setting of bulky tumors that adhere to the pelvic sidewall, and in reoperative cases. Bleeding from presacral veins can generally be controlled by direct pressure with hemostatic agents, packing, bipolar cautery, or suture. Thumbtacks placed into the sacral cortex are rarely required, but may be effective for tamponade of vessels bleeding from the lower sacral foramina [34]. Perineal wound dehiscence is a major complication that can be minimized by careful avoidance of enteric contamination, good drainage of the pelvis and deep perineal space, secure closure of the perineal skin, and placement of myocutaneous flaps to reconstruct large skin, vaginal, or soft tissue deficits.

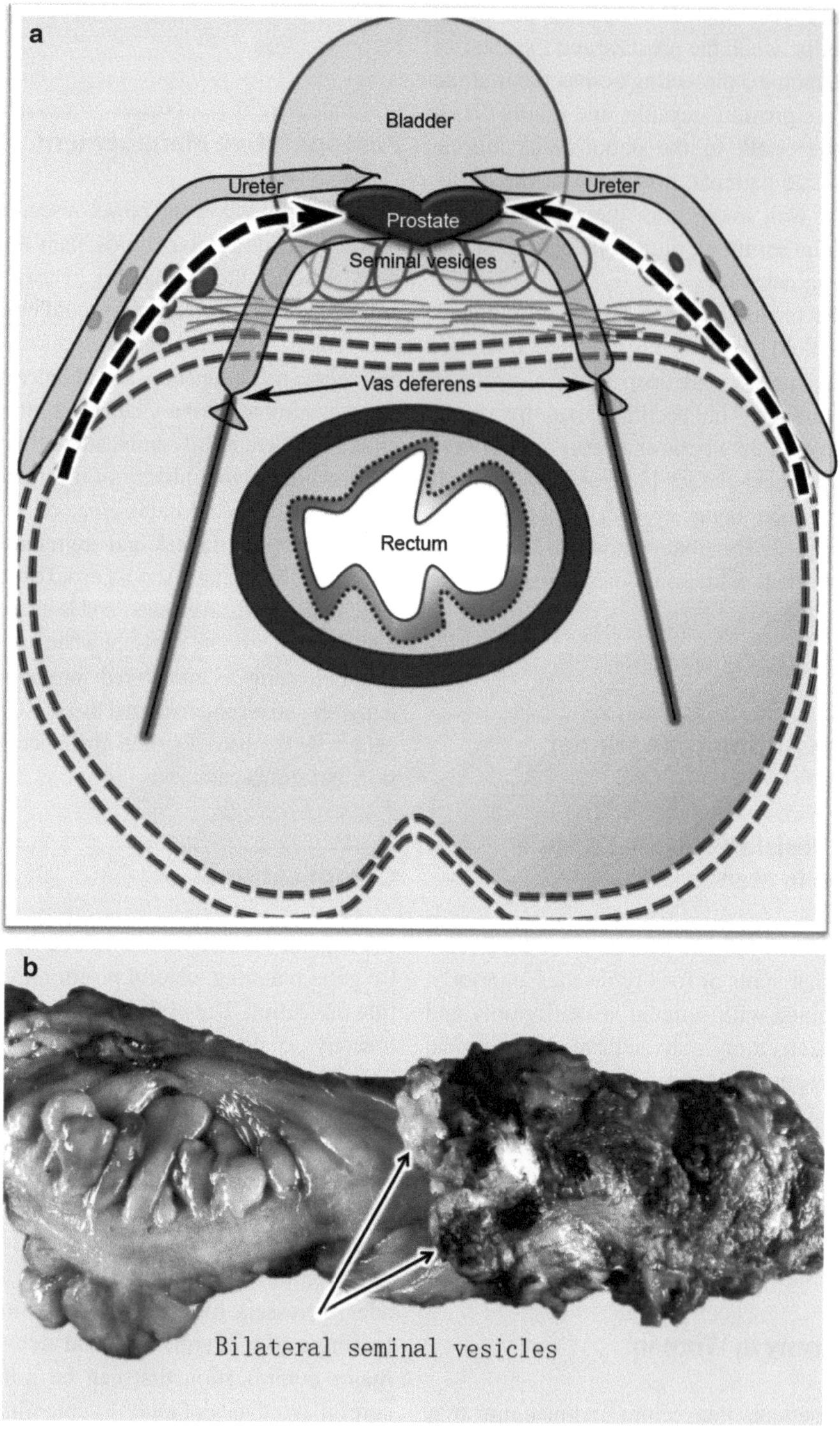


**Fig. 24.4** (**a**) Surgical planes for APR with seminal vesicle resection (*heavy black dashed lines*). The vas deferens are divided and ligated as retraction to expose the plane between the base of bladder/bilateral ureters and seminal vesicle/upper prostate. (**b**) Operative specimen following APR with seminal vesicle resection

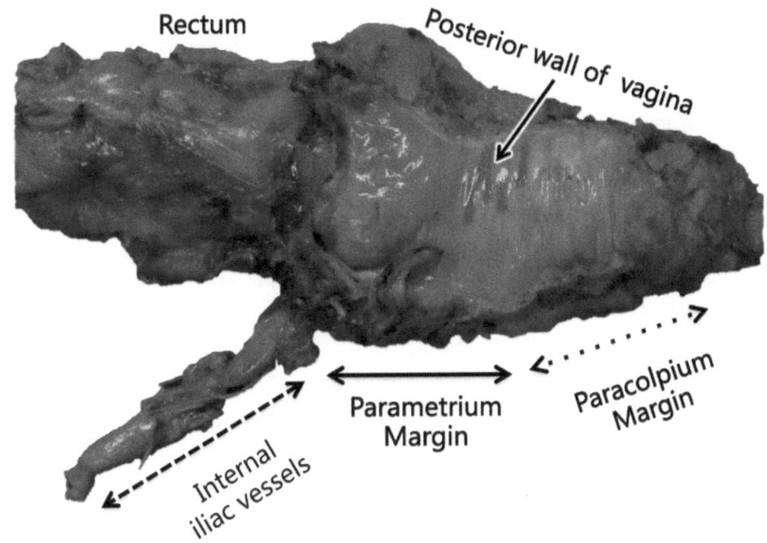


**Fig. 24.5** Operative specimen following APR with vaginectomy and resection of the right iliac vessels. Composition of the resection margin on the tumor side was labeled

## References


1. Lange MM, Rutten HJ, van de Velde CJ. One hundred years of curative surgery for rectal cancer: 1908–2008. Eur J Surg Oncol. 2009;35(5):456–63. doi:10.1016/j.ejso.2008.09.012.
2. Lefevre JH, Corte H, Tiret E, Boccara D, Chaouat M, Touboul E, et al. Abdominoperineal resection for squamous cell anal carcinoma: survival and risk factors for recurrence. Ann Surg Oncol. 2012;19(13):4186–92. doi:10.1245/s10434-012-2485-1.
3. Marr R, Birbeck K, Garvican J, Macklin CP, Tiffin NJ, Parsons WJ, et al. The modern abdominoperineal excision: the next challenge after total mesorectal excision. Ann Surg. 2005;242(1):74–82.
4. Watanabe T, Kazama S, Nagawa H. A 1cm distal bowel margin is safe for rectal cancer after preoperative radiotherapy. Hepatogastroenterology. 2012;59(116):1068–74.
5. Holm T, Ljung A, Haggmark T, Jurell G, Lagergren J. Extended abdominoperineal resection with gluteus maximus flap reconstruction of the pelvic floor for rectal cancer. Br J Surg. 2007;94(2):232–8. doi:10.1002/bjs.5489.
6. Guo M, Gao C, Li D, Guo W, Shafik AA, Zbar AP, et al. MRI anatomy of the anal region. Dis Colon Rectum. 2010;53(11):1542–8. doi:10.1007/DCR.0b013e3181f05256.
7. Shihab OC, How P, West N, George C, Patel U, Quirke P, et al. Can a novel MRI staging system for low rectal cancer aid surgical planning? Dis Colon Rectum. 2011;54(10):1260–4. doi:10.1097/DCR.0b013e31822abd78.
8. Bretagnol F, Panis Y, Rullier E, Rouanet P, Berdah S, Dousset B, et al. Rectal cancer surgery with or without bowel preparation: the French GRECCAR III multicenter single-blinded randomized trial. Ann Surg. 2010;252(5):863–8. doi:10.1097/SLA.0b013e3181fd8ea9.
9. Stelzner S, Koehler C, Stelzer J, Sims A, Witzigmann H. Extended abdominoperineal excision vs. standard abdominoperineal excision in rectal cancer–a systematic overview. Int J Colorectal Dis. 2011;26(10):1227–40.
10. West NP, Finan PJ, Anderin C, Lindholm J, Holm T, Quirke P. Evidence of the oncologic superiority of cylindrical abdominoperineal excision for low rectal cancer. J Clin Oncol. 2008;26(21):3517–22. doi:10.1200/JCO.2007.14.5961.
11. de Campos-Lobato LF, Stocchi L, Dietz DW, Lavery IC, Fazio VW, Kalady MF. Prone or lithotomy positioning during an abdominoperineal resection for rectal cancer results in comparable oncologic outcomes. Dis Colon Rectum. 2011;54(8):939–46. doi:10.1097/DCR.0b013e318221eb64.
12. Keller DS, Lawrence JK, Delaney CP. Prone jackknife position is not necessary to achieve a cylindrical abdominoperineal resection: demonstration of the lithotomy position. Dis Colon Rectum. 2014;57(2):251. doi:10.1097/DCR.0000000000000047.
13. Tayyab M, Sharma A, Ragg JL, Macdonald AW, Gunn J, Hartley JE, et al. Evaluation of the impact of implementing the prone jackknife position for the perineal phase of abdominoperineal excision of the rectum. Dis Colon Rectum. 2012;55(3):316–21. doi:10.1097/DCR.0b013e31823e2424.
14. Shihab OC, Heald RJ, Holm T, How PD, Brown G, Quirke P, et al. A pictorial description of extralevator abdominoperineal excision for low rectal cancer. Colorectal Dis. 2012. doi:10.1111/j.1463-1318.2012.03181.x.

15. Han JG, Wang ZJ, Wei GH, Gao ZG, Yang Y, Zhao BC. Randomized clinical trial of conventional versus cylindrical abdominoperineal resection for locally advanced lower rectal cancer. Am J Surg. 2012;204(3): 274–82. doi:10.1016/j.amjsurg.2012.05.001.
16. Holm T. Controversies in abdominoperineal excision. Surg Oncol Clin N Am. 2014;23(1):93–111. doi:10.1016/j.soc.2013.09.005.
17. Ramsay G, Parnaby C, Mackay C, Hanlon P, Ong S, Loudon M. Analysis of outcome using a levator sparing technique of abdominoperineal excision of rectum and anus. Cylindrical ELAPE is not necessary in all patients. Eur J Surg Oncol. 2013;39(11):1219–24. doi:10.1016/j.ejso.2013.08.004.
18. Campos FG, Habr-Gama A, Nahas SC, Perez RO. Abdominoperineal excision: evolution of a centenary operation. Dis Colon Rectum. 2012;55(8):844–53. doi:10.1097/DCR.0b013e31825ab0f7.
19. Finan P, Haboubi N. The Miles operation—extralevator abdominoperineal excision. Colorectal Dis. 2012;14(10):1171–2. doi:10.1111/j.1463-1318.2012.03191.x.
20. Han JG, Wang ZJ, Gao ZG, Yang Y, Du YF. Human acellular dermal matrix for pelvic floor reconstruction after cylindrical abdominoperineal resection. Hepatogastroenterology. 2011;58(109):1205–7. doi:10.5754/hge10809.
21. Bebenek M, Wojnar A. Infralevator lymphatic drainage of low-rectal cancers: preliminary results. Ann Surg Oncol. 2009;16(4):887–92. doi:10.1245/s10434-009-0324-9.
22. Ngamprasertwong P, Phupong V, Uerpairojkit K. Brachial plexus injury related to improper positioning during general anesthesia. J Anesth. 2004;18(2):132–4. doi:10.1007/s00540-003-0220-6.
23. Ikeya E, Taguchi J, Ohta K, Miyazaki Y, Hashimoto O, Yagi K, et al. Compartment syndrome of bilateral lower extremities following laparoscopic surgery of rectal cancer in lithotomy position: report of a case. Surg Today. 2006;36(12):1122–5. doi:10.1007/s00595-006-3313-7.
24. Lange MM, Buunen M, van de Velde CJ, Lange JF. Level of arterial ligation in rectal cancer surgery: low tie preferred over high tie. A review. Dis Colon Rectum. 2008;51(7):1139–45. doi:10.1007/s10350-008-9328-y.
25. Clinical Practice Guidlines of rectal cancer 2014. v2. Available at http://www.nccn.org/professionals/physician_gls/pdf/rectal.pdf.
26. Barabouti DG, Wong WD. Current management of rectal cancer: total mesorectal excision (nerve sparing) technique and clinical outcome. Surg Oncol Clin N Am. 2005;14(2):137–55. doi:10.1016/j.soc.2004.11.003.
27. Heald RJ, Moran BJ, Brown G, Daniels IR. Optimal total mesorectal excision for rectal cancer is by dissection in front of Denonvilliers' fascia. Br J Surg. 2004;91(1):121–3. doi:10.1002/bjs.4386.
28. Chi P, Chen ZF, Lin HM, Lu XR, Huang Y. Laparoscopic extralevator abdominoperineal resection for rectal carcinoma with transabdominal levator transection. Ann Surg Oncol. 2013;20(5):1560–6. doi:10.1245/s10434-012-2675-x.
29. Simunovic M, Pinthus J, Coates AJ, DeNardi F. Anterior-entry abdominoperineal resection: a variation in the method of perineal dissection. Ann Surg Oncol. 2012;19(3):794–800. doi:10.1245/s10434-011-2016-5.
30. Fingerhut A, Hay JM, Delalande JP, Paquet JC. Passive vs. closed suction drainage after perineal wound closure following abdominoperineal rectal excision for carcinoma. A multicenter, controlled trial. The French Association for Surgical Research. Dis Colon Rectum. 1995;38(9):926–32.
31. Komori K, Hirai T, Kanemitsu Y, Shimizu Y, Sano T, Ito S, et al. Pathology studies of combined radical resection of seminal vesicle in the treatment of rectal cancer. Int Surg. 2011;96(1):51–5.
32. How P, West NP, Brown G. An MRI-based assessment of standard and extralevator abdominoperineal excision specimens: time for a patient tailored approach? Ann Surg Oncol. 2013;21(3):822–8. doi:10.1245/s10434-013-3378-7.
33. Ruo L, Paty PB, Minsky BD, Wong WD, Cohen AM, Guillem JG. Results after rectal cancer resection with in-continuity partial vaginectomy and total mesorectal excision. Ann Surg Oncol. 2003; 10(6):664–8.
34. Timmons MC, Kohler MF, Addison WA. Thumbtack use for control of presacral bleeding, with description of an instrument for thumbtack application. Obstet Gynecol. 1991;78(2):313–5.


## Key Operative Steps

1. The patient is placed in lithotomy position.
2. The abdomen is opened and explored to rule out metastatic disease.
3. The sigmoid colon is mobilized and the left ureter and gonadal vessels are identified and preserved.
4. Incise the right lateral peritoneum from the sacral promontory to the origin of the IMA.
5. Perform low ligation of the IMA including the superior rectal vessels and the first trunk of sigmoid vessels.
6. Divide the sigmoid colon with a linear stapler ensuring adequate mobilization for tension-free, well-vascularized colostomy.
7. Retract sigmoid and rectum anteriorly for posterior dissection and proceed with anterior and lateral dissection.
8. Establish plane of extralevator resection and complete levator dissection.
9. Begin perineal phase with an elliptical incision around the anus.
10. The incision is carried anteriorly to the perineal body and laterally and posteriorly through the ischiorectal fossa until the anococcygeal ligament and the posterior/lateral levator muscles are exposed.
11. Proceed with dissection circumferentially around the rectum until it is completely free.
12. Remove the specimen transanally and close the perineal defect. Drain the pelvis and perineal space.
13. Create and mature an end colostomy.

# 25 Robotic Abdominoperineal Resection

Brian K. Bednarski and George J. Chang

## Introduction

Abdominoperineal resection (APR) historically was the operation of choice for any rectal cancer within 5 cm of the anal verge. Given the improvements of surgical technology and better oncologic understanding of the behavior of primary tumors of the rectum, the technique for standard APR has evolved in practice, although the principles have remained the same. In the era of minimally invasive surgery, the robotic approach has quickly gained traction as a reliable technique for complex pelvic procedures including total mesorectal excision and APR for rectal cancer [1].

Electronic supplementary material: Supplementary material is available in the online version of this chapter at 10.1007/978-1-4939-1893-5_25. Videos can also be accessed at http://www.springerimages.com/videos/978-1-4939-1892-8.

B.K. Bednarski, M.D. • G.J. Chang, M.D., M.S., F.A.C.S., F.A.S.C.R.S. (✉)
Department of Surgical Oncology, The University of Texas MD Anderson Cancer Center, 1515 Holcombe Blvd., Unit 1484, Houston, TX 77030, USA
e-mail: gchang@mdanderson.org

## Anatomical Highlights

Whether an operation is conducted in a traditional open fashion or with newer technology, the importance of anatomical knowledge and the understanding of common anatomical variants remain critical to operative and oncologic success. For cancers of the rectum, treating the disease in a manner that minimizes morbidity requires a good fundamental understanding of pelvic and perineal anatomy.

### Vascular Supply and Drainage

For adenocarcinoma of the rectum, understanding the vascular supply and lymphatic drainage is crucial to an oncologically sound resection. The primary blood supply to the rectum comes from the inferior mesenteric artery (IMA) and its terminal vessel, the superior hemorrhoidal artery. Additionally, there are mid-rectal and pudendal vessels arising from the internal iliac artery that also provide additional blood supply to the middle and lower rectum. Similarly, the venous drainage for the rectum includes the pudendal, middle rectal, and inferior mesenteric veins. Given the fact that lymphatic drainage mirrors the vascular supply, an oncologic resection for rectal tumors should include all of the lymphovascular tissue comprising the mesorectum (a total mesorectal excision) as well as the lymphovascular

J. Kim and J. Garcia-Aguilar (eds.), *Surgery for Cancers of the Gastrointestinal Tract: A Step-by-Step Approach*, DOI 10.1007/978-1-4939-1893-5_25, © Springer Science+Business Media New York 2015 

pedicle extending up to the origin of the IMA at the aorta. In distal rectal cancer, the presence of lateral pelvic nodal metastasis (internal iliac or obturator nodes) may be identified on preoperative imaging and should be removed at surgery.

## Planes of Pelvic Dissection

In addition to the vascular supply of the rectum, a comprehensive knowledge of the relationship of the rectum to additional pelvic organs is critical to successful extirpation of the tumor while minimizing morbidity. This can best be understood by considering the three planes of pelvic dissection required for this operation, including the posterior, lateral, and anterior planes.

### Posterior Plane

The posterior plane of dissection lies in the avascular space between Waldeyer's fascia and the enveloping fascia propria of the mesorectum. This is best identified by mobilization of the sigmoid colon mesentery following the vascular dissection. By following the IMA down toward the pelvic brim, one can safely identify several critical structures to avoid injury, including the ureters, the superior hypogastric plexus containing sympathetic fibers, and the hypogastric nerve trunks. Once the total mesorectal excision (TME) plane has been identified, safe posterior dissection toward the pelvic floor can be performed while avoiding injury to the nerves innervating the genitourinary tract and the sacral venous plexus. By maintaining meticulous techniques in the proper plane, one can minimize the risk of urinary retention, retrograde ejaculation, erectile dysfunction, and hemorrhage.

### Lateral Plane

During the lateral dissection, the critical structures include the lateral stalks of the rectum, which contain the middle rectal vessels. Variation exists in the size of these vessels and their contribution to the blood supply of the rectum. Also important is the autonomic innervation of the pelvic viscera. The inferior hypogastric plexus is located medial to the internal iliac vessels and contains the parasympathetic innervation (S2–4) to the pelvic viscera and the cavernous nerves (nervi erigentes) to erectile tissue of the penis and clitoris. This nerve bundle travels in the posterolateral wall of the pelvis before reaching its terminal anatomic structures and can be at risk for injury with extensive lateral dissection. Additionally, the nervi erigentes are perhaps at greatest risk at the junction of the lateral and anterior dissection planes in the male pelvis as the nerves coalesce at the seminal vesicles to become the periprostatic neurovascular bundle which runs posterolateral to the base of the prostate and anterolateral to the rectum. Lastly, while not typically of great concern unless an extensive lateral resection is required, the ureters also run in the lateral compartment of the pelvis.

### Anterior Plane

When considering the anterior dissection of the rectum, understanding the close proximity of the anterior border of the rectum to the genitourinary structures in men and women is critical for preoperative planning and intraoperative execution. In the male pelvis, electrocautery for control of bleeding near the seminal vesicles can lead to injury to the nervi erigentes. In the female pelvis, there is a thin avascular plane between the anterior rectum and the posterior wall of the vagina. A locally advanced tumor may extend to involve these adjacent structures, necessitating extended en bloc resection. This should be preceded by appropriate preoperative planning to include multidisciplinary reconstruction as necessary.

## Pelvic Floor

Finally, while the aforementioned anatomic principles can impact any pelvic procedure, the anatomy of the perineum and the pelvic floor is unique to APRs. The pelvic floor musculature which must be divided to adequately resect the anal canal and sphincter complex and to ensure a wide circumferential margin includes the anococcygeal ligament posteriorly, the levator ani muscles laterally, and the puborectalis, pubococcygeus, and rectourethralis muscles anteriorly.

For females, the rectovaginal septum is the target for anterior dissection. In males it is important to understand the relationship of the urethra, the prostate, and the periprostatic neurovascular bundles to the anterior rectum.

## Historical Perspective

APR was first described by Sir Ernest Miles in 1908 as a means to treat cancers of the rectum [2]. Although the initial report was associated with high surgical morbidity and mortality, variations of this procedure remained the gold standard for middle and low rectal cancers for the better part of the century. The widespread adoption of TME technique was one such modification that improved the ability of the surgeon to continue the dissection into the distal pelvis [3]. However, the tapering mesorectum can result in an increased risk for a positive circumferential radial margin at the level of the tumor with the TME technique or even with APR [4, 5]. More recently, the principle of wide resection of the pelvic floor around the tumor has been again highlighted with the concept of the cylindrical APR. Whether performed using either open or minimally invasive technique, the approach and oncologic principles are the same. However, modern videoscopic approaches (e.g., laparoscopy or robotics) permit direct visualization of the pelvic floor to permit wide division of the levator ani without the need for prone positioning. In fact, the COlorectal cancer Laparoscopic or Open Resection (COLOR II) trial compared laparoscopic to open resection for rectal cancer and observed a lower rate of radial margin positivity in the laparoscopic arm among patients with distal rectal cancers [6].

## Indications

While APR has been the standard of care for low rectal cancers for nearly a century, advances in stapling devices, surgical technique, and the incorporation of multidisciplinary treatment strategies have facilitated sphincter-preserving surgery. Moreover, surgeons around the world continue to explore the limits of sphincter preservation with coloanal anastomoses and intersphincteric resection [7].

In addition to the technical aspects, advances in knowledge regarding minimum distal mucosal margins have greatly influenced the frequency of APRs [8–10]. In the era of neoadjuvant chemoradiotherapy, APR is indicated for a patient with rectal adenocarcinoma in whom a negative margin resection requires removal of the anal sphincter complex or for patients in whom poor sphincter function would result in unacceptable functional outcomes. Similar rules apply to some of the other less common rectal malignancies including neuroendocrine tumors and gastrointestinal tumors. APR is also indicated for patients with recurrent or persistent squamous cell carcinoma after definitive chemoradiotherapy [11–13].

Similar to other minimally invasive procedures, patient selection is critical to successful robotic APR. While the only absolute contraindication to using robotic-laparoscopic approach to any surgery is hemodynamic instability or inability to tolerate laparotomy, there are several relative contraindications that should be considered. These include extensive prior abdominal surgery, severe obesity, cardiopulmonary insufficiency, or locally advanced pathology for which margin negative resection with a minimally invasive approach cannot be achieved [14, 15]. As relative contraindications, minimally invasive procedures under these circumstances may be technically more demanding and may portend higher risk of conversion and complications.

## Perioperative Preparation

Workup should include a complete history and physical examination to ensure that the patient will be able to tolerate the physiologic demands of pneumoperitoneum and Trendelenburg position. Additionally, a digital rectal exam, pelvic exam, and an endoscopic visualization of the tumor will help the surgeon determine the best operative approach. It will help identify adjacent pelvic structures that are involved by direct extension of the tumor, and enable preoperative planning for en bloc resection. Lastly, a repeat exam following neoadjuvant therapy will help to reconfirm the appropriate surgical procedure given that significant tumor response may permit select patients to avoid APR and be considered for a sphincter-sparing procedure.

Adequate preparation for success in the operating room extends to the radiographic assessment of the extent of disease. When considering a minimally invasive approach to surgical resection for malignancy, preoperative imaging not only serves to identify patients with distant disease, but also can help to anticipate and plan for the extent of surgical resection. For rectal tumors, high-resolution pelvic magnetic resonance imaging (MRI) is the primary staging modality of choice. It provides detailed anatomic information about the extent of the tumor, invasion into adjacent structures, margins at risk, and the potential for lymphatic spread [16, 17]. Lastly, an evaluation of the perineum after radiotherapy will help identify patients that may need vascularized flap reconstruction (e.g., vertical rectus abdominal myocutaneous flap).

Each patient should be evaluated by a wound ostomy continence nurse to assure that the patient will have the best opportunity to have a well-placed, easily pouched colostomy, which is critical to minimizing the impact of the ostomy on the patient postoperatively. The preoperative evaluation provides an early opportunity for ostomy education and simultaneously enables the patient to undergo assessment and marking for optimal siting of the colostomy.

The role for bowel preparation in colon and rectal surgery is a topic of debate. Recent data suggests that it is safe to proceed with colon and rectal surgery without a bowel preparation [18]. Laparoscopic surgery is no different in terms of the relationship between infectious complications and mechanical bowel preparation. However, for minimally invasive surgery, there is the potential benefit of improved visibility and greater maneuverability of the intestine during laparoscopy following bowel preparation [19, 20].

Prior to incision, prophylaxis against deep venous thrombosis (DVT) and antibiotic prophylaxis for wound infection should be administered [21, 22]. Chemical prophylaxis with subcutaneous heparin should be administered given the magnitude of abdominal operation, the duration of the procedure, the presence of malignancy, and the need for lithotomy position. In addition to chemoprophylaxis, sequential compression devices (SCDs) are advocated throughout the procedure.

## Operative Procedure

### Patient Positioning

As for all surgical cases, the first step of the operation is patient positioning. For robotic-assisted procedures, it is critical to not only consider appropriate positioning of the patient to provide adequate anatomical access, but to also allow for docking of the robotic surgical cart. Attention should be paid to ensuring that the patient is adequately protected from potential contact by the robotic arms. The patient is placed in low lithotomy position with the robotic surgical cart positioned between the legs in order to gain the best access/range of motion for pelvic surgery. Maintaining the legs in moderately flexed position permits more flexibility and range of motion for robotic/laparoscopic instruments. The arms are tucked at the patient's side and the patient should be secured to the bed adequately to enable severe tilting of the bed into steep Trendelenburg position in order to gain access to the pelvis. In addition to placing security straps across the chest, it is important to consider padded support to the shoulders to prevent the patient from sliding when the bed is tilted.

### Trocar Placement

With the patient anesthetized and adequately positioned, the trocars are placed. A 12-mm camera port is typically placed above the umbilicus to maintain an adequate distance from the surgical target (10–20 cm). It is critical to perform a thorough laparoscopic exploration to assess the peritoneal surfaces and the liver as well as the ovaries for evidence of distant spread of disease. The remaining trocars are then placed in a slightly downward curving horizontal line from the supraumbilical port. The set-up uses three robotic ports: arm 1 on the patient's right mid abdomen and arms 2 and 3 on the left abdomen side of the patient. It is important to maintain a distance of 8–10 cm between robotic arm trocars to enable the greatest range of motion for the robotic instruments, while minimizing collision. Arm 2 port may sometimes be placed at the site marked for the colostomy, however if the port is placed too low, it will not be possible to perform the IMA dissection. This approach also keeps the outer trocars from encroaching on the pelvis, maintaining greater access for those trocars to the sidewalls of the pelvis. Finally, an additional 5-mm assistant port is placed in the right upper quadrant and 12-mm utility port is placed in the right lateral abdomen.

The patient is then placed in steep Trendelenburg position, slightly tilted with the left side up to facilitate exposure of the retroperitoneum. The omentum and transverse colon are reflected cephalad and placed over the liver and stomach to facilitate retraction of the small bowel towards the right upper quadrant to expose the retroperitoneum. The robot is then docked between the legs (Fig. 25.1). The instruments for the surgical robot are then introduced under direct visualization. Our preferred instruments include the curved monopolar scissors for arm 1, the Maryland or fenestrated bipolar instrument for arm 2 and the Prograsp (Intuitive) instrument for arm 3. Arm 1 is also used for the robotic clip applier or energy device. The utility port can provide access for a stapler, clip applier, or additional retraction as needed.

## Inferior Mesenteric Artery Dissection

With the robot docked the operation is performed using a zero-degree camera. The lymphovascular dissection is performed at the base of the IMA. Including this nodal tissue up to at least the origin of the superior rectal artery with the specimen is crucial to a successful oncologic resection. Identification of the IMA begins by using arm 3 to help retract the sigmoid colon or sigmoid mesentery anteriorly and laterally toward the pelvic sidewall to tent up the base of the mesentery. Given the lack of tactile feedback with minimally invasive instruments, it is important to avoid grasping the viscera, which can result in a crush injury. Rather the retraction can be done by sweeping the colon, or if grasping is required this should be limited to the peritoneum or the epiploicae. Identification of the IMA is facilitated by incising the peritoneum along the medial aspect of the rectosigmoid mesentery to expose the areolar retrovascular plane that can be followed cephalad to the origin of the IMA.

Once the retroperitoneum is incised, the superior rectal vessels can be elevated and the dissection to elevate the mesocolon from the retroperitoneum in a medial-to-lateral fashion continues. The ureter and gonadal vessels should be visualized below the plane of dissection and the use of cautery should be judicious until the ureter is clearly visualized to avoid injury. Once the plane has been established, it can be carried cephalad to visualize the base of the IMA. This step is crucial to the oncologic quality of the resection and is important because it is also a point of potential nerve injury. The sympathetic nerves innervating the pelvis form a plexus along the aorta at the IMA and are at risk for injury during the IMA dissection. Elevating the lymphatic tissue surrounding the base of the IMA up towards the surgical specimen rather than dissecting down toward the retroperitoneum will help delineate the anatomy and ensure complete lymphadenectomy. A window can then be created on the superior aspect of the IMA allowing space to divide the vessel with a stapling device, vessel sealing device, or clips (Fig. 25.2).

One alternative to the IMA dissection described above is to divide the superior hemorrhoidal artery and vein just distal to the origin of the ascending left colic artery. The lymphatic tissue along the IMA out to the left colic branches can easily be mobilized onto the specimen to

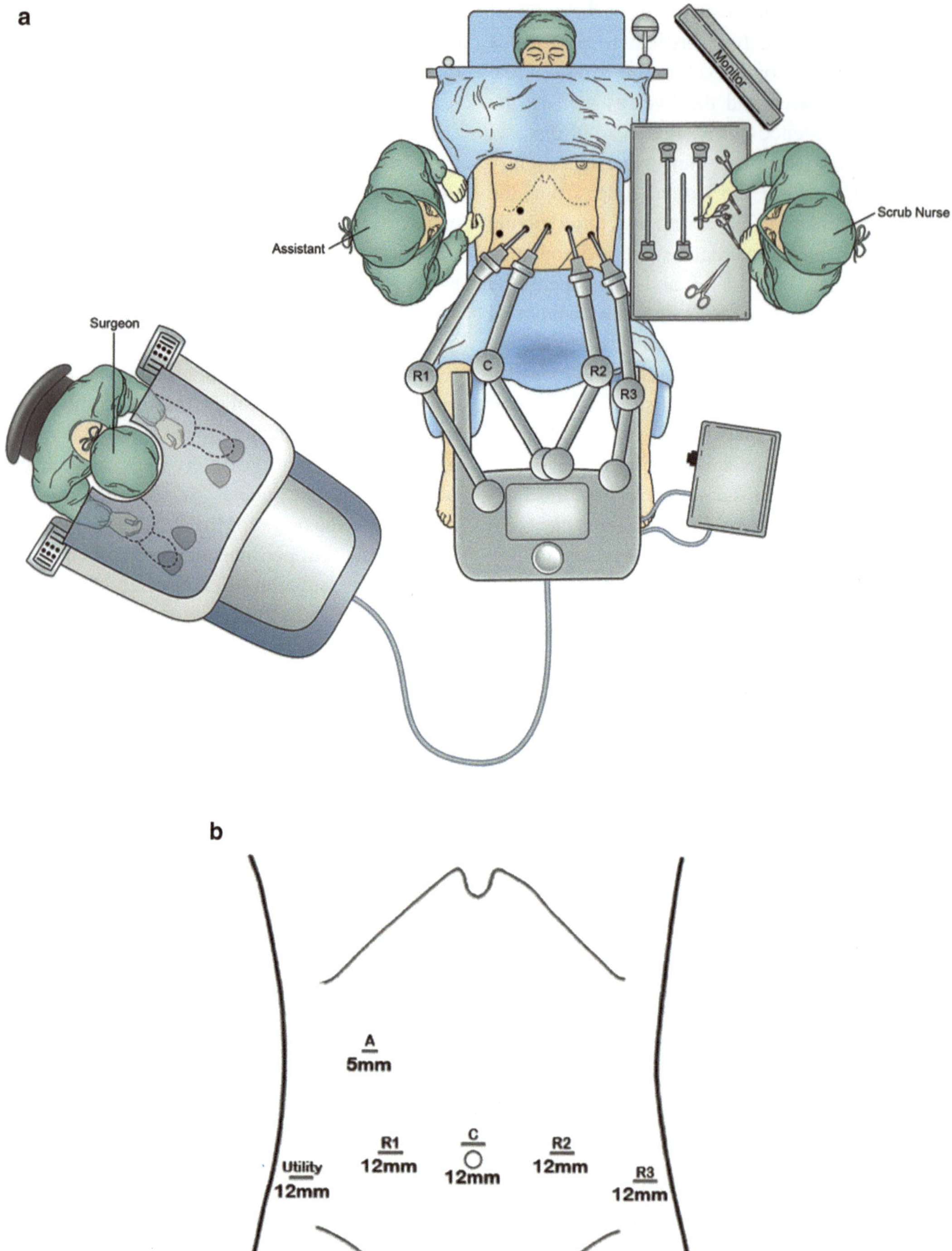


**Fig. 25.1** (**a**) Operative positioning of the patient in modified lithotomy position. The robot is docked between the legs. (**b**) The placement of trocars is depicted for robotic abdominoperineal resection. Maintaining the lateral trocars in a slightly downward curve across the abdomen permits greater access to the pelvis for distal dissection. The spacing between robotic ports is critical to avoid collision between robotic arms

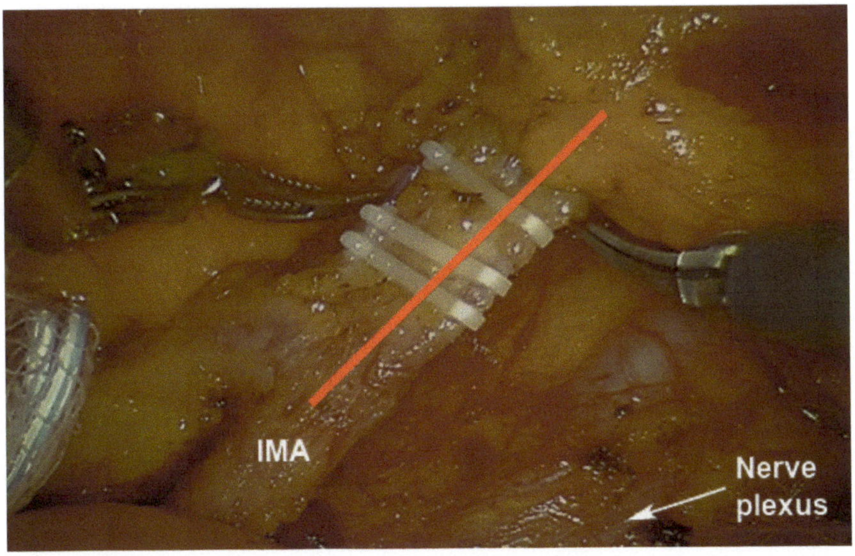


**Fig. 25.2** During dissection of the inferior mesenteric artery (*red line*), identifying the correct plane between the mesocolon and the retroperitoneum can help avoid injury to the hypogastric nerve plexus (*white arrow*). Clips have been placed across the inferior mesenteric artery prior to dividing the vessel

clearly delineate the anatomy. The vessels can then be ligated distal to the take-off of the left colic artery, providing additional blood supply to the colon via the IMA. This approach has been associated with a lower rate of anastomotic complications among patients undergoing low anterior resection (LAR) but may be less critical during APR [23]. However, in order to use this technique, one must first ensure that an adequate lymphadenectomy has been performed. This technique can be very useful in patients who may have issues with peripheral colonic perfusion through the usual collateral vessels.

## Completing the Mesocolic Dissection

The dissection of the mesocolon from the retroperitoneum is then continued laterally as far as possible. By completing this dissection and the vascular isolation, the plane naturally continues down to the areolar tissue between the mesorectum and the presacral fascia (Fig. 25.3). Accessing this plane is critical to preserve the autonomic nerve function, avoid excessive bleeding, and complete an oncologic TME. The lateral mobilization of the sigmoid and descending colon is then performed by gently retracting the sigmoid colon away from the retroperitoneum and incising Toldt's fascia to meet the medial retromesocolic dissection plane. Injury to the ureter or gonadal vein or inadvertent mobilization of the perinephric fat are potential pitfalls during this step which may be avoided by careful attention to the plane of dissection.

## Pelvic Dissection

The circumferential pelvic dissection is then performed. Effective retraction of the rectum is a critical during this step. The instrument in arm 2 is used to retract the mesorectum anteriorly and laterally exposing the presacral areolar mesorectal fascial plane (Fig. 25.4). It is helpful to control the rectum by wrapping the rectosigmoid with either a gauze sponge or umbilical tape. The knot is then grasped with a locking grasper by the surgical assistant through the right upper quadrant accessory port. This enables the assistant to generate traction to pull the rectum out of the pelvis and aids in the manipulation for continued

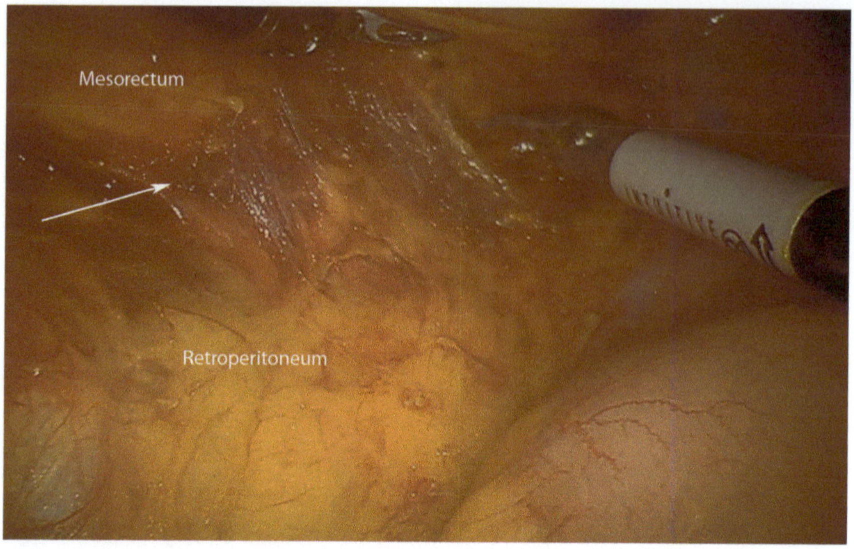


**Fig. 25.3** As the dissection into the retroperitoneum begins, the proper plane (*marked with arrow*) is the areolar tissue between the mesorectum and the retroperitoneum. Once the peritoneum is incised the pneumoperitoneum helps to dissect along the areolar tissues

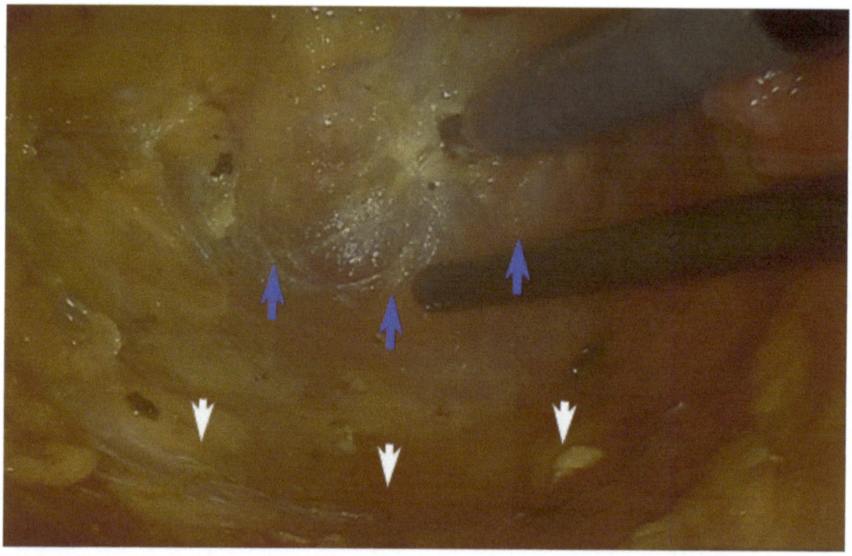

**Fig. 25.4** Posterior dissection is performed between the fascia propria of the mesorectum and the presacral fascia (*white arrows*) along the avascular plane (*blue arrows*)

circumferential rectal dissection. The posterior and right lateral dissection is first performed using sharp electrocautery in a posterior-to-anterior manner similar to open TME. The rectum can then be retracted towards the right to complete the dissection along the left side to the level of the pelvic floor. Care should be taken to avoid inadvertent cautery injury to the pelvic parasympathetic nerve fibers along the internal iliac artery branches. A grasper through arm 3 is now brought

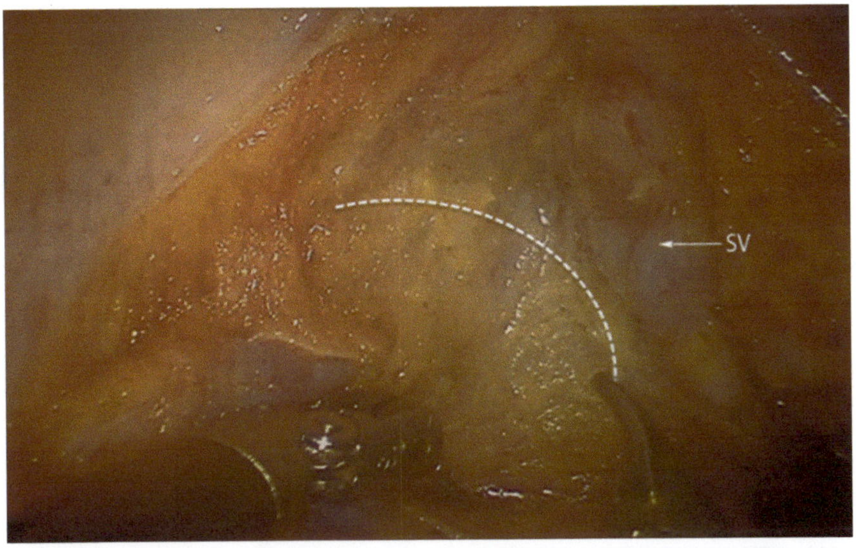


**Fig. 25.5** The plane of dissection with the right seminal vesicle (SV) in view. Staying within the appropriate plane (*dashed line*) minimizes bleeding and damage to the nervi erigentes in the lateral most aspect of the dissection

into the pelvis to provide anterior counter-retraction of the base of the bladder, seminal vesicles, and prostate while arm 2 is used to retract the distal rectum towards the sacrum to expose Denonvillier's fascia. The plane of dissection may be taken either anterior or posterior to Denonvillier's depending on the location of the tumor; however the nervi erigentes course along the anterolateral aspect of this layer and are at risk for injury during this step (Fig. 25.5).

## Mobilization of Distal Mesorectum

Now that the rectum has been mobilized to the pelvic floor, the levator ani muscles can be incised laterally before the distal mesorectum is mobilized to maintain a wide margin. It is important not to follow the TME plane along the pelvic floor, as this will risk a positive margin. Rather the levator ani should be incised widely away from the area of the tumor to expose the underlying ischiorectal fossa fat that marks the end of this phase of the dissection (Fig. 25.6a). Anteriorly the dissection can be taken to the level of the prostatic apex anal sphincter complex; and posteriorly the sacrococcygeal ligament can be divided with en bloc coccygectomy when indicated. At the completion of the abdominal portion of the procedure, the last step is to divide the mesocolon to the proximal sigmoid colon. Finally, the colon is divided with a linear stapler.

## Perineal Dissection

The perineal excision is then performed in the typical fashion by making an elliptical incision around the anus from the mid-perineal body anteriorly to a distance approximately halfway between the coccyx and the anus posteriorly. Laterally, the skin is incised to access the ischiorectal fat. With the levators incised during the abdominal approach, the pelvis is entered laterally (generally on the opposite side of the tumor) and the posterior dissection is then performed either anterior to the coccyx by dividing the anococcygeal ligament or en bloc with the coccyx after mobilizing the posterior attachments. The anterior dissection is performed last and is facilitated by dividing the anterior fibers of the levator ani to expose the posterior aspect of the prostate gland along its sides. Here, the prostate gland itself can be inadvertently mobilized placing the neurovascular bundles at

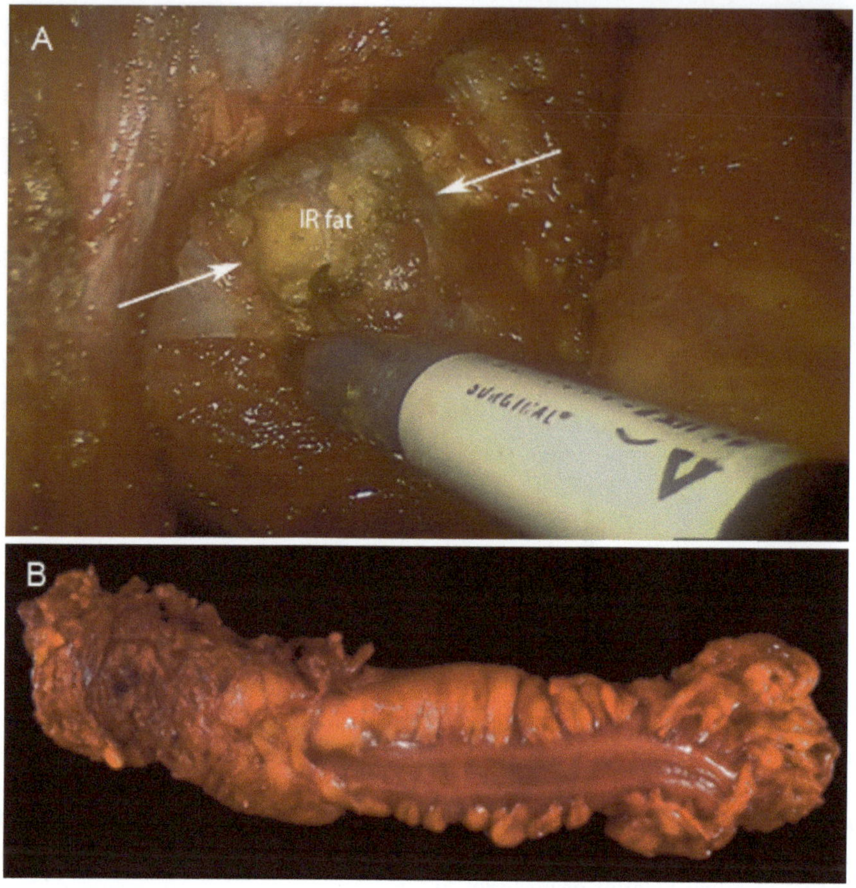


**Fig. 25.6** (**a**) Intraoperative photo showing the transabdominal division of the levator ani (*white arrows*) to expose the ischiorectal (IR) fat. (**b**) Photograph of the operative specimen showing a cylindrical resection of the pelvic floor

risk for injury. While this dissection may also be performed in the prone position, by dividing the levator ani widely during the transabdominal approach, a cylindrical excision can be achieved minimizing the risk for a positive radial margin (Fig. 25.6b). The specimen is then extracted through the perineal wound.

The abdomen and perineal wound are copiously irrigated and hemostasis is achieved. Whenever possible, the pelvic defect should be filled with vascularized soft tissue to reduce the potential for severe complications from a pelvic abscess or perineal hernia. In a narrow pelvis, employing a pedicled omental flap is an excellent option. However, if the skin resection was large, vascularized soft tissue flaps such as gluteus or rectus muscle flaps may be utilized even with a minimally invasive approach. Given the empty space that is created, a closed suction drain serves to prevent fluid accumulation and aid in wound healing. The pelvic drain can be brought out through one of the trocar access sites and should remain in place postoperatively until the output has diminished or the perineal wound has sufficiently healed to avoid breakdown due to fluid accumulation.

## Colostomy Creation

To complete the procedure, the colostomy site is prepared by excising a disc of skin and dissecting down to the rectus fascia. The anterior fascia is incised and the rectus muscle fibers are separated bluntly. The posterior sheath is then incised gaining access to the peritoneum. It can be helpful to incise the posterior sheath under laparoscopic vision to facilitate creation of the ostomy site defect. The proximal colon can then be delivered through the ostomy site and matured. Proper siting of the colostomy is critical since it will be permanent and adequate pouching of the stoma is a very important part of patient satisfaction and quality of life. Patients should be marked preoperatively by an enterostomal therapist; and if appropriate, one of the robotic port sites can be placed at the colostomy site.

## Postoperative Management

The postoperative management of patients following minimally invasive procedures requires the same diligence and attention to detail that are hallmarks of patient care following traditional open operations. While there is no strict dogma that governs postoperative care, there are a few important management principles that are important following all major abdominal operations. Some of the key components for patients following robotic APR include fluid management, diet, mobilization, ostomy management, and venous thromboembolism prophylaxis.

Fluid management following surgical procedures has evolved. The implementation and research into enhanced recovery after surgery has demonstrated that excessive fluid can result in prolonged hospital stay and delayed return of bowel function. It is thus important to communicate with the anesthesia team to optimize fluid management intraoperatively and this strategy is carried through the postoperative period. The type of fluids is also important and should be a balanced electrolyte solution, as opposed to isotonic saline [24]. The minimization of narcotic usage is facilitated by the minimally invasive approach.

Following robotic APR, early feeding may be initiated; typically liquids on postoperative day #1 and advancement as tolerated [24]. Like many perioperative management principles, dietary intake should be individualized based on the patient's clinical progress. In our practice oral gastric tubes are used intraoperatively to decompress the stomach and increase the working space for robotic surgery and removed at the conclusion of the procedure.

Early mobilization is another essential part of postoperative care for patients undergoing robotic APR. Akin to other major abdominal surgeries, encouraging and enabling patients to ambulate is a major factor in accelerating the recovery from surgery and minimizing complications. Even if rotational flaps are used to assist with perineal wound closure, it is critical to begin ambulating early in the postoperative course. This will enhance recovery and increase mobility providing some protection against venous thromboembolism. In addition to ambulation, the use of pharmacologic venous thromboembolic prophylaxis with or without mechanical prophylaxis should be included.

Lastly, it is important to institute education regarding proper ostomy care following the operation. Education regarding ostomy management should be initiated early in the preoperative evaluation, once the need for colostomy has been determined. Following surgery, ostomy care teaching should begin immediately as the patient may be ready for discharge as early as 2–3 days following surgery.

## Complications and Management

Robotic APR, while minimally invasive, remains a complex operation with significant risks that should be reviewed with all patients during informed consent. Complications that are relevant to any abdominal operation, such as pneumonia, myocardial infarction, postoperative bowel obstruction, or venous thromboembolism, are not reviewed here. However, there are complications that are specific to complex pelvic surgery whether done open or through a minimally invasive approach. These morbidities can be categorized as wound complications and neurogenic complications.

Despite smaller abdominal incisions, wound complications remain a common problem following robotic APR. Wound problems can range from superficial surgical site infections to wound dehiscence to hernia formation, including the rare port-site hernia. Most frequently, the perineal wound is the culprit for wound related issues. Routine wound infections should be managed with incision and drainage and antibiotics for patients with evidence for cellulitis. Perineal wound complications are not uncommon with reported incidence rates of 25–46 % [25–28]. Early drainage and debridement are keys to successful management.

In addition to superficial surgical site infections, deep space infections are also a concern occurring in up to 35 % of patients [28]. Given the large space created in the pelvis, it is easy and common to accumulate fluid that can then become secondarily infected. This is the reason to use closed suction drains in the pelvis. In the event of a deep space infection, percutaneous drainage remains the standard of care with or without the addition of antibiotics. However, the abscess cavity may be difficult to collapse and early operative intervention should be considered if percutaneous drainage does not resolve the abscess. Moreover, perineal wound dehiscence also occurs frequently (>30 % of patients with primary closure). Negative pressure wound therapy can be highly effective in appropriately selected patients either as definitive treatment or in preparation for flap reconstruction.

While various potential wound complications make up the majority of morbidity risk, other potential complications are unique to rectal cancer pathology, specifically damage to the nerves supplying the genitourinary organs. As outlined above, the critical nerves at risk include the sympathetic nerves (controlling ejaculation) and the pelvic plexus or nervi erigentes (controlling erectile function in males and sexual function in women). The common pitfalls during robotic APR that can result in nerve damage include excessive use of cautery during dissection of the IMA, dissection with cautery anterior to Denonvillier's fascia, and excessive use of cautery in the anterolateral dissection.

The collective incidence of sexual dysfunction in patients treated for rectal cancer varies widely from 10–70 % [29, 30]. Fortunately, it is not always a permanent injury and recovery of sexual function can occur. Studies have reported that over a period of 6–12 months, 60–85 % of male patients can obtain erections either spontaneously or with pharmacologic therapy, specifically, sildenafil [31, 29, 30]. Unfortunately, these complications are not well studied in females.

In addition to sexual dysfunction, patients are also at risk for bladder dysfunction. Urinary dysfunction has been reported to occur in up to 50 % of patients undergoing APR [32]. In the era of enhanced recovery after surgery and minimally invasive surgery, patients are being discharged from the hospital earlier. This requires early removal of the Foley catheter. In this situation understanding the risk of urinary retention is important and postvoid residual volumes should be examined after discontinuing the foley to ensure that the patient is completely emptying their bladder. Generally, recovery of bladder function can be anticipated although it may take up to a year [32, 29].

Last, patient positioning during these operations (low lithotomy) places patients at risk for common peroneal nerve palsy. This injury is rare, occurring in less than 0.5 % of patients in the lithotomy position, but can arise from pressure on the nerve while the patient is in stirrups or as a result of the rare development of compartment syndrome [33]. These complications are easily identified by a physical exam following the surgery but are preventable with attention to positioning and avoiding leaning on the legs during surgery. Compression injury to the common peroneal nerve results in foot drop. Treatment includes physical therapy and strengthening exercises as well as education regarding close observation of the foot for traumatic injuries in cases of decreased sensation. A full recovery can generally be anticipated.

## References


1. Park IJ, You YN, Schlette E, Nguyen S, Skibber JM, Rodriguez-Bigas MA, et al. Reverse-hybrid robotic mesorectal excision for rectal cancer. Dis Colon Rectum. 2012;55(2):228–33. doi:10.1097/DCR.0b013e31823c0bd2.
2. Lange MM, Rutten HJ, van de Velde CJ. One hundred years of curative surgery for rectal cancer: 1908–2008. Eur J Surg Oncol. 2009;35(5):456–63. doi:10.1016/j.ejso.2008.09.012.
3. Kapiteijn E, Marijnen CA, Nagtegaal ID, Putter H, Steup WH, Wiggers T, et al. Preoperative radiotherapy combined with total mesorectal excision for resectable rectal cancer. N Engl J Med. 2001; 345(9):638–46. doi:10.1056/NEJMoa010580.
4. Adam IJ, Mohamdee MO, Martin IG, Scott N, Finan PJ, Johnston D, et al. Role of circumferential margin involvement in the local recurrence of rectal cancer. Lancet. 1994;344(8924):707–11.
5. Nagtegaal ID, van de Velde CJ, Marijnen CA, van Krieken JH, Quirke P, Dutch Colorectal Cancer Group. Low rectal cancer: a call for a change of approach in abdominoperineal resection. J Clin Oncol. 2005; 23(36):9257–64. doi:10.1200/JCO.2005.02.9231.
6. van der Pas MH, Haglind E, Cuesta MA, Furst A, Lacy AM, Hop WC, et al. Laparoscopic versus open surgery for rectal cancer (COLOR II): short-term outcomes of a randomised, phase 3 trial. Lancet Oncol. 2013;14(3):210–8. doi:10.1016/S1470-2045(13)70016-0.
7. Silberfein EJ, Kattepogu KM, Hu CY, Skibber JM, Rodriguez-Bigas MA, Feig B, et al. Long-term survival and recurrence outcomes following surgery for distal rectal cancer. Ann Surg Oncol. 2010;17(11):2863–9. doi:10.1245/s10434-010-1119-8.
8. Bujko K, Rutkowski A, Chang GJ, Michalski W, Chmielik E, Kusnierz J. Is the 1-cm rule of distal bowel resection margin in rectal cancer based on clinical evidence? A systematic review. Ann Surg Oncol. 2012;19(3):801–8. doi:10.1245/s10434-011-2035-2.
9. Kim TG, Park W, Choi DH, Kim SH, Kim HC, Lee WY, et al. The adequacy of the distal resection margin after preoperative chemoradiotherapy for rectal cancer. Colorectal Dis. 2014;16(8):O257–63. doi:10.1111/codi.12554.
10. Rutkowski A, Nowacki MP, Chwalinski M, Oledzki J, Bednarczyk M, Liszka-Dalecki P, et al. Acceptance of a 5-mm distal bowel resection margin for rectal cancer: is it safe? Colorectal Dis. 2012;14(1):71–8. doi:10.1111/j.1463-1318.2010.02542.x.
11. Eng C, Chang GJ, You YN, Das P, Xing Y, Delclos M, et al. Long-term results of weekly/daily cisplatin-based chemoradiation for locally advanced squamous cell carcinoma of the anal canal. Cancer. 2013; 119(21):3769–75. doi:10.1002/cncr.28296.
12. Flam M, John M, Pajak TF, Petrelli N, Myerson R, Doggett S, et al. Role of mitomycin in combination with fluorouracil and radiotherapy, and of salvage chemoradiation in the definitive nonsurgical treatment of epidermoid carcinoma of the anal canal: results of a phase III randomized intergroup study. J Clin Oncol. 1996;14(9):2527–39.
13. Mullen JT, Rodriguez-Bigas MA, Chang GJ, Barcenas CH, Crane CH, Skibber JM, et al. Results of surgical salvage after failed chemoradiation therapy for epidermoid carcinoma of the anal canal. Ann Surg Oncol. 2007;14(2):478–83. doi:10.1245/s10434-006-9221-7.
14. Bretagnol F, Dedieu A, Zappa M, Guedj N, Ferron M, Panis Y. T4 colorectal cancer: is laparoscopic resection contraindicated? Colorectal Dis. 2011;13(2):138–43. doi:10.1111/j.1463-1318.2010.02380.x.
15. Marks JH, Kawun UB, Hamdan W, Marks G. Redefining contraindications to laparoscopic colorectal resection for high-risk patients. Surg Endosc. 2008;22(8):1899–904. doi:10.1007/s00464-008-9828-9.
16. Samdani T, Garcia-Aguilar J. Imaging in rectal cancer: magnetic resonance imaging versus endorectal ultrasonography. Surg Oncol Clin N Am. 2014;23(1):59–77. doi:10.1016/j.soc.2013.09.011.
17. Torkzad MR, Kamel I, Halappa VG, Beets-Tan RG. Magnetic resonance imaging of rectal and anal cancer. Magn Reson Imaging Clin N Am. 2014; 22(1):85–112. doi:10.1016/j.mric.2013.07.007.
18. van't Sant HP, Weidema WF, Hop WC, Lange JF, Contant CM. Evaluation of morbidity and mortality after anastomotic leakage following elective colorectal surgery in patients treated with or without mechanical bowel preparation. Am J Surg. 2011;202(3):321–4. doi:10.1016/j.amjsurg.2010.10.018.
19. Slieker JC, van't Sant HP, Vlot J, Daams F, Jansen FW, Lange JF. Bowel preparation prior to laparoscopic colorectal resection: what is the current practice? J Laparoendosc Adv Surg Tech A. 2011;21(10):899–903. doi:10.1089/lap.2011.0064.
20. Zmora O, Lebedyev A, Hoffman A, Khaikin M, Munz Y, Shabtai M, et al. Laparoscopic colectomy without mechanical bowel preparation. Int J Colorectal Dis. 2006;21(7):683–7. doi:10.1007/s00384-005-0044-y.
21. Douketis JD, Spyropoulos AC, Spencer FA, Mayr M, Jaffer AK, Eckman MH, et al. Perioperative management of antithrombotic therapy: Antithrombotic Therapy and Prevention of Thrombosis, 9th ed: American College of Chest Physicians Evidence-Based Clinical Practice Guidelines. Chest. 2012;141(2 Suppl):e326S–50. doi:10.1378/chest.11-2298.
22. Stulberg JJ, Delaney CP, Neuhauser DV, Aron DC, Fu P, Koroukian SM. Adherence to surgical care improvement project measures and the association with postoperative infections. JAMA. 2010;303(24):2479–85. doi:10.1001/jama.2010.841.
23. Fegiz G, Tonelli F, Rossi P, Di Paola M, De Masi E, Simonetti G. Preservation of the superior hemorrhoidal artery in resection of the colon and rectum. Surg Gynecol Obstet. 1976;143(6):919–25.
24. Lassen K, Soop M, Nygren J, Cox PB, Hendry PO, Spies C, et al. Consensus review of optimal perioperative care

in colorectal surgery: Enhanced Recovery After Surgery (ERAS) Group recommendations. Arch Surg. 2009;144(10):961–9. doi:10.1001/archsurg.2009.170.
25. Hawkins AT, Berger DL, Shellito PC, Sylla P, Bordeianou L. Wound dehiscence after abdominoperineal resection for low rectal cancer is associated with decreased survival. Dis Colon Rectum. 2014;57(2): 143–50. doi:10.1097/DCR.0000000000000027.
26. Welsch T, Mategakis V, Contin P, Kulu Y, Buchler MW, Ulrich A. Results of extralevator abdominoperineal resection for low rectal cancer including quality of life and long-term wound complications. Int J Colorectal Dis. 2013;28(4):503–10. doi:10.1007/s00384-012-1611-7.
27. West NP, Anderin C, Smith KJ, Holm T, Quirke P, European Extralevator Abdominoperineal Excision Study Group. Multicentre experience with extralevator abdominoperineal excision for low rectal cancer. Br J Surg. 2010;97(4):588–99. doi:10.1002/bjs.6916.
28. Butler CE, Gundeslioglu AO, Rodriguez-Bigas MA. Outcomes of immediate vertical rectus abdominis myocutaneous flap reconstruction for irradiated abdominoperineal resection defects. J Am Coll Surg. 2008;206(4):694–703. doi:10.1016/j.jamcollsurg.2007.12.007.
29. Lange MM, van de Velde CJ. Urinary and sexual dysfunction after rectal cancer treatment. Nat Rev Urol. 2011;8(1):51–7. doi:10.1038/nrurol.2010.206.
30. Sartori CA, Sartori A, Vigna S, Occhipinti R, Baiocchi GL. Urinary and sexual disorders after laparoscopic TME for rectal cancer in males. J Gastrointest Surg. 2011;15(4):637–43. doi:10.1007/s11605-011-1459-0.
31. Kim JY, Kim NK, Lee KY, Hur H, Min BS, Kim JH. A comparative study of voiding and sexual function after total mesorectal excision with autonomic nerve preservation for rectal cancer: laparoscopic versus robotic surgery. Ann Surg Oncol. 2012;19(8):2485–93. doi:10.1245/s10434-012-2262-1.
32. Delacroix Jr SE, Winters JC. Voiding dysfunction after pelvic colorectal surgery. Clin Colon Rectal Surg. 2010;23(2):119–27. doi:10.1055/s-0030-1254299.
33. Warner MA, Warner DO, Harper CM, Schroeder DR, Maxson PM. Lower extremity neuropathies associated with lithotomy positions. Anesthesiology. 2000;93(4):938–42.

## Key Operative Steps

1. The patient is placed in low lithotomy position with the robot docked between the legs.
2. Trocars are placed for robotic abdominoperineal resection.
3. Lymphovascular dissection and high vascular ligation of the inferior mesenteric artery is performed.
4. Lateral mobilization of the descending and sigmoid colon joins the medial retromesocolic dissection plane.
5. Total mesorectal excision is performed.
6. Transabdominal incision of the levator ani muscles.
7. Perineal resection and specimen extraction.
8. Maturation of end colostomy.

# Open Technique for Transanal Resection

# 26

Vitaliy Poylin and James Yoo

## Introduction

Tumors in the lower third of the rectum present unique challenges for the surgeon. Local excision has long been a technique used as an alternative to radical surgery for these low rectal polyps and tumors. Radical resection in this location often requires a low rectal or colo-anal anastomosis or even an abdominoperineal excision, procedures that carry significant morbidity and mortality. For that reason, local excision has always been an appealing alternative with lower morbidity and preservation of function. However, improved functional outcomes have to be balanced with proper oncologic outcomes.

## Historical Perspective

Local excision of rectal lesions has been performed since the 1800s as an alternative to radical resection. The posterior approaches, the paracoccygeal approach described by Kraske [1, 2] or the transsphincteric approach introduced by York-Mason [3], probably provide a better exposure of the distal rectum, compared to the conventional or transanal approach. However, they are associated with higher morbidity, such as fistula with the Kraske [4, 5], compared to the open transanal approach popularized by Parks. Therefore, open transanal resection remains a viable option for the local treatment of low to mid-rectal tumors.

Historically, transanal resection of tumors was used for all lower rectal masses amenable to this approach. This often included tumors that were located more proximal in the rectum by utilizing sutures to bring the tumor into view. However, the advent of Transanal Endoscopic Microsurgery (TEM) and Transanal Minimally Invasive Surgery (TAMIS) have provided an easier way to reach almost anywhere in the rectum with both good visualization and a better ability to achieve negative margins and closure. These techniques are described elsewhere.

## Indications

A number of options are available today to deal with low rectal tumors. There should be a thoughtful preoperative discussion with the patient about the advantages and disadvantages of a local approach vs. radical surgery, both from functional and oncologic standpoints. In addition,

V. Poylin, M.D.
Division of Colon and Rectal Surgery, Beth Israel Deaconess Medical Center, Boston, MA, USA

Harvard Medical School, Boston, MA, USA

J. Yoo, M.D. (✉)
Division of Colon and Rectal Surgery, Department of Surgery, Tufts Medical Center, Tufts University School of Medicine, 800 Washington St, Box 6190, Boston, MA 02111, USA
e-mail: jyoo@tuftsmedicalcenter.org

J. Kim and J. Garcia-Aguilar (eds.), *Surgery for Cancers of the Gastrointestinal Tract: A Step-by-Step Approach*, DOI 10.1007/978-1-4939-1893-5_26, © Springer Science+Business Media New York 2015

a variety of transanal approaches (open technique, TEM, or TAMIS) are currently available to the surgeon. The choice of transanal approach depends on a careful assessment of the patient, the location of the lesion, and the skill set and expertise of the operating surgeon.

Before deciding on a local excision, the tumor must be appropriately staged, including a digital rectal exam to determine its location in the rectum, mobility, and relationship to the sphincter. As with any colorectal cancer, a full colonoscopy with biopsy of the tumor is mandatory. Lesions that penetrate beyond the submucosa or have aggressive histological features (i.e., poor differentiation, lymphovascular invasion, or major mucinous component) are generally not appropriate for transanal resection with curative intent [6, 7]. Imaging should include evaluation of the extent of local disease with magnetic resonance imaging (MRI) or endorectal ultrasound (ERUS) and distant disease with computed tomography (CT). Transanal excision rarely provides appropriate lymph node sampling and has been associated with a higher chance of recurrence [8, 9]; therefore adequate imaging to assess the depth of tumor invasion and the presence of nodal metastasis is essential in the decision-making process. Once an appropriate workup has been completed, the decision to proceed with transanal excision is based on the tumor location and features and patient-related factors.

Only tumors located in the lower rectum (i.e., 6–7 cm above dentate line or occasionally higher in select patients based on individual anatomy) can safely and reliably be removed using the open transanal approach. Ideally, tumors feasible for transanal excision should be movable. Tis and T1 tumors are generally considered appropriate for local excision since the risk of lymph node positivity in the absence of negative features is low [6, 10, 11]. Patients with adenomas are also good candidates for transanal excision. Traditionally, tumors less than 3–4 cm and less than 40 % of the circumference of the rectal lumen have been considered amenable to transanal resection. However, better staging and techniques make these criteria less important. The most important factor is the absence of negative histological features.

## Operative Considerations

### Preparation for Surgery

Prior to local excision, patients should receive a bowel preparation. Generally, full mechanical bowel preparation is not necessary. A Fleets enema to clear the distal colon and rectum is usually adequate. Diluted betadine solution can be used to further wash out the distal rectum prior to beginning the procedure. Immediately prior to incision, appropriate antibiotics covering both gram-negative and anaerobic bacteria should be administered. Most of the transanal excisions can be accomplished with combination of monitored anesthesia care and local anesthesia. However, the anticipated degree of difficulty, patient positioning, and patient characteristics (e.g., body habitus) may call for general anesthesia to be utilized.

### Positioning and Anatomic Considerations

After induction, patients should be placed in the prone-jackknife position with buttocks taped apart. For lesions located directly in the posterior midline, the high lithotomy position may provide better visualization of the tumor. In women, preparation should include the vagina in case there is an injury to the vaginal wall. With the exception of very distal and small tumors, a Foley catheter should be used to decompress the bladder and be removed at the end of the case.

There are a few anatomical considerations that make the transanal approach feasible as well as define the possible pitfalls. The ability to perform transanal resection relies on the ability to dilate/distend the anal sphincters. This generally can be accomplished by a combination of anesthesia (both local and systemic) and careful dilatation. Everting sutures can also be placed into the distal anal canal, providing better exposure by simultaneously widening the anal canal and shortening the distance between the distal rectal cancer and the operating surgeon (Fig. 26.1).

The rectum, especially its lowest part, is wider than most other parts of the colon and also has a

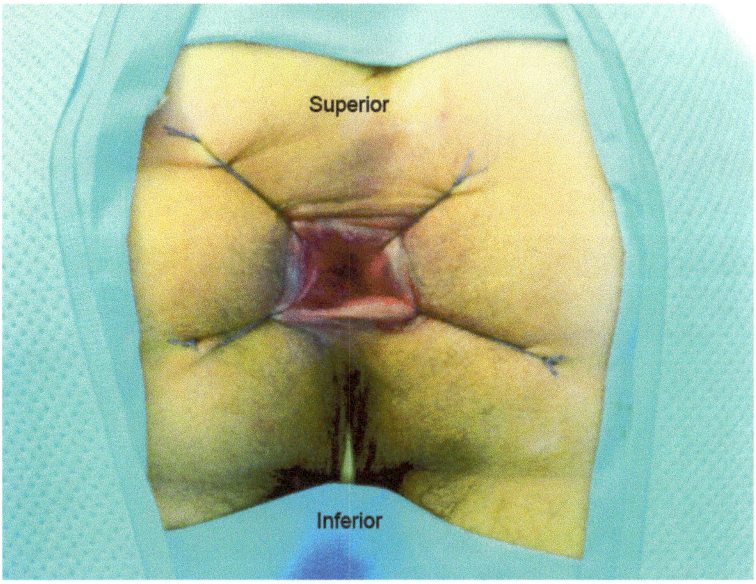


**Fig. 26.1** Everting sutures in the distal anal canal widen the anal canal and shorten the distance between surgeon and tumor

thicker wall. This allows for tumors to grow to a larger size without becoming symptomatic, but it also allows for the rectum to be stretched. That helps with visualization as well as closure at the end of the procedure. The rectum starts bending posteriorly a few centimeters above the dentate line. This anatomy may, in some situations, limit visualization and the ability to reach higher lesions. This can be partly overcome by placing the patient in lithotomy position, which is the preferred position for patients with posterior lesions.

In the anterior projection the lower rectum borders the prostate in men and the posterior vaginal wall in women. In addition, the anterior peritoneal reflection can be quite low, especially in thin older women. Entry into the peritoneal cavity should be avoided to limit the systemic inflammatory response. A prone-jackknife position (Fig. 26.2) would be more appropriate for anterior or laterally based lesions.

## Nerve Blocks and Retraction

Perianal and pudendal nerve blocks should be performed with a local anesthetic (e.g., combination of short-acting lidocaine and long-acting bupivicaine with epinephrine). This decreases bleeding during the procedure, helps to relax the sphincter complex, and provides good pain control after surgery. Since good visualization is the key to a successful transanal resection, a headlight or a lighted retractor is extremely important. For lower tumors, a variety of retractors may be used, e.g., Pratt-bivalve, Fansler, Sawyer, or Hill-Furguson retractor anal speculum. For deeper lesions, everting sutures, along with a LoneStar retractor, can be used to provide better exposure and to pull the anorectal junction distally.

## Examination and Marking

After a thorough exam to make sure that the mass is accessible by the transanal approach, the margins of resection should be marked. At least a 1-cm margin from the border of the tumor should be taken in all directions. Electrocautery can be used to mark the margin. Occasionally, traction sutures can be placed both distal and proximal to the tumor to pull a high tumor down within reach. These sutures will help control the proximal resection margin, which may retract after removal of the specimen. However, the presence of multiple sutures in a

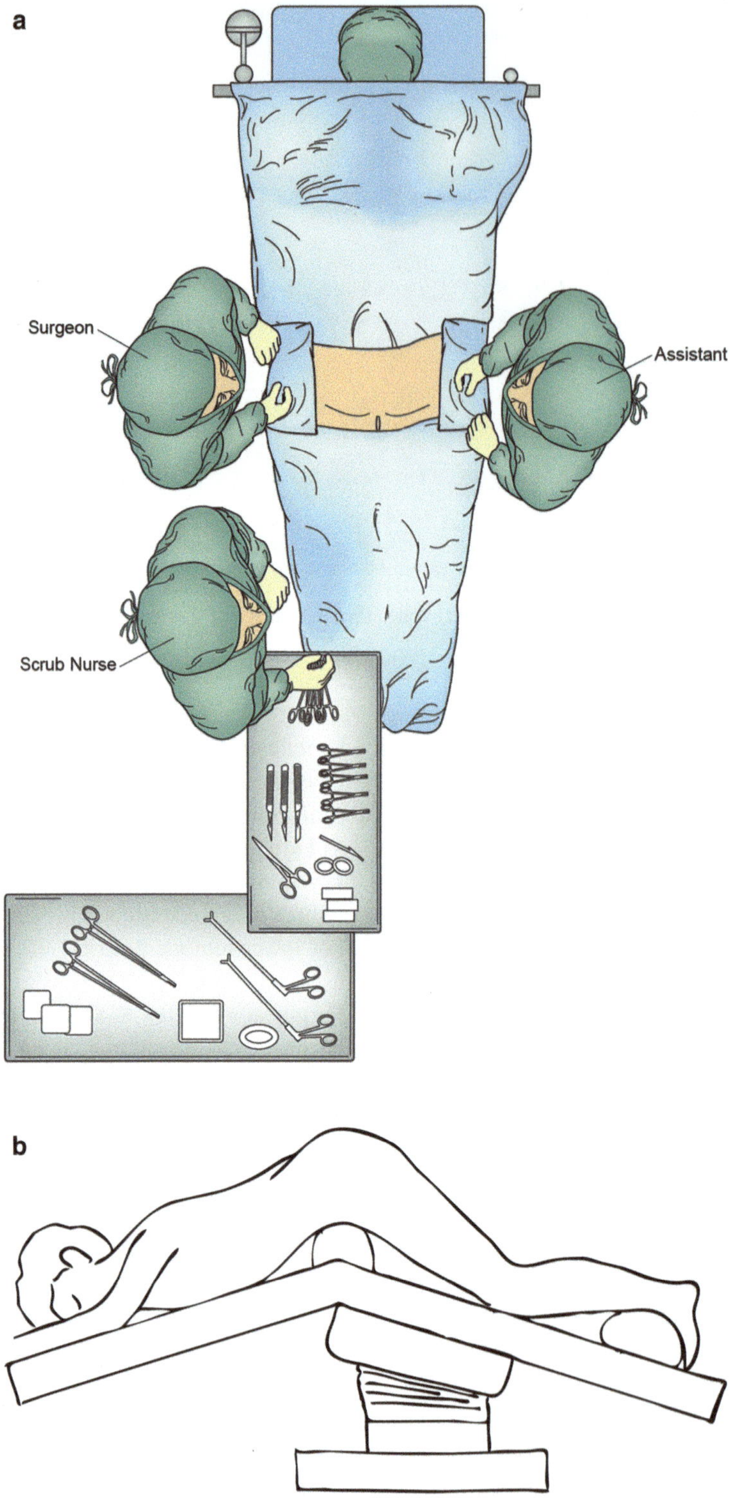


**Fig. 26.2** Patient positioning and operating room setup. The patient is placed in prone-jackknife position

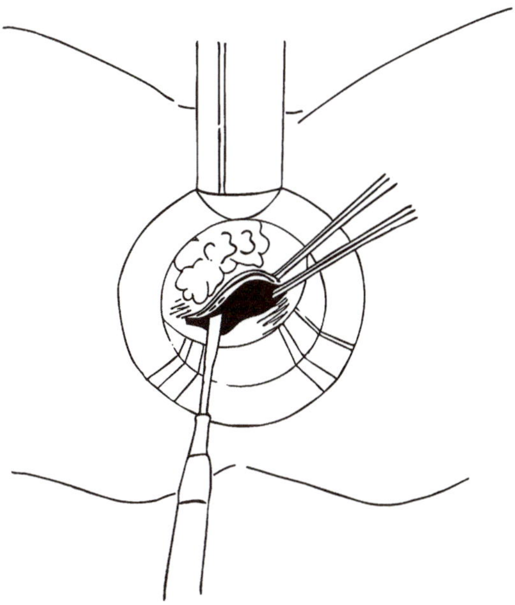

**Fig. 26.3** Operative diagram showing the resection of the specimen with electrocautery beginning at the distal margin

narrow operative field can be bothersome; an Allis clamp can also be used to pull down the rectal wall and grasp the specimen. An alternative approach for lesions in the mid-rectum involves making an elliptical incision distal to the lesion and then continuing the dissection behind the rectal wall as the proximal margin is approached.

## Resection of the Specimen

Electrocautery can be used to perform a full-thickness resection along the previously marked margin (Fig. 26.3). Special care should be taken not to grasp the tumor or damage its margin. The key to successful resection is slow, meticulous incision of the bowel wall and mesorectal tissue with proper control of the submucosal and mesorectal blood vessels. Upon completion, the perirectal fat should be visualized to confirm a complete full-thickness excision (Fig. 26.4).

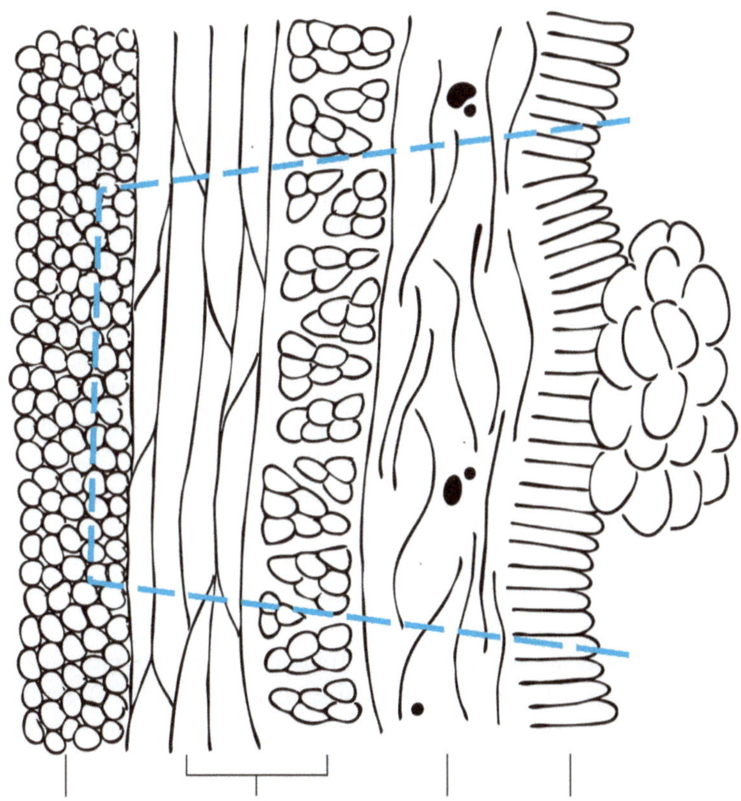


**Fig. 26.4** Diagram indicating the extent of a full-thickness resection of a rectal lesion

Once the specimen is removed, it should be carefully oriented on a pin board clearly marking its orientation (proximal, distal, left, and right). The use of pins also helps to keep the margins from shrinking during processing of the specimen. Since careful orientation of the specimen is critically important, pathologists should be called if possible to explain the specimen and its orientation. In our institution, all transanal excisions are processed with a "rectal cancer protocol," which includes inking the resection in quadrants (four colors) with deep and peripheral mucosal margins inked the same colors and then fixing the specimen prior to submitting it for histologic examination. Frozen section exam of the margins may also be considered.

## Closure of the Defect

Once the specimen is removed, the area is irrigated and hemostasis is ensured. The defect should be closed if possible. Although most transanal lesions will be below the peritoneal reflection and closure is not mandatory, the defect should be closed to decrease the rates of postoperative bleeding and expedite recovery. The defect should be closed transversely to prevent stricturing and obstruction. Absorbable sutures such as 2-0 and 3-0 vicryl should be used for this full-thickness closure. The wound can be closed in either a continuous running or interrupted fashion. Other absorbable sutures may be used.

## Postoperative Recovery

Most patients after transanal excision can be safely sent home from the recovery room, unless the excision was extensive, the peritoneal cavity was entered, or significant bleeding was encountered. We may observe patients with significant comorbidities. For procedures above the dentate line, there should be minimal pain, and we recommend multimodal pain regimen with acetaminophen, nonsteroidal antiinflammatory drugs, and a mild oral narcotic. A bowel regimen may be considered, starting with docusate sodium twice daily or metamucil powder daily, and expanding to milk of magnesia if the patient feels constipated after 36–48 h and to avoidance of significant straining after the procedure. It is often helpful to set expectations with patients by explaining that bloody and mucus discharge is common during the initial stages of healing.

## Potential Pitfalls and Complications

When resecting anterior tumors in both men and women, extra care should be taken at the deep margin to avoid injuring the prostate capsule or the urethra in men or the posterior wall of the vagina in women. In addition, the pouch of Douglas can be very deep, especially in older, thin females, and can be entered. If the peritoneum is entered, it is important to ensure that intraperitoneal organs are not injured and then close the defect with interrupted absorbable sutures. If indicated, patients can be observed in the hospital overnight.

Overall, the risk of complications after transanal excision is quite low. Urinary retention, urinary tract infection, bleeding, and infection of perirectal and ischiorectal spaces are potential complications. Occasionally, more significant infections (especially from posterior resections) can be encountered when an infection extends into retroperitoneal planes all the way to the thoracic cavity. As with all anorectal procedures, early warning signs for infection include urinary retention after initial normal urination, high fever, and increased pain after the first few days. These early signs are then followed by systemic symptoms and drainage. Patients should be advised to watch for the above symptoms and should be promptly evaluated if they arise.

## Conclusion

Transanal excision of rectal tumors is an alternative to radical surgery. Overall, worse oncologic outcomes need to be carefully balanced with better functional outcomes. Careful patient selection and thorough discussion and meticulous technique are the keys to better patient outcomes.

## References


1. Classic articles in colonic and rectal surgery. Paul Kraske 1851–1930. Extirpation of high carcinomas of the large bowel. Dis Colon Rectum. 1984;27(7):499–503.
2. Hargrove 3rd WC, Gertner MH, Fitts Jr WT. The Kraske operation for carcinoma of the rectum. Surg Gynecol Obstet. 1979;148(6):931–3.
3. Kilpatrick FR, Mason AY. Post-operative recto-prostatic fistula. Br J Urol. 1969;41(6):649–54.
4. Christiansen J. Excision of mid-rectal lesions by the Kraske sacral approach. Br J Surg. 1980;67(9):651–2.
5. Westbrook KC, Lang NP, Broadwater JR, Thompson BW. Posterior surgical approaches to the rectum. Ann Surg. 1982;195(6):677–85.
6. Beck DEASoC, Rectal S. The ASCRS textbook of colon and rectal surgery. New York: Springer; 2011.
7. Friel CM. Local excision of T1 rectal cancer: where are we now? Dis Colon Rectum. 2010;53(9):1231–3. doi:10.1007/DCR.0b013e3181e1a1ff.
8. Garcia-Aguilar J, Mellgren A, Sirivongs P, Buie D, Madoff RD, Rothenberger DA. Local excision of rectal cancer without adjuvant therapy: a word of caution. Ann Surg. 2000;231(3):345–51.
9. Mellgren A, Sirivongs P, Rothenberger DA, Madoff RD, Garcia-Aguilar J. Is local excision adequate therapy for early rectal cancer? Dis Colon Rectum. 2000;43(8):1064–71; discussion 71–4.
10. Nash GM, Weiser MR, Guillem JG, Temple LK, Shia J, Gonen M, et al. Long-term survival after transanal excision of T1 rectal cancer. Dis Colon Rectum. 2009;52(4):577–82. doi:10.1007/DCR.0b013e3181a0adbd.
11. Gopaul D, Belliveau P, Vuong T, Trudel J, Vasilevsky CA, Corns R, et al. Outcome of local excision of rectal carcinoma. Dis Colon Rectum. 2004;47(11):1780–8.


## Key Operative Steps

1. Bowel prep with Fleets enema.
2. Place patient in prone-jackknife position.
3. Perform perianal and pudendal nerve blocks.
4. Place retaining sutures, if necessary.
5. Insert retractor into anus. For deeper lesions, everting sutures may be used.
6. Mark 1-cm margins of resection around the tumor.
7. Perform full-thickness resection along the margins. Must visualize perirectal fat to confirm adequacy of resection.
8. Close the defect transversely using absorbable sutures.

# 27 Transanal Minimally Invasive Surgery for Rectal Cancer

Avo Artinyan

## Introduction

Surgery is the most critical component of the curative-intent treatment of rectal cancer, a fact that has been recognized for almost 200 years. The surgical treatment of rectal cancer has evolved significantly in that time, from Lisfranc's description of perineal rectal excision [1], to Miles' description of abdominoperineal resection (APR) in 1908 [2], and to Heald's description of total mesorectal excision (TME) in 1982 [3].

In recent years, there has been a growing focus on sphincter-preservation, functional outcomes, and quality of life after treatment for rectal cancer; and rates of APR have seen a measurable decrease [4]. Yet, early malignant and premalignant lesions of the rectum are still commonly treated with radical operations that compromise function and quality of life, in some instances without added oncologic benefit. It is within this context that organ-preserving approaches, such as local excision and watch-and-wait [5], have seen increasing popularity.

Electronic supplementary material: Supplementary material is available in the online version of this chapter at 10.1007/978-1-4939-1893-5_27. Videos can also be accessed at http://www.springerimages.com/videos/978-1-4939-1892-8.

A. Artinyan, M.D., M.S. (✉)
Division of Surgical Oncology, Department of Surgery, Baylor College of Medicine, 2002 Holcombe Blvd., Houston, TX 77030, USA
e-mail: artinyan@bcm.edu

Local excision for rectal adenoma and cancer is not a new concept. A.G. Parks and colleagues first described transanal excision (TAE) in the mid-1960s using the now ubiquitous Parks' anal retractor and standard open surgical instruments [6]. While relatively effective for lesions of the low rectum, TAE is significantly more difficult for lesions extending into the mid rectum and above. To overcome the difficulties of TAE for proximal lesions, Gerhard Buess and colleagues described transanal endoscopic microsurgery (TEM) in the early 1980s using a binocular operating proctoscope, gas insufflation, and specialized instruments that facilitate bimanual dissection and suture repair [7]. The technique of TEM has since been modified with the incorporation of modern endoscopic equipment, but still remains an important modality for the local excision of rectal adenomas and early rectal cancers.

Largely driven by the prohibitive cost of standard TEM instrumentation, a more recent modification has involved the use of disposable single-incision laparoscopic ports or dedicated transanal ports along with standard laparoscopic instrumentation. This technique, termed transanal minimally invasive surgery (TAMIS) [8], is the focus of this chapter. Although slightly varied in approach, TAMIS shares with TEM a number of common features including: (1) endoscopic visualization of the rectum, (2) gas/$CO_2$ insufflation, and (3) the use of laparoscopic and other specialized instrumentation for bimanual surgical dissection and suture repair.

J. Kim and J. Garcia-Aguilar (eds.), *Surgery for Cancers of the Gastrointestinal Tract: A Step-by-Step Approach*, DOI 10.1007/978-1-4939-1893-5_27, © Springer Science+Business Media New York 2015

## Indications

Prior to proceeding with TAMIS for rectal cancer, especially if treatment is to be of curative intent, it is critical to perform a thorough history, physical exam, and workup. A detailed discussion with the patient regarding the oncologic risks of local excision compared to radical resection, as well as potential functional benefits should be documented. The surgeon must understand the patient's expectations and wishes, particularly with respect to permanent colostomy.

TAMIS can serve as both a diagnostic or therapeutic procedure and the multiple indications are highlighted below. The technical success, postoperative outcomes, and long-term oncologic results of TAMIS are highly dependent on proper patient selection. Factors that should be taken into account in selecting patients for TAMIS fall into two general categories: (1) disease-specific/oncologic considerations and (2) anatomic considerations. Poor patient selection within these respective categories can often result in the improper inclusion of patients with unrecognized nodal disease, or surgical margin positivity, both of which will contribute to oncologic failure.

## Disease-Specific/Oncologic Considerations

The indications for local excision of rectal cancer as curative-intent therapy continue to evolve, particularly with the recent completion of multimodality trials such as the American College of Surgeons Oncology Group (ACOSOG) Z6041 trial [9]. Because local excision of rectal cancer only treats disease that is present in the rectal wall and lumen, the degree to which the procedure is oncologically successful is directly proportional to the likelihood of nodal metastasis.

The most important pathologic predictor of nodal disease is T stage. The risk of nodal metastasis by T stage varies between 5 and 10 % for T1 lesions, 15–25 % for T2 disease, and 35–75 % for T3 disease in the combined literature. Other pathologic factors are also useful in predicting risk of nodal disease and recurrence, and these should be taken into account for patient selection.

## Indications

- Adenomatous rectal polyps not amenable to colonoscopic resection, particularly lesions demonstrating high-grade dysplasia or adenocarcinoma in situ.
- Invasive rectal adenocarcinoma with low-risk T1 disease, without any high-risk factors. This is the current position of both the National Comprehensive Cancer Network (NCCN) [10] and the American Society of Colon and Rectal Surgeons (ASCRS) [11], who consider local excision to be an acceptable alternative to radical resection only in this setting. Because they are not reliable risk factors for nodal disease [12], size and circumferential extent alone are not absolute contraindications.
- Nonstandard indications include high-risk T1 or any T2 disease with multimodality therapy in patients who refuse radical resection or in patients enrolled in a clinical trial; T3 lesions in patients who refuse radical resection; rectal adenocarcinomas of any stage for palliative purposes; and Stage II or III rectal adenocarcinomas with complete clinical response to neoadjuvant therapy in highly selected and individualized circumstances.
- Less common indications for TAMIS include carcinoids, endometriomas, angiodysplasia, ulcers, strictures, and other benign pathologies.

## Anatomic Considerations

The selection of patients with rectal lesions that are too distal, too proximal, or too large can lead to both poor oncologic result (e.g., margin positivity and recurrence) and unnecessary morbidity. From the technical standpoint, TAMIS is ideally suited for lesions confined to the mid-upper rectum, involving less than 1/3 of the rectal circumference.

Lesions in the distal rectum are more appropriately treated with transanal excision (TAE). Excision of lesions proximal to 15 cm greatly increases the risk of peritoneal entry and radical resection should be considered in these cases. The likelihood of peritoneal entry is highly dependent on the circumferential location of the lesion, with anterior excisions presenting the greatest risk. Although there is significant individual anatomic variation based on body habitus, Najarian and colleagues have provided useful estimates of the distance of the peritoneal reflection from the anal verge using intraoperative rigid proctoscopy [13].

## Anatomic Indications

- Posterior lesions that are 5–15 cm from the anal verge.
- Anterior, anterolateral, and lateral lesions that are 5–10 cm from the anal verge.
- More proximal lesions (both anteriorly and posteriorly) may be approached with planned peritoneal entry. Defects that communicate with the peritoneum can be repaired either transanally, laparoscopically, or a combination of both. With posterior rectosigmoid lesions proximal to 15 cm, it is possible (though difficult) to avoid peritoneal entry by confining the transanal dissection to the space within the visceral peritoneal boundaries of the rectosigmoid mesentery [14].

## Diagnosis and Workup

Patients with rectal lesions generally present with clinically evident or occult lower gastrointestinal bleeding or a rectal lesion discovered on screening colonoscopy. Before reaching the surgeon, these patients often have been evaluated by a primary physician and gastroenterologist, and a pathologic diagnosis has already been established. Regardless, a thorough history and physical examination should be performed by the surgeon with specific attention to detailed oncologic history, presence of rectal pain and/or tenesmus, presence of obstructive symptoms, assessment of anorectal function, and assessment of urinary and erectile function/dysfunction. The surgeon should perform rigid proctoscopy documenting proximal and distal extent of the lesion, circumferential position of the lesion within the rectal wall (anterior, posterior, or lateral), and an approximation of the total diameter and circumferential extent of the lesion.

## Additional Diagnostic Studies

- Complete colonoscopy.
- Transrectal ultrasound (TRUS) or high-resolution rectal magnetic resonance imaging to stage all rectal neoplasms (≤15 cm from anal verge on rigid proctoscopy). Although there is some debate as to which modality is superior, we prefer TRUS given its ability to better discriminate between T1 and T2 disease, along with comparable sensitivity and specificity with respect to nodal involvement [11].
- Complete staging computed tomography (CT) scan of the chest, abdomen, and pelvis to rule out metastatic disease.
- Positron emission topography (PET)/CT can be used selectively for patients with suspected metastatic disease or in patients in whom intravenous contrast is contraindicated.
- Anal physiologic studies with manometry should be considered in patients with physical evidence of anorectal dysfunction to document preoperative sphincter function.

## Preoperative Considerations

The operative field in TAMIS is the lumen of the rectum. Therefore, thorough mechanical bowel preparation is essential for visualization and exposure. We ask our patients to eat a normal lunch the day before surgery with clear liquids thereafter and nothing by mouth after midnight. Our preferred mechanical bowel preparation consists of one bottle of magnesium citrate orally during the afternoon before surgery, with a Fleet's enema the night before and the morning of the procedure.

## Equipment

- Disposable transanal access port. Single-incision laparoscopic surgery (SILS) ports from multiple manufacturers have been used to obtain transanal access. More recently, dedicated disposable transanal access ports have become commercially available. We have used a number of these ports and currently prefer the GelPoint Path system (Applied Medical). All of these ports have their limitations. The most notable issue is that in obese patients placed in prone-jackknife position, the ports are sometimes too short to traverse the entire length of the external sphincter/levators. Although we have devised improvised methods of circumventing this particular shortcoming, traditional TEM may be a better option in these circumstances.
- Standard laparoscopic equipment including laparoscopic tower, insufflator, monitors, camera, and a 10-mm 30° laparoscope.
- Laparoscopic/articulating instruments including graspers, dissectors/energy devices, and needle driver. Our preferred grasper at present is the standard Maryland dissector held in the nondominant hand. We have used both straight and articulating hooks with cautery for dissection, as well as ultrasonic shears. We currently use both an articulating SILS hook (Covidien) as well as a harmonic scalpel (Ethicon) for dissection. We prefer standard laparoscopic needle drivers for suture repair of the excision defect.

## Surgical Technique

### Positioning and Preparation

The patient is placed under general anesthesia with endotracheal intubation. A Foley catheter is routinely inserted. A minimal sterile preparation of the perineum is performed and the patient is draped in standard fashion. Abdominal preparation may be performed if peritoneal entry is expected. Careful patient positioning is critical to ensure technical success of TAMIS. Although some groups perform TAMIS exclusively in lithotomy, we prefer to adjust patient positioning in order to keep the lesion down at the 6 o'clock position as much as possible. For posterior lesions, the patient is placed in a high-lithotomy position with the surgeon standing in the center and the assistant standing on either side of the surgeon (Fig. 27.1a). For anterior lesions, the patient is placed in the prone-jackknife position on a split-leg table, with the surgeon positioned between the legs (Fig. 27.1b). In case of inadequate flexion/jackknife, the ischial tuberosities will hinder the proper insertion of currently available transanal ports beyond the levators, which will result in poor visualization and exposure.

For lateral lesions, the patient is positioned either in prone-jackknife or lithotomy and turned in either direction such that the lesion is as close to the 6 o'clock position as possible. If the lesion cannot be placed directly at the midline, it is preferentially oriented toward the surgeon's dominant hand to facilitate suture repair. The patient must be firmly secured to the table, which we accomplish with towels and circumferential tape at the level of the chest.

### Port Placement and Exposure

The anal sphincter is manually dilated with 2–3 fingers. We no longer perform intersphincteric injections of any kind. The transanal access channel/port is heavily lubricated and inserted into the anal canal with the lip of the port placed proximal to the sphincters and levator. If the lip of the port does not completely traverse the levators, visualization will invariably be obstructed by internal hemorrhoidal tissue. Insertion of the port can be facilitated by internally folding and grasping the port with a ring clamp. After initial insertion, gentle pressure can be applied with the introducer supplied by the manufacturer to push the lip of the port past the levators. There is no need to suture the port to the skin, given that it is fairly stable if placed in the appropriate position (Fig. 27.2).

a

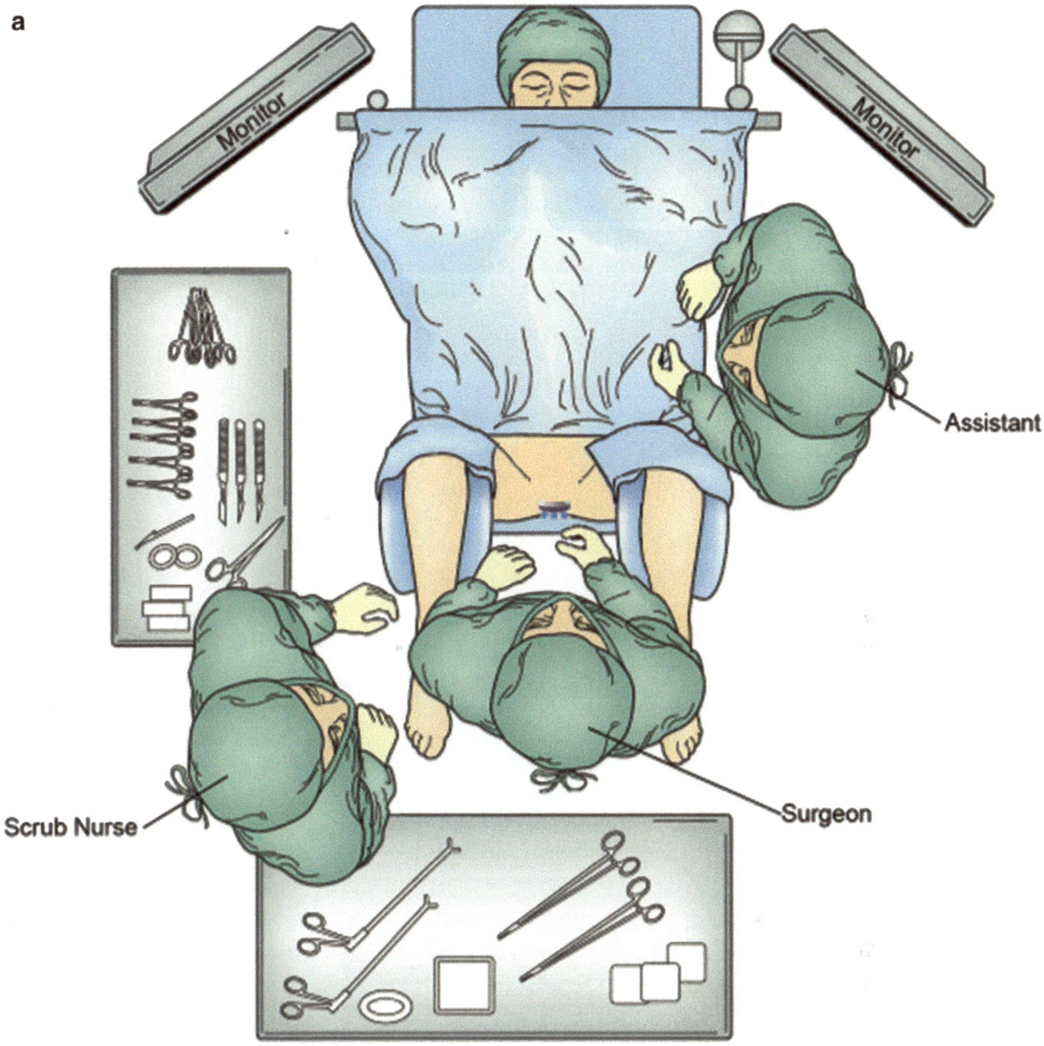


**Fig. 27.1** Operative positioning for TAMIS. (**a**) The patient is placed in high lithotomy position for posterior lesions. (**b**) The patient is placed in prone-jackknife position on a split-leg table for anterior lesions

A lightly moistened sponge is inserted into the rectum, to be pushed into the proximal lumen during insufflation. This helps prevent insufflation of the proximal colon and may also limit periodic collapse of the pneumorectum during the case. The instrument sleeves are then placed into the gel cap and the gel cap is then fixed to the transanal port.

## Identification of Excision Margins of at Least 1 cm

We routinely mark 1-cm margins using a hook cautery device. As the dissection proceeds, tissue distortion and retraction are encountered and these cautery marks are invaluable in preventing disorientation and assuring adequate margins of excision (Fig. 27.3).

## Full-Thickness Incision of the Rectal Wall

A full-thickness incision is made into the perirectal tissue beginning 1 cm distal to the lesion. This is usually accomplished by lifting the rectal wall with a grasper and incising the rectum with a hook cautery device. Distal incision allows

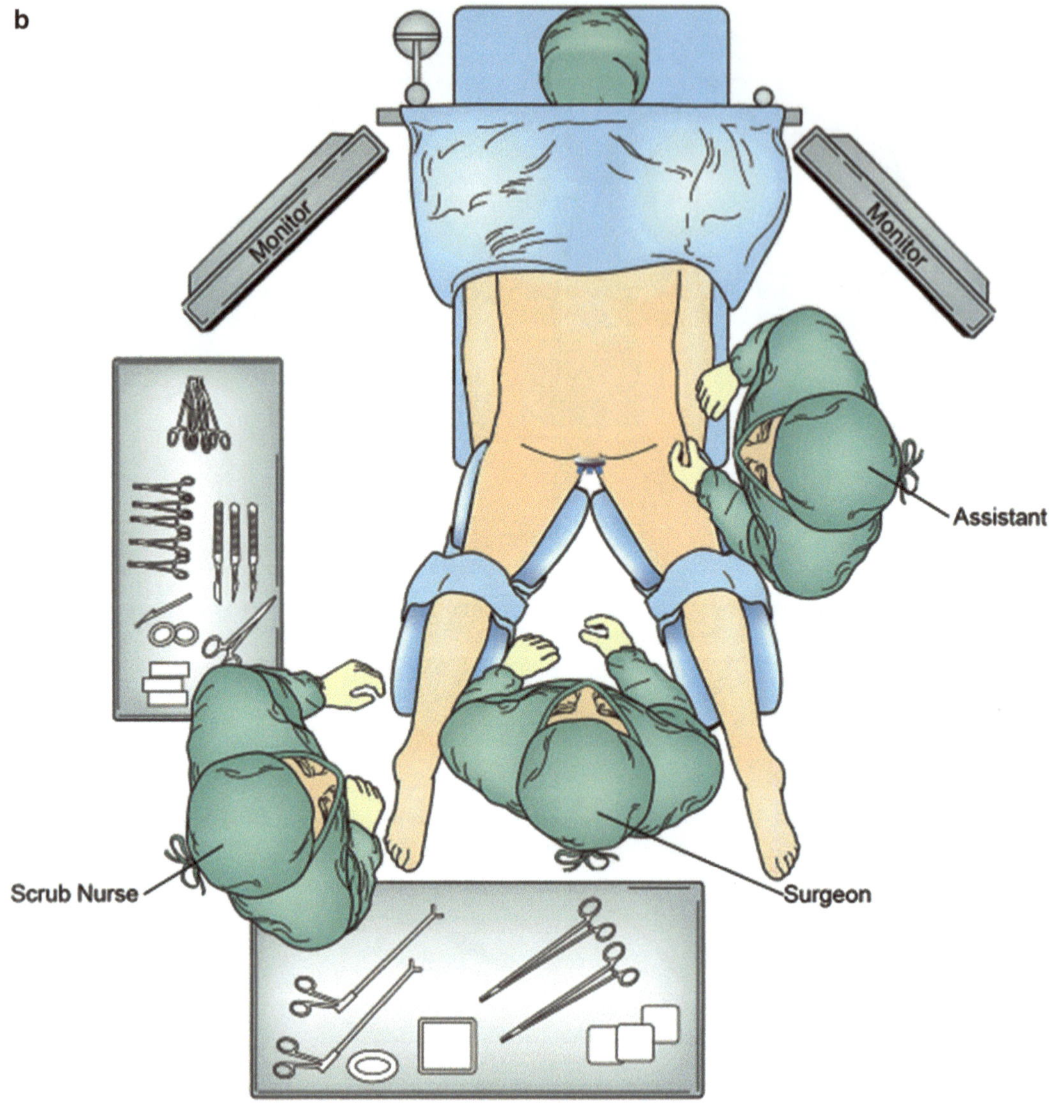


**Fig. 27.1** (continued)

complete visualization of the tissue planes during the course of the dissection (Fig. 27.4).

Posteriorly, the perirectal tissue is usually easily recognized by the presence of perirectal fat. While there is often some fat anteriorly as well, the correct plane generally consists of loose, relatively avascular areolar tissue between the rectal wall and the urogenital structures. This initial step should be performed with extreme caution for anterior and lateral excisions to avoid injury to major vascular and urogenital structures.

We do not perform partial-thickness excisions given that this alternative is not oncologically appropriate in the setting of a suspected cancer, and because (in our experience) benign adenomas are almost always appropriately treated with endoscopic mucosal resection by our gastroenterology colleagues.

## Circumferential Dissection

The perirectal tissue is dissected first by bluntly spreading the tissue in the appropriate plane and by taking the perirectal tissue sharply with cautery. The overlying rectal wall is then taken

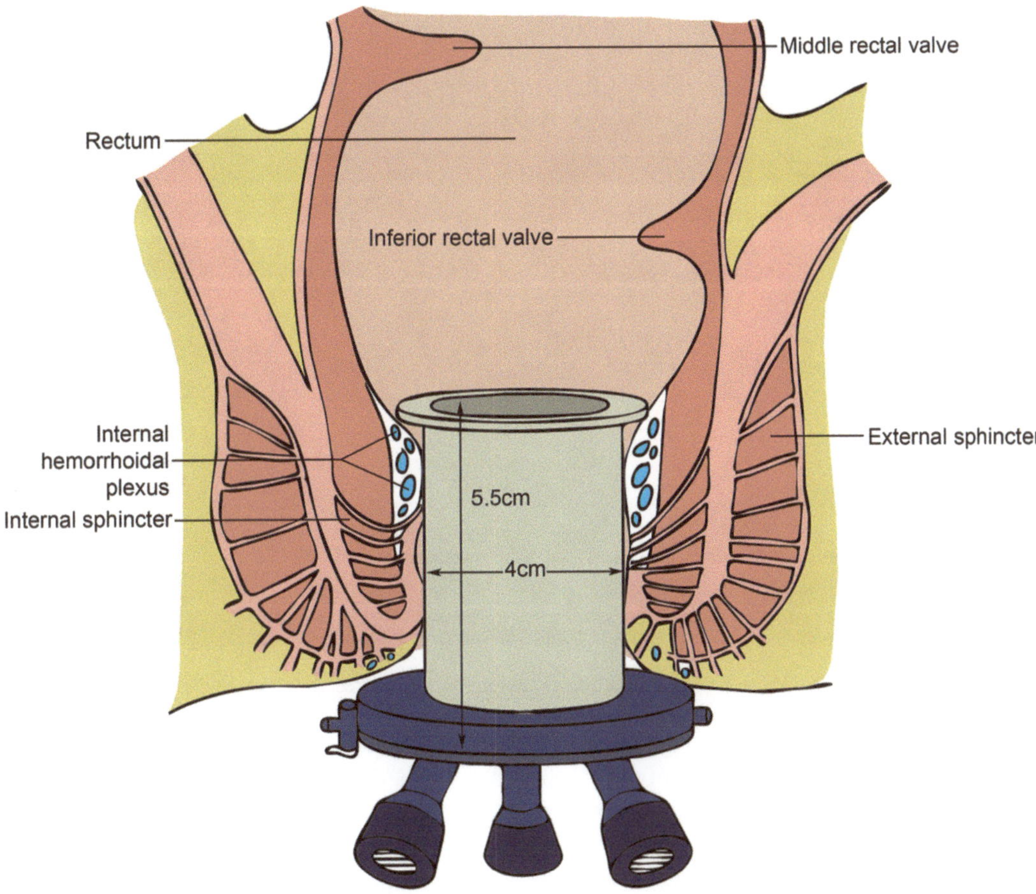


**Fig. 27.2** Diagram illustrating proper seating of the transanal port in the anal canal. The body of the port is approximately 4 cm wide and is properly inserted at 5.5 cm

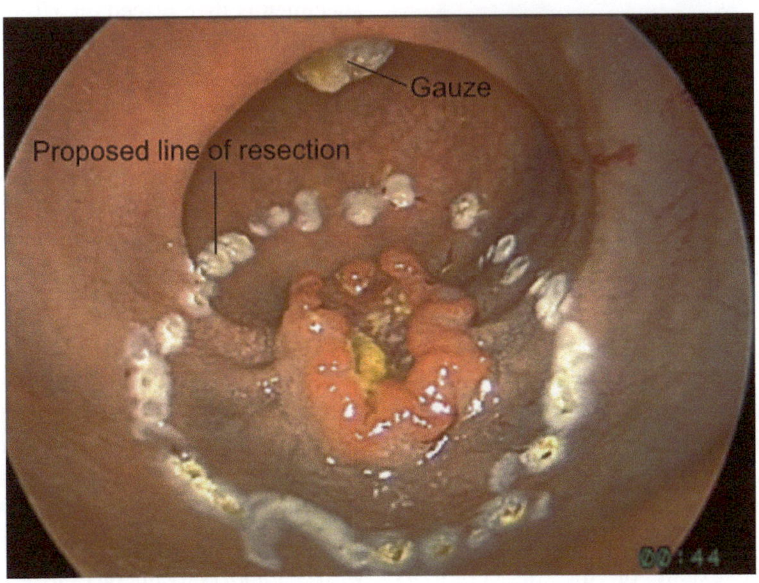


**Fig. 27.3** Marking 1-cm margin of excision of rectal lesion marked with hook cautery

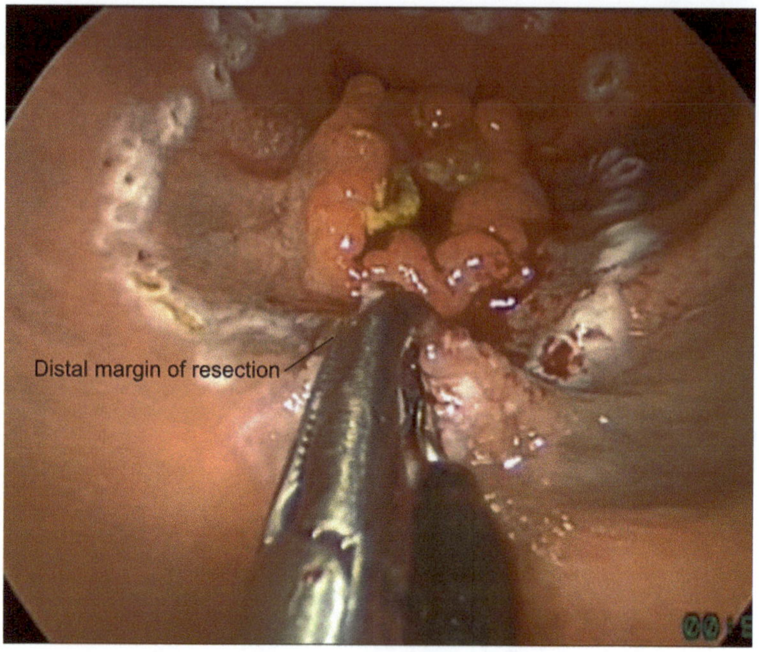


**Fig. 27.4** Excision of rectal lesion begins with full-thickness incision of the rectal wall at the distal margin

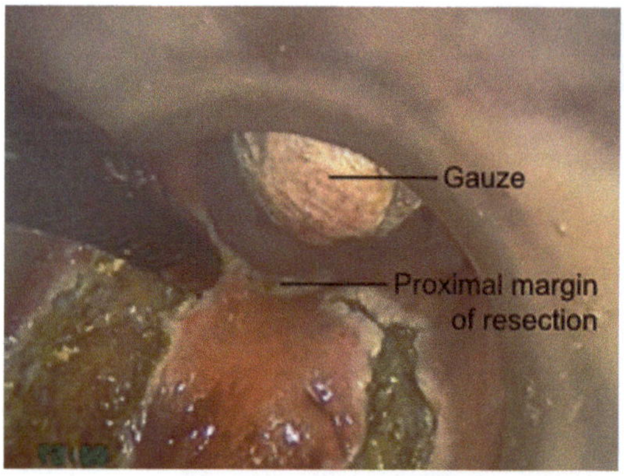


**Fig. 27.5** Intraoperative photo demonstrates circumferential dissection of the lesion with 1-cm margin. A Ray-tec sponge has been inserted in the proximal rectum to limit insufflations of the colon and preserve the pneumorectum

progressively with cautery or ultrasonic shears. Dissection in this manner is especially important as the peritoneal reflection is approached and minimizes the risk of injury to perirectal structures (Fig. 27.5). The dissection is carried circumferentially in this manner on both sides. The proximal extent of the dissection is approached in the deep plane first, with the overlying rectal wall and mucosa taken with energy immediately thereafter.

Once free, the specimen is securely grasped to maintain orientation, and removed after unclamping the gelcap of the transanal port. The specimen is then placed on a Telfa dressing and oriented for pathologic examination. The surgeon routinely accompanies the specimen to the pathology room to assure orientation. Gross examination is routinely performed. Frozen section analysis is performed selectively if margin involvement is suspected.

## Suture Repair

The pneumorectum often causes the excision defect to appear impressively large in size. This effect can be reduced by decreasing insufflation pressure in order to facilitate repair, though we generally find this unnecessary. We repair the defect using a multifilament absorbable suture with a LapraTy (Ethicon) on one end to avoid

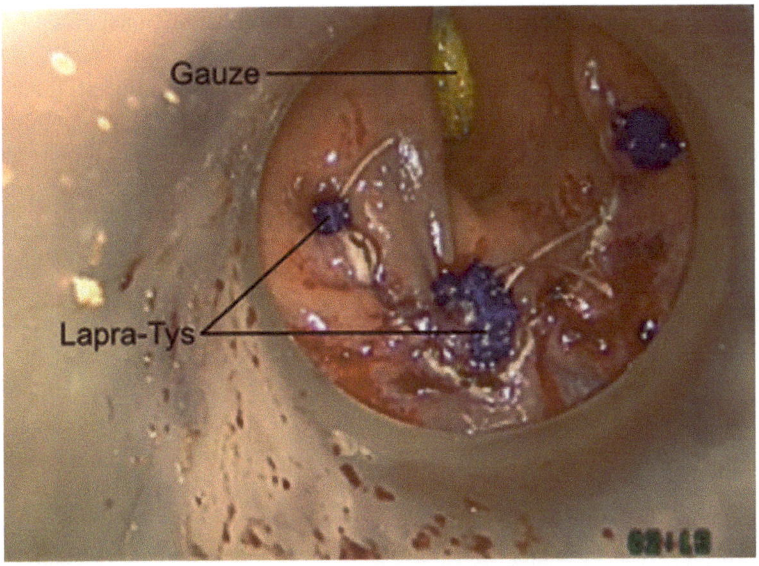


**Fig. 27.6** Intraoperative photo demonstrates suture repair of the resulting rectal defect with running multifilament suture. LapraTys (Ethicon) have been placed to secure the sutures in place of knot-tying

tying in a confined space (Fig. 27.6). Locking monofilament absorbable suture is now commercially available and is also a good option.

The repair proceeds in a running fashion with large full-thickness bites from the side of the surgeon's dominant hand towards the nondominant side. Depending on the size of the defect, 2 or 3 separate running sutures may be use to traverse the entire defect. This limits the amount of redundant suture that is in the lumen at any given time. Once the last bite is taken, a LapraTy (Ethicon) is placed and the suture divided to complete the repair. The gauze and transanal port are then gently removed.

## Postoperative Care

The patient is admitted overnight for observation and diet is advanced as tolerated. Analgesics are usually unnecessary. In the absence of significant pain, fever, bleeding, or urinary retention the patient is discharged home on postoperative day #1. If fevers are noted, pelvic and abdominal sepsis should be ruled out. In the presence of a benign abdominal exam, empiric antibiotics may be used and the patient may be observed until resolution.

If fevers persist, imaging studies such as abdominal plain-films and/or CT scan of the abdomen and pelvis with rectal contrast should be considered. Free abdominal air should immediately raise concern for unrecognized peritoneal entry and should prompt laparoscopy and/or laparotomy in the setting of persistent abdominal pain and/or fevers.

With large transanal excisions, CT scan may demonstrate fluid within the excision defect, which in the absence of clinical findings is likely to be inconsequential. However, in the setting of persistent fevers refractory to antibiotics, consideration should be given to either transanal or percutaneous drainage. Diverting ileostomy should be considered if pelvic sepsis persists or is severe.

## Complications

The primary benefits of both TEM and TAMIS are the avoidance of most of the complications encountered from low anterior and abdominoperineal resections, including surgical site infections, anastomotic leak, and other morbidity related to abdominal surgery. In addition, the relatively frequent and severe functional complications of radical resection, such as erectile dysfunction, urinary retention, low anterior resection syndrome, and fecal soilage, are almost completely obviated by TEM/TAMIS.

Because TAMIS is a relatively new modification of TEM, the combined worldwide experience is relatively small. However, given the similarity between the two procedures, morbidity data for TAMIS can in most instances be extrapolated from TEM data. Complications from both TEM/TAMIS tend to be relatively infrequent, minor, and self-limited. Overall morbidity rate in most series is <15 % for TEM [15], and is likely the same or lower for TAMIS [16]. The risk of perioperative mortality is extremely low (<<1 % in major series). The risk of major morbidity requiring admission and/or significant intervention is also low at <5 % in most series [15, 16]. Specific complications include:

- Rectal bleeding. This complication is relatively rare and, in the majority of cases, self-limited. It can occur intraoperatively, early in the postoperative course, or several days after discharge. The need for operative reintervention is exceedingly rare.
- Suture dehiscence. This may occur in as many as 15 % of patients and is likely more common with large excisions [17]. In most instances, suture dehiscence is likely to be subclinical, though dehiscence of the extraperitoneal rectum may present with fever. While transanal repair can be performed, most cases can be managed nonoperatively with systemic antibiotics. Conversely, intraperitoneal dehiscence after planned or unplanned peritoneal entry will result in intraabdominal contamination and peritonitis mandating urgent exploration. Signs of refractory and progressive sepsis should prompt consideration of abdominal exploration with fecal diversion and possibly radical resection.
- Functional complications. Transient urinary retention is among the more commonly encountered complications of TEM. A brief period of anal leakage has also been reported in rare cases, but is almost always temporary. Significant functional complications have not been reported with TAMIS and we have not encountered significant functional issues in our experience. Both complications may be related to traction injury from the transanal access device, which is potentially mitigated by the somewhat smaller disposable TAMIS platforms.
- Peritoneal entry. We do not consider planned peritoneal entry a complication. Unintended peritoneal entry, however, is more common with anterior, lateral, and upper rectal lesions. Dissection into the peritoneal cavity should be recognized intraoperatively, and may result in abdominal insufflation and collapse of the pneumorectum. With intraoperative recognition and adequate visualization, transanal repair may be sufficient. If transanal repair is not possible, primary repair via laparoscopy or laparotomy can also be accomplished. If repair is impossible or inadequate, resection and/or diversion should be considered.
- Relatively rare complications include intraoperative injury to genitourinary structures; rectovaginal, rectourethral, and rectovesical fistulae; rectal stricture; and complications related to positioning.

## Surveillance

There are no standardized protocols for oncologic surveillance after TAMIS. We have been very aggressive with surveillance, particularly in our early experience. Given the concern for local recurrence, our protocol has been to perform flexible sigmoidoscopy every 3 months for the first 6 months, then every 6 months for 2 years, followed by routine endoscopy and cancer screening for a total of 5 years. In patients with invasive cancer, we perform CT scans of the chest, abdomen, and pelvis every 6–12 months for the first 3 years and yearly thereafter for a total of 5 years. Less aggressive surveillance protocols, however, are likely adequate.

## References


1. Lisfranc J. Memoire sur l'excision de la partie inferieure du rectum devenue carcinomateuse. Mem Ac R Chir. 1833;3:291–302.
2. Miles W. A method of performing abdomino-perineal excision for carcinoma of the rectum and of the terminal portion of the pelvic colon. Lancet. 1908;2:1812–3.
3. Heald RJ, Husband EM, Ryall RD. The mesorectum in rectal cancer surgery—the clue to pelvic recurrence? Br J Surg. 1982;69(10):613–6.
4. Tilney HS, Heriot AG, Purkayastha S, Antoniou A, Aylin P, Darzi AW, et al. A national perspective on the decline of abdominoperineal resection for rectal cancer. Ann Surg. 2008;247(1):77–84. doi:10.1097/SLA.0b013e31816076c3.
5. Habr-Gama A, Sabbaga J, Gama-Rodrigues J, Sao Juliao GP, Proscurshim I, Bailao Aguilar P, et al. Watch and wait approach following extended neoadjuvant chemoradiation for distal rectal cancer: are we getting closer to anal cancer management? Dis Colon Rectum. 2013;56(10):1109–17. doi:10.1097/DCR.0b013e3182a25c4e.
6. Parks AG. A technique for the removal of large villous tumours in the rectum. Proc R Soc Med. 1970; 63(Suppl):89–91.
7. Buess G, Hutterer F, Theiss J, Bobel M, Isselhard W, Pichlmaier H. [A system for a transanal endoscopic rectum operation] Der Chirurg; Zeitschrift fur alle Gebiete der operativen Medizen. Chirurg. 1984; 55(10):677–80.
8. Atallah S, Albert M, Larach S. Transanal minimally invasive surgery: a giant leap forward. Surg Endosc. 2010;24(9):2200–5. doi:10.1007/s00464-010-0927-z.
9. Garcia-Aguilar J, Shi Q, Thomas Jr CR, Chan E, Cataldo P, Marcet J, et al. A phase II trial of neoadjuvant chemoradiation and local excision for T2N0 rectal cancer: preliminary results of the ACOSOG Z6041 trial. Ann Surg Oncol. 2012;19(2):384–91. doi:10.1245/s10434-011-1933-7.
10. Benson 3rd AB, Bekaii-Saab T, Chan E, Chen YJ, Choti MA, Cooper HS, et al. Rectal cancer. J Natl Compr Canc Netw. 2012;10(12):1528–64.
11. Monson JR, Weiser MR, Buie WD, Chang GJ, Rafferty JF, Buie WD, et al. Practice parameters for the management of rectal cancer (revised). Dis Colon Rectum. 2013;56(5):535–50. doi:10.1097/DCR.0b013e31828cb66c.
12. Salinas HM, Dursun A, Klos CL, Shellito P, Sylla P, Berger D, et al. Determining the need for radical surgery in patients with T1 rectal cancer. Arch Surg. 2011;146(5):540–3. doi:10.1001/archsurg.2011.76.
13. Najarian MM, Belzer GE, Cogbill TH, Mathiason MA. Determination of the peritoneal reflection using intraoperative proctoscopy. Dis Colon Rectum. 2004;47(12):2080–5. doi:10.1007/s10350-004-0740-7.
14. Hussein Q, Artinyan A. Pushing the limits of local excision for rectal cancer: transanal minimally invasive surgery for an upper rectal/rectosigmoid lesion. Ann Surg Oncol. 2014. doi:10.1245/s10434-013-3457-9.
15. Kumar AS, Coralic J, Kelleher DC, Sidani S, Kolli K, Smith LE. Complications of transanal endoscopic microsurgery are rare and minor: a single institution's analysis and comparison to existing data. Dis Colon Rectum. 2013;56(3):295–300. doi:10.1097/DCR.0b013e31827163f7.
16. Albert MR, Atallah SB, deBeche-Adams TC, Izfar S, Larach SW. Transanal minimally invasive surgery (TAMIS) for local excision of benign neoplasms and early-stage rectal cancer: efficacy and outcomes in the first 50 patients. Dis Colon Rectum. 2013;56(3): 301–7.
17. Schafer H, Baldus SE, Holscher AH. Giant adenomas of the rectum: complete resection by transanal endoscopic microsurgery (TEM). Int J Colorectal Dis. 2006;21(6):533–7. doi:10.1007/s00384-005-0025-1.


## Key Operative Steps

1. Dilate the anal sphincter with 2–3 fingers.
2. Insert the transanal access channel/port into the anal canal.
3. Insert a sponge/gauze into the proximal rectum.
4. Mark 1-cm margin with hook cautery.
5. Make a full-thickness incision into the perirectal tissue at the distal margin.
6. Dissect the perirectal tissue with blunt and sharp maneuvers.
7. Divide the rectal wall with cautery or ultrasonic shears.
8. Complete dissection circumferentially until resection is complete.
9. Secure the specimen to maintain orientation for pathologic examination.
10. Repair the defect with a single layer of full-thickness multifilament suture(s). May close defect with a single running suture or 2–3 serial running sutures. LapraTys (Ethicon) may be used to secure sutures to obviate knot-tying.

# Transanal Endoscopic Surgery for Rectal Cancer

# 28

Xavier Serra-Aracil and Laura Mora-Lopez

## Introduction

Total mesorectal excision (TME) is an effective operation for most patients with rectal cancer, achieving locoregional tumor control in almost 95 % of patients [1]. Whether performed with sphincter preservation or with permanent colostomy, TME is associated with 2 % mortality [2], up to 33 % morbidity, and 20–30 % genitourinary alterations and sexual dysfunction [3, 4].

Local excision (LE), in theory, can cure tumors that have not penetrated beyond the muscularis propria and not metastasized to the regional lymph nodes [5]. However, LE using the conventional transanal approach is only an option for tumors located in the distal rectum. LE using transsphincteric exposure, described by Mason [6], has been used to treat lesions in the middle third of the rectum and located in the anterior rectal wall; however, dividing the sphincters can cause fecal incontinence. Kraske's transsacral rectal excision [7] allows the removal of tumors located in the mid and even upper third of the rectum, but it has also been abandoned due to its high morbidity and mortality.

Transanal endoscopic microsurgery (TEM) equipment (Richard Wolf GMBH, Knittlingen, Germany), first described by Buess in the 1980s [8], permits access to rectal tumors located as far as 20 cm from the anal verge. TEM facilitates dissection, cutting, coagulation, and suturing by providing excellent 3-dimensional (3-D) viewing and by using specially designed instrumentation. The rate of resection with negative margins is high, postoperative morbidity is usually below 10 %; and bowel, genitourinary, and sexual function are preserved [9, 10]. Transanal endoscopic operation (TEO) equipment (Karl Storz GMBH, Tütlingen, Germany) is somewhat simpler compared to TEM. However, the incorporation of high-resolution cameras and panoramic screens into the laparoscopic armamentarium results in image quality as good as in TEM.

## Selection of Patients: Treatment Groups

The success of all forms of LE for rectal cancer is based upon adequate patient selection. All possible candidates for TEM/TEO must undergo full

Electronic supplementary material: Supplementary material is available in the online version of this chapter at 10.1007/978-1-4939-1893-5_28. Videos can also be accessed at http://www.springerimages.com/videos/978-1-4939-1892-8.

X. Serra-Aracil, M.D. (✉)
Coloproctology Unit, Department of General and Digestive Surgery, Parc Tauli University Hospital, Universitat Autònoma de Barcelona,
Parc Tauli 1 Sabadell, Barcelona 08208, Spain
e-mail: jserraa@tauli.cat

L. Mora-Lopez, M.D.
Coloproctology Unit, Department of General and Digestive Surgery, Parc Tauli University Hospital, Barcelona, Spain

J. Kim and J. Garcia-Aguilar (eds.), *Surgery for Cancers of the Gastrointestinal Tract: A Step-by-Step Approach*,
DOI 10.1007/978-1-4939-1893-5_28, © Springer Science+Business Media New York 2015

preoperative staging of the tumor. A full colonoscopy with multifocal biopsy is mandatory. A rigid proctoscopy prior to endorectal ultrasound (ERUS) is important to confirm tumor size, the distance of the tumor's lower and upper edge from the anal verge, and its location according to quadrant (anterior, posterior, and right or left lateral). ERUS allows staging of the lesion according to Hildebrandt's criteria [11]. Rectal magnetic resonance imaging (MRI) is an important complement. MRI is less accurate than ERUS in distinguishing between T1 and T2 tumors, but it is useful in detecting nodal metastasis.

In patients with invasive adenocarcinoma, an abdominal and chest computed tomography (CT) scan should be performed to rule out distant metastasis. The levels of the tumor markers carcino-embryonic antigen (CEA) and carbohydrate antigen (CA) 19-9 should also be measured before starting treatment. All patients are administered validated questionnaires assessing bowel, urinary, and sexual function [12]. If there are signs of fecal incontinence, anorectal manometry is performed to obtain baseline parameters. In our experience, TEM/TEO causes manometric alterations but does not affect clinical continence scores [13]. After these complementary examinations, patients are classified into one of four preoperative groups [10, 14].

## Group I (Curative Intent)

This group includes adenoma staged as T0N0 by ERUS and pelvic MRI. Colorectal adenomatous polyps are considered to be premalignant lesions with a risk of developing into adenocarcinoma [15]. Early detection and removal are the best means of avoiding the development of adenocarcinoma [16]. In our series [17], and in the study by Absar and Haboubi [18], more than 18 % of patients diagnosed with adenomatous polyps were ultimately found to have invasive adenocarcinoma after surgical excision. For this reason, a piecemeal endoscopic resection or less than a full-thickness transanal excision is considered insufficient treatment for patients with large rectal villous adenomas. In the case of large rectal adenomas we advocate full-thickness rectal wall resection using TEM/TEO, leaving adequate safety margins for correct staging by the pathologist [19]. In our series [17], half of the infiltrating adenocarcinomas resulting from adenomas were pT1 lesions. This means that with adequate resection and in the absence of unfavorable histological features (high grade or lymphovascular or perineural invasion), these patients will not require additional radical surgery [14, 20, 21].

## Group II (Curative Intent)

Group II includes adenocarcinomas with favorable histological features (G1 or G2, no lymphovascular or perineural invasion) and staged as T0-1N0 by ERUS and pelvic MRI. LE is considered an alternative to TME for treatment of these tumors. However, retrospective case series of patients who had conventional transanal LE have reported local recurrence rates as high as 29 % [9, 22, 23]. The initial local recurrence rates for similar patients treated with TEM were below 10 %. However, more recent series have reported local recurrence rates as high as 20 % for patients with T1 tumors treated with TEM [24–27]. These discrepancies between older and newer series have been explained by differences in patient selection, with newer series including patients with high-grade tumors [28]. Thus, Tytherleigh et al. have reported that the risk of local recurrence for T1 tumors with favorable histology, no fragmentation, and negative resection margins is lower than 5 % [28], compared to 29 % in patients with T1 tumors with poor histological features, tumor fragmentation, or positive resection margins [14].

## Group III (Indication by Consensus)

Group III includes adenocarcinomas with favorable histological features staged as T2N0 by ERUS and pelvic MRI. According to the National Comprehensive Cancer Network Rectal Cancer Guidelines [29], the standard treatment of rectal adenocarcinoma T2N0M0 is TME without adjuvant therapy. However, recent evidence suggests that chemoradiation (CRT) and LE can be an alternative to TME in patients with adequately staged T2N0 tumors. The risk of recurrence and metastasis in these patients seems to be related to the final pathology of the surgical specimen. In a review of the literature on the use of CRT followed by LE in patients with clinical stage T2N0 rectal adenocarcinoma, Borschitz observed no local recurrence (LR) and 4 % systemic recurrence (SR) in patients with ypT0 tumors; 2 % LR and 7 % SR in ypT1 tumors; and 7 % both LR and SR in ypT2 tumors [30]. Patients with ypT3 tumors had LR rate of 21 % and SR rate of 12 %. These data suggest that CRT and LE is a viable alternative for selected patients with clinically staged T2N0 rectal adenocarcinoma, in particular those lesions smaller than 4 cm in diameter, involving less than 40 % of the circumference of the rectum, and G1-2 [31]. However, the evidence is still based mainly on retrospective case series, and these findings need to be confirmed in prospective randomized controlled trials.

### Group IV (Palliative)

Group IV includes palliative indications, regardless of the tumor stage. In expert hands, certain rectal and pelvic pathologies are habitually treated by laparotomy or laparoscopy via an abdominal approach. In expert hands, TEM/TEO is a less aggressive approach that is suitable for some of these surgeries and achieves lower morbidity rates [32, 33].

## Preparation of the Patient and Surgical Technique

### Preoperative Preparation of the Patient

On the day prior to surgery, all patients should undergo full mechanical preparation. We use thromboembolism prophylaxis and standard intravenous antibiotic prophylaxis. All patients have a bladder catheter inserted in order to avoid bladder distension.

### Positioning and Preoperative Rectoscopy

Although the surgeon should know the location of the tumor prior to the operation, it is important to confirm the location in the operating theater. This is done using rigid rectoscopy to determine the tumor's location, size, and distance from the anal verge (Fig. 28.1a). In TEM/TEO the surgeon works best with the tumor visible in the lower portion of the field. Therefore, the positioning of the patient depends on the location of the tumor. When the tumor is located posteriorly, the patient is placed in lithotomy (Fig. 28.1b); for anterior tumors, the patient should be placed prone (Fig. 28.1c); and for lateral tumors, the patient should be placed in the corresponding lateral decubitus position. The positioning of the legs is important to allow the surgeon to move the TEM/TEO rectoscope.

### Anesthesia

We recommend general anesthesia. The patient should be paralyzed, as any increase in the intraabdominal pressure will collapse the rectum and impede proper visualization of the lesion. These patients do not require high levels of analgesia during surgery.

### TEM Equipment

The instrumentation required for TEM includes a 4-cm diameter rectoscope, in two different lengths (12 and 20 cm) (Fig. 28.2a). The choice of length depends on the site of the tumor. The rectoscope is secured to the operating table by a polyarticulated U-shaped holding system with a mechanical central clamp (Fig. 28.2b). The proximal part of the rectoscope contains a working attachment with four channels. Through one of these channels the vision system is inserted. This system incorporates a 10-mm 3-D stereoscopic telescope for the surgeon and a video-camera connection for the screen, which allows the rest of the team to follow the procedure. The other TEM instruments

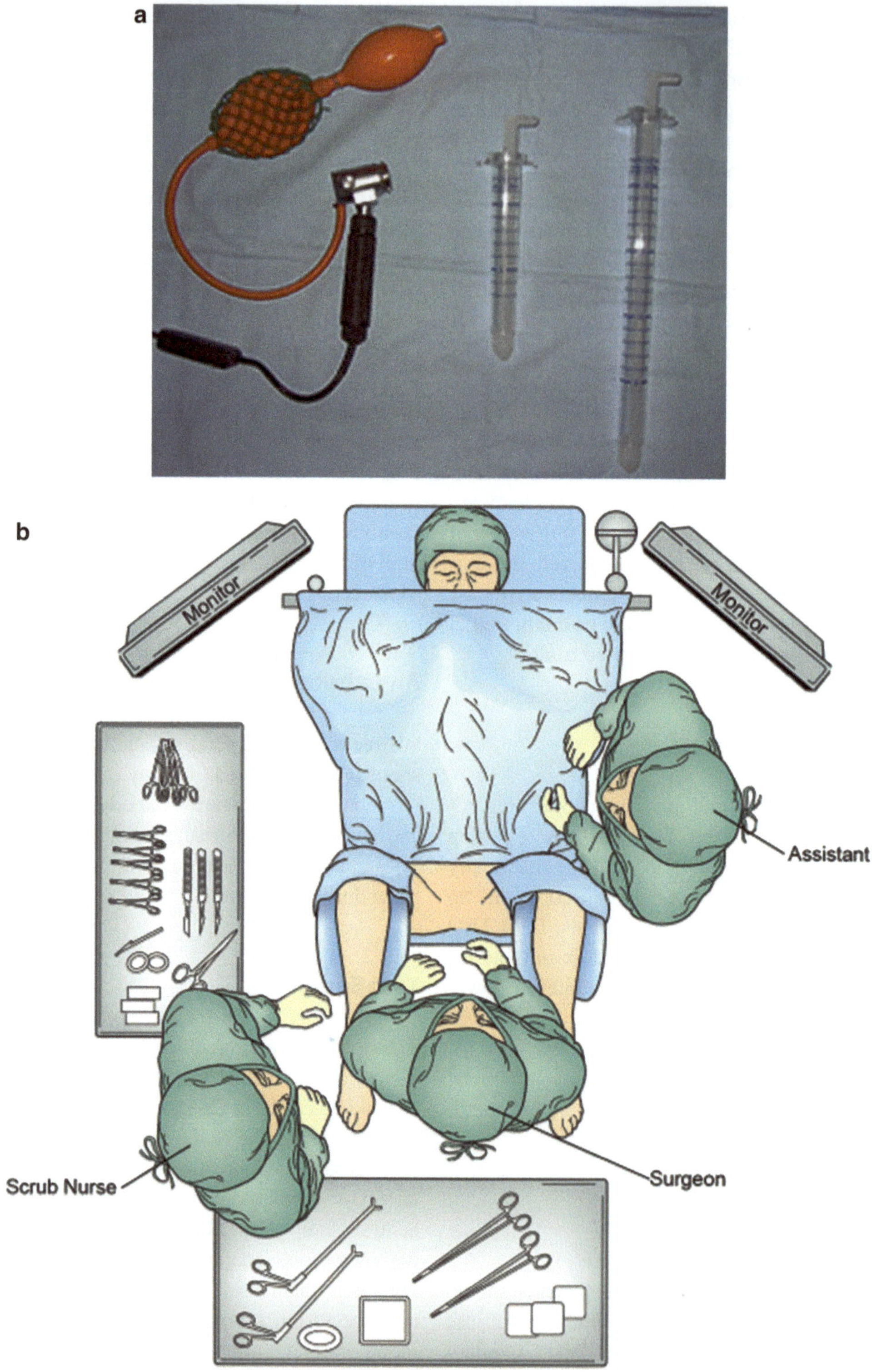


**Fig. 28.1** Operative equipment and positioning. (**a**) Preoperative rectoscope. (**b**) Supine lithotomy position. (**c**) Prone position

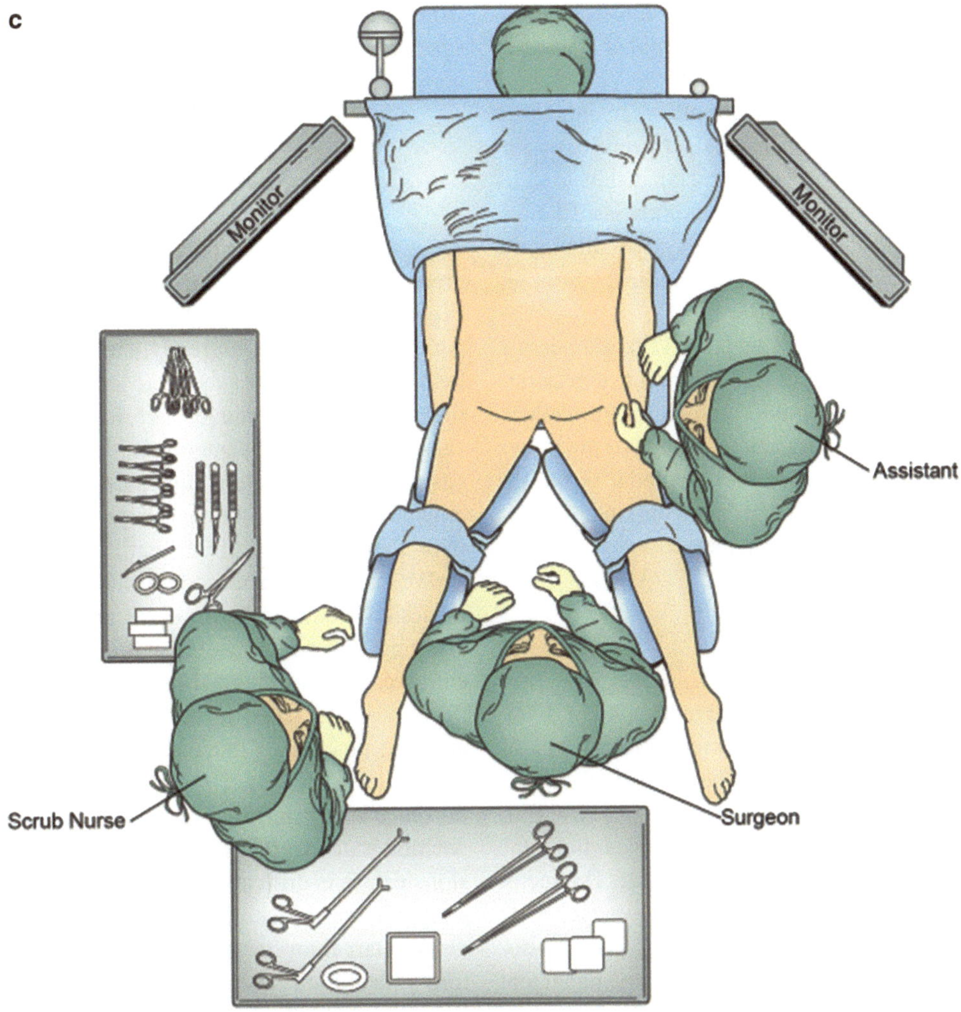


**Fig. 28.1** (continued)

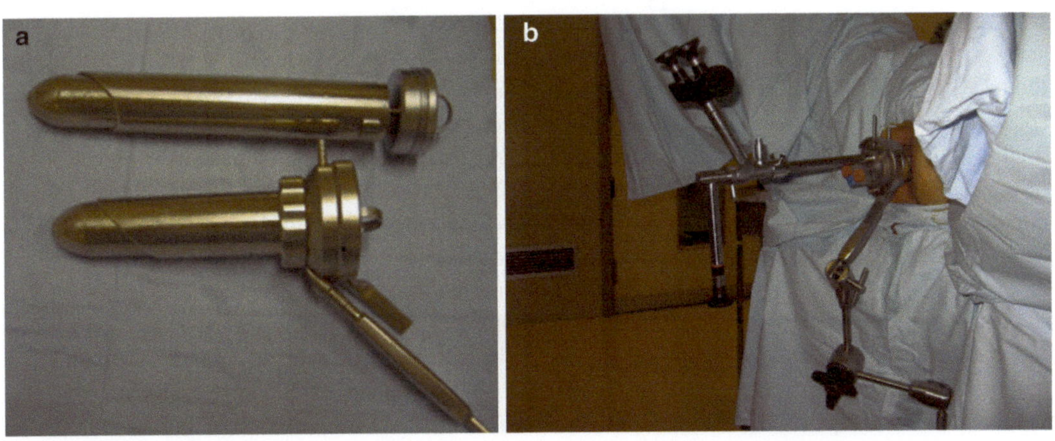


**Fig. 28.2** TEM equipment. (**a**) Rectoscopes of two different lengths (12 and 20 cm). (**b**) TEM equipment in position with the U-shaped holding system

are introduced through the other three channels. These channels are sealed by rubber valves to prevent air leakage (Fig. 28.2b).

The TEM $CO_2$ insufflator allows maintenance of a stable pneumorectum (10–12 mmHg) without the risk of excessive rectal distension. Its mechanism is based on continuous insufflation-aspiration in the rectum. The system allows the irrigation of the lens to obtain optimal vision via the TEM telescope [10].

The essential instruments for TEM all measure 5 mm in diameter: grasping forceps, ergonomic aspirator, a monopolar scalpel, needle-holder, clip-holder, and surgical scissors. We place two pedals on the ground: the left pedal is for the aspiration-irrigation system and the right pedal is for the bipolar electric scalpel.

## TEO Equipment

The TEO equipment also includes a 4 cm diameter rectoscope. There are three different lengths (7.5, 15, and 22 cm). The choice of model depends on the site of the tumor. As in TEM, after draping and preparing the surgical field, the U-shaped holding system is mounted. The rectoscope is then introduced gently and attached to the holding system. The obturator of the rectoscope is withdrawn and the working attachment is secured in position. The silicon leaflet valves are checked to ensure that there is no air leak. The working attachment contains three more channels for instruments. The telescope guide measures 5 mm in diameter, compared with 10 mm in the case of TEM; this means that there is more space inside the rectoscope. The high-resolution digital camera is fitted to the 30° telescope. Then the cold light cable is inserted and the two tubes, one for insufflations and the other for smoke aspiration, are connected. The most recent models incorporate a new tube, which allows irrigation of the camera. In the new system, the smoke aspiration tube is fitted to the end of the rectoscope handle. On the ground there is only one pedal, which is for the bipolar electric scalpel. It is usually placed beneath the surgeon's right foot. The high-definition screen is placed as directly in front of the surgeon as possible. The insufflation system is the same as the one used in any laparoscopy cart.

## Standard Surgical Strategy

We work with a pneumorectum under a constant pressure of 10–12 mmHg. The rectal distension exposes the tumor and the rectal wall. If the patient is positioned correctly, the lesion should be in the lower part of the rectoscopic view. The first important maneuver before initiation of surgery is the mobilization of the rectoscope, ensuring that the rectal lumen is visible at all times. Then, we place the rectoscope over the lesion in order to gain access to the entire perimeter.

We place the rectoscope around 2 cm from the lesion. Before initiating dissection, we use the grasping forceps to check that we can reach the entire periphery of the lesion, or at least two-thirds of it. We assess its mobility by moving the adjacent mucosa. We stress that the TEM/TEO technique is dynamic: the rectoscope will be moved as many times as is necessary to achieve a position that facilitates the maneuver. On occasion, lesions in difficult locations can be accessed simply by repositioning the rectoscope.

We start the procedure by marking a dotted line with the electrocautery 10–15 mm around the tumor. We then open the mucosa along the dotted line and initiate the dissection of the lesion. The ultrasonic scalpel (UltraCision, Ethicon Endo-Surgery, Cincinnati, OH, USA) [34] is our instrument of choice for cutting the bowel wall. The curved tip of the ultrasound scalpel facilitates lateral dissection when working in parallel to the camera in a narrow field. With the setting in "low speed" the ultrasonic scalpel cuts through the rectal wall and mesorectal tissue without bleeding. The thin jaws allow a view of the tissue being sectioned, facilitating gradual advance. The grasping forceps are used to hold the healthy rectal mucosa, but never the tumor.

We begin the dissection at the most distal edge of the tumor in caudal-cephalo direction; that is, in the area closest to the rectoscope. Full-thickness excision of the rectal wall is performed

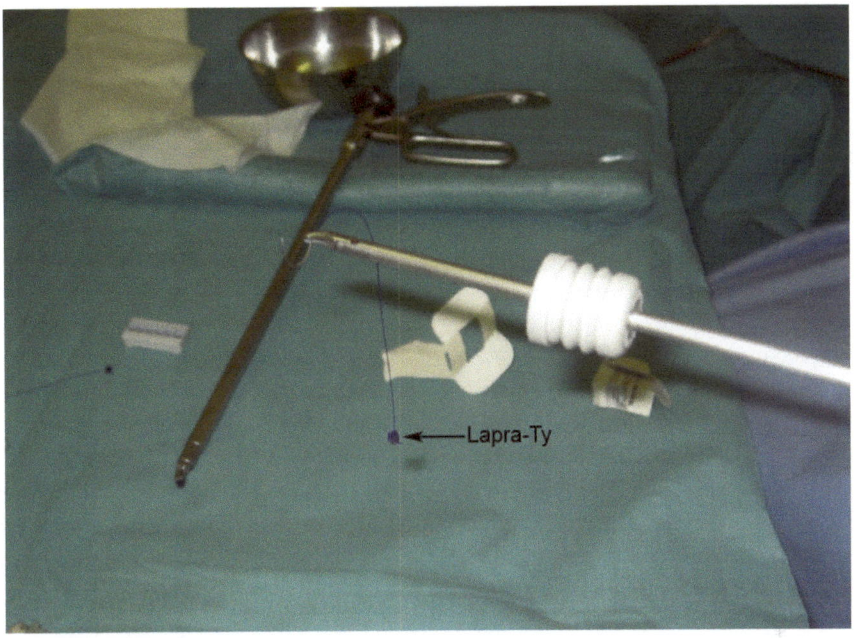


**Fig. 28.3** The suture is held with the needle-holder as close to the end of the needle as possible and is then introduced into the rectoscope. A Lapra-Ty (Ethicon) has been placed on the end of the suture

in all cases, in search of the perirectal fat, known as "the yellow plane." We continue laterally, then excise underneath and finish in the proximal area. The proximal area is usually the most difficult because it is impossible to lateralize the lesion, as we always work in parallel. After completing the excision, we irrigate with povidone-iodine solution diluted to 1 % using saline solution to induce cytolysis of any exfoliated cancer cells [10].

After excision, the surgeon or nurse attaches the specimen to a cork board and keeps the resection margins in place with pins to avoid retraction. The piece should also be oriented anatomically. In the case of broad margin resections, we indicate the correct position with respect to the specimen and also pin them in place.

The defect in the rectal wall must be sutured to avoid the risk of stenosing the rectal lumen (in large defects) and postoperative bleeding due to the traumatic effect of the tools. For suture, we use a 3-0 reabsorbable monofilament suture with an atraumatic cylindrical curved needle. A thread approximately 10 cm long is cut and inserted inside the rectoscope [10]. A silver clip or a LAPRA-TY (Suture Clip Applier, Ethicon Endo-Surgery, Cincinnati, OH, USA) is placed at the end of the suture to act as an anchor and avoid tying a knot (Fig. 28.3). A curved clip-holder is used, if possible, for suturing. Its ergonomic handle, which is easy to open and close, facilitates the maneuver. To introduce the suture into the rectoscope, first a rubber valve of the working channel is placed in the needle-holder (Fig. 28.3). Then the suture is held with the needle-holder as close to the needle as possible, and introduced into the rectoscope. With the suture inside the rectoscope, the needle is placed in the needle-holder with the help of the grasping forceps. The defect should be closed so as not to compromise the rectal lumen. The defect is closed from end to end with full-thickness stitches. The end of the suture is then secured with a second silver clip or Lapra-Ty. Occasionally, the rectoscope must be repositioned to achieve the optimal view. In large excisions it is helpful to begin suturing by placing one or two stitches in the center of the defect, so as to bring together its margins. We then perform two lateral running sutures. After finishing the suture, we again irrigate with a povidone-iodine solution diluted to 1 % with saline solution and the equipment is withdrawn.

In a comparative study of our experience with TEO and TEM, we found similar results with respect to surgical difficulty, postoperative morbidity, and quality of surgical resection, but lower economic cost with TEO [35].

## Postoperative Management

We remove the Foley catheter in the operating theater or the recovery room. Patients are encouraged to ambulate and take a regular diet within 12 h of surgery, and they are usually discharged 2 days after surgery. Little postoperative analgesia is required: only nonsteroidal antiinflammatory drugs are typically needed. Thromboembolism prophylaxis is maintained for a month, as is standard practice in colorectal cancer surgery.

## Technical Limitations of TEM

The distance of the upper edge of the lesion from the anal verge is of vital importance. Conventional endoanal excision is limited to lesions located at distances up to 7–8 cm. With TEM/TEO, the limits were set initially by the need to avoid penetrating into the peritoneal cavity. The risk of entering the peritoneal cavity was considered low in the setting of posterior tumors located up to 18–20 cm, and for anterior or lateral tumors located 15 cm or below. Today, perforation of the peritoneal cavity is not considered a contraindication for TEM/TEO [36]. There are no limits in terms of the location of the lesion (i.e., anterior, posterior, or lateral), as long as it can be technically removed. The real limit with respect to removal of the tumor is determined by the length of the rectoscope, and occasionally by other anatomical features such as the width of the rectosigmoidal junction or the rectal ampulla (below 10 cm), or a history of pelvic surgery that may impede the progression of the rectoscope. The limit for low lesions is the anal verge itself.

It is possible to excise adenomatous lesions that cover up to three quadrants of the circumference (10–12 cm). In fact, circumferential lesions, especially villous tumors, can sometimes be removed if they are not excessively long. The problem presented by large lesions is the need to suture the defect and the associated risk of stenosis.

## Postoperative Morbidity and Mortality After TEM/TEO

Mortality rate among patients treated with TEM/TEO is low, and almost always occurs in patients with severe comorbid conditions who are treated for palliation. Postoperative morbidity ranges between 4 and 24 % [10, 37–40]. In contrast to TME, the vast majority of these complications are defined as minor; that is, they are complications that can be resolved with conservative treatment. In our series and in previous studies, the most frequent complication associated with TEM/TEO is postoperative bleeding (2–5 %). This bleeding tends to be self-limited, and only on very few occasions is colonoscopy with hemostatic intention or repeat TEM/TEO required.

Another minor complication is postoperative fever above 38 °C (5–10 %), which is well-tolerated by the patient and remits with conventional antipyretics within 24–48 h. This is usually self-limiting and does not require intervention. Suture dehiscence occurs in about 10–15 %, but this does not require change in postoperative management. Acute urinary retention is another rare complication in these patients, occurring in 2–7 %.

Among major complications, the most important is perineal sepsis due to rectal manipulation, principally in excision of the lower third of the rectum. It occurs in fewer than 2 % of cases. In this situation the initial treatment is antibiotic therapy with debridement. Only in exceptional cases is a terminal colostomy required to control the perineal sepsis. In our series of 523 cases, this was necessary in only two patients, both of whom were immunosuppressed.

A special situation is the risk of rectovaginal fistula in women, in the setting of tumors of the anterior wall of the rectum. In this setting, particular care is required when performing full-thickness wall excision, due to the risk of rectovaginal perforation. To avoid this complication, continuous digital vaginal examination should be performed. We have had three cases of rectovaginal fistula. Even though the perforation was sutured after TEM/TEO, the fistula persisted and required terminal colostomy and subsequent repair.

In our experience, if perforation into the peritoneal cavity is observed during surgery and can be sutured using TEM/TEO, it does not represent a postoperative complication. Prior to surgery, surgeons can gain a reasonable idea of the risk of perforation involved in resecting a particular lesion from the results of rectal MRI and by identifying the peritoneal reflection and its relation to the lesion [36, 41]. Perforations during surgery that pass unnoticed and are not properly sutured may cause intraabdominal sepsis and in these cases represent a major complication [10, 42–44].

## References


1. Heald RJ, Ryall RD. Recurrence and survival after total mesorectal excision for rectal cancer. Lancet. 1986;1(8496):1479–82.
2. Law WL, Chu KW. Anterior resection for rectal cancer with mesorectal excision: a prospective evaluation of 622 patients. Ann Surg. 2004;240(2):260–8.
3. Kneist W, Junginger T. Residual urine volume after total mesorectal excision: an indicator of pelvic autonomic nerve preservation? results of a case-control study. Colorectal Dis. 2004;6(6):432–7. doi:10.1111/j.1463-1318.2004.00711.x.
4. Shah EF, Huddy SP. A prospective study of genito-urinary dysfunction after surgery for colorectal cancer. Colorectal Dis. 2001;3(2):122–5.
5. Mellgren A, Sirivongs P, Rothenberger DA, Madoff RD, Garcia-Aguilar J. Is local excision adequate therapy for early rectal cancer? Dis Colon Rectum. 2000;43(8):1064–71; discussion 71–4.
6. Mason AY. Surgical access to the rectum—a trans-sphincteric exposure. Proc R Soc Med. 1970;63 (Suppl):91–4.
7. Kraske P, Perry EG, Hinrichs B. A new translation of professor Dr P. Kraske's Zur Exstirpation Hochsitzender Mastdarmkrebse 1885. Aust N Z J Surg. 1989;59(5):421–4.
8. Buess G, Hutterer F, Theiss J, Bobel M, Isselhard W, Pichlmaier H. [A system for a transanal endoscopic rectum operation]. Chirurg. 1984;55(10):677–80.
9. Lee W, Lee D, Choi S, Chun H. Transanal endoscopic microsurgery and radical surgery for T1 and T2 rectal cancer. Surg Endosc. 2003;17(8):1283–7. doi:10.1007/s00464-002-8814-x.
10. Serra Aracil X, Bombardo Junca J, Mora Lopez L, Alcantara Moral M, Ayguavives Garnica I, Navarro SS. Transanal endoscopic microsurgery (TEM). Current situation and future expectations. Cir Esp. 2006;80(3):123–32.
11. Hildebrandt U, Feifel G. Preoperative staging of rectal cancer by intrarectal ultrasound. Dis Colon Rectum. 1985;28(1):42–6.
12. Jorge JM, Wexner SD. Etiology and management of fecal incontinence. Dis Colon Rectum. 1993;36(1): 77–97.
13. Mora Lopez L, Serra Aracil J, Rebasa Cladera P, Puig Divi V, Hermoso Bosch J, Bombardo Junca J, et al. [Anorectal disorders in the immediate and late postoperative period after transanal endoscopic microsurgery]. Cir Esp. 2007;82(5):285–9.
14. Serra-Aracil X, Mora-Lopez L, Alcantara-Moral M, Caro-Tarrago A, Gomez-Diaz CJ, Navarro-Soto S. Transanal endoscopic surgery in rectal cancer. World J Gastroenterol. 2014 Sep 7;20(33):11538–11545.
15. Winawer SJ, Zauber AG, Ho MN, O'Brien MJ, Gottlieb LS, Sternberg SS, et al. Prevention of colorectal cancer by colonoscopic polypectomy. The National Polyp Study Workgroup. N Engl J Med. 1993;329(27):1977–81. doi:10.1056/nejm199312303292701.
16. Zheng S, Liu XY, Ding KF, Wang LB, Qiu PL, Ding XF, et al. Reduction of the incidence and mortality of rectal cancer by polypectomy: a prospective cohort study in Haining County. World J Gastroenterol. 2002;8(3):488–92.
17. Serra-Aracil X, Caro-Tarrago A, Mora-Lopez L, Casalots C, Rebasa P, Navarro-Soto S. Transanal endoscopic surgery with total wall excision is required in rectal adenomas due to the high frequency of adenocarcinoma. Dis Colon Rectum. 2014;57(7): 823–9.
18. Absar MS, Haboubi NY. Colonic neoplastic polyps: biopsy is not efficient to exclude malignancy. The Trafford experience. Tech Coloproctol. 2004;8 Suppl 2:s257–60. doi:10.1007/s10151-004-0172-3.
19. Barendse RM, van den Broek FJ, Dekker E, Bemelman WA, de Graaf EJ, Fockens P, et al. Systematic review of endoscopic mucosal resection versus transanal endoscopic microsurgery for large rectal adenomas. Endoscopy. 2011;43(11):941–9. doi:10.1055/s-0030-1256765.
20. Borschitz T, Gockel I, Kiesslich R, Junginger T. Oncological outcome after local excision of rectal carcinomas. Ann Surg Oncol. 2008;15(11):3101–8. doi:10.1245/s10434-008-0113-x.
21. De Graaf EJ, Doornebosch PG, Tollenaar RA, Meershoek-Klein Kranenbarg E, de Boer AC, Bekkering FC, et al. Transanal endoscopic microsurgery versus total mesorectal excision of T1 rectal adenocarcinomas with curative intention. Eur J Surg Oncol. 2009;35(12):1280–5. doi:10.1016/j.ejso.2009.05.001.
22. Garcia-Aguilar J, Mellgren A, Sirivongs P, Buie D, Madoff RD, Rothenberger DA. Local excision of

rectal cancer without adjuvant therapy: a word of caution. Ann Surg. 2000;231(3):345–51.
23. Madbouly KM, Remzi FH, Erkek BA, Senagore AJ, Baeslach CM, Khandwala F, et al. Recurrence after transanal excision of T1 rectal cancer: should we be concerned? Dis Colon Rectum. 2005;48(4):711–9. doi:10.1007/s10350-004-0666-0; discussion 9–21.
24. Christoforidis D, Cho HM, Dixon MR, Mellgren AF, Madoff RD, Finne CO. Transanal endoscopic microsurgery versus conventional transanal excision for patients with early rectal cancer. Ann Surg. 2009;249(5):776–82. doi:10.1097/SLA.0b013e3181a3e54b.
25. Lezoche G, Paganini AM, Campagnacci R, Ghiselli R, Pelloni M, Rombini A, et al. Treatment of rectal cancer by transanal endoscopic microsurgery: review of the literature. Minerva Chir. 2013;68(1):1–9.
26. Doornebosch PG, Ferenschild FT, de Wilt JH, Dawson I, Tetteroo GW, de Graaf EJ. Treatment of recurrence after transanal endoscopic microsurgery (TEM) for T1 rectal cancer. Dis Colon Rectum. 2010;53(9):1234–9. doi:10.1007/DCR.0b013e3181e73f33.
27. Serra Aracil X, Bombardo Junca J, Mora Lopez L, Alcantara Moral M, Ayguavives Garnica I, Darnell Marti A, et al. Site of local surgery in adenocarcinoma of the rectum T2N0M0. Cir Esp. 2009;85(2):103–9. doi:10.1016/j.ciresp.2008.09.007.
28. Tytherleigh MG, Warren BF, Mortensen NJ. Management of early rectal cancer. Br J Surg. 2008;95(4):409–23. doi:10.1002/bjs.6127.
29. National Comprehensive Cancer Network. Rectal Cancer (Version 3.2014). www.nccn.org/professionals/physician_gls/PDF/rectal.pdf. Accessed 26 Apr 2014.
30. Borschitz T, Wachtlin D, Mohler M, Schmidberger H, Junginger T. Neoadjuvant chemoradiation and local excision for T2-3 rectal cancer. Ann Surg Oncol. 2008;15(3):712–20. doi:10.1245/s10434-007-9732-x.
31. Garcia-Aguilar J, Shi Q, Thomas Jr CR, Chan E, Cataldo P, Marcet J, et al. A phase II trial of neoadjuvant chemoradiation and local excision for T2N0 rectal cancer: preliminary results of the ACOSOG Z6041 trial. Ann Surg Oncol. 2012;19(2):384–91. doi:10.1245/s10434-011-1933-7.
32. Saclarides TJ. TEM/local excision: indications, techniques, outcomes, and the future. J Surg Oncol. 2007;96(8):644–50. doi:10.1002/jso.20922.
33. Serra-Aracil X, Mora-Lopez L, Alcantara-Moral M, Corredera-Cantarin C, Gomez-Diaz C, Navarro-Soto S. Atypical indications for transanal endoscopic microsurgery to avoid major surgery. Tech Coloproctol. 2014;18(2):157–64. doi:10.1007/s10151-013-1040-9.
34. Langer C, Markus P, Liersch T, Fuzesi L, Becker H. Ultra Cision or high-frequency knife in transanal endoscopic microsurgery (TEM)? Advantages of a new procedure. Surg Endosc. 2001;15(5):513–7. doi:10.1007/s004640090015.
35. Gavagan JA, Whiteford MH, Swanstrom LL. Full-thickness intraperitoneal excision by transanal endoscopic microsurgery does not increase short-term complications. Am J Surg. 2004;187(5):630–4. doi:10.1016/j.amjsurg.2004.01.004.
36. Serra-Aracil X, Mora-Lopez L, Alcantara-Moral M, Caro-Tarrago A, Navarro-Soto S. Transanal endoscopic microsurgery with 3-D (TEM) or high-definition 2-D transanal endoscopic operation (TEO) for rectal tumors. A prospective, randomized clinical trial. Int J Colorectal Dis. 2014;29(5):605–10.
37. Floyd ND, Saclarides TJ. Transanal endoscopic microsurgical resection of pT1 rectal tumors. Dis Colon Rectum. 2006;49(2):164–8. doi:10.1007/s10350-005-0269-4.
38. Guerrieri M, Baldarelli M, Morino M, Trompetto M, Da Rold A, Selmi I, et al. Transanal endoscopic microsurgery in rectal adenomas: experience of six Italian centres. Dig Liver Dis. 2006;38(3):202–7. doi:10.1016/j.dld.2005.11.01439.
39. Endreseth BH, Wibe A, Svinsas M, Marvik R, Myrvold HE. Postoperative morbidity and recurrence after local excision of rectal adenomas and rectal cancer by transanal endoscopic microsurgery. Colorectal Dis. 2005;7(2):133–7. doi:10.1111/j.1463-1318.2004.00724.x.
40. Stipa F, Burza A, Lucandri G, Ferri M, Pigazzi A, Ziparo V, et al. Outcomes for early rectal cancer managed with transanal endoscopic microsurgery: a 5-year follow-up study. Surg Endosc. 2006;20(4):541–5.
41. Beets-Tan RG, Beets GL, Vliegen RF, Kessels AG, Van Boven H, De Bruine A, et al. Accuracy of magnetic resonance imaging in prediction of tumour-free resection margin in rectal cancer surgery. Lancet. 2001;357(9255):497–504.
42. Kumar AS, Coralic J, Kelleher DC, Sidani S, Kolli K, Smith LE. Complications of transanal endoscopic microsurgery are rare and minor: a single institution's analysis and comparison to existing data. Dis Colon Rectum. 2013;56(3):295–300. doi:10.1097/DCR.0b013e31827163f7.
43. Ramwell A, Evans J, Bignell M, Mathias J, Simson J. The creation of a peritoneal defect in transanal endoscopic microsurgery does not increase complications. Colorectal Dis. 2009;11(9):964–6. doi:10.1111/j.1463-1318.2008.01719.x.
44. Baatrup G, Borschitz T, Cunningham C, Qvist N. Perforation into the peritoneal cavity during transanal endoscopic microsurgery for rectal cancer is not associated with major complications or oncological compromise. Surg Endosc. 2009;23(12):2680–3. doi:10.1007/s00464-008-0281-6.

## Key Operative Steps

1. Place Foley catheter and decompress the bladder.
2. Position the patient according to the location of the tumor.
3. Place the rectoscope over the lesion to gain access to the entire perimeter.

4. Initiate dissection by marking a circumferential dotted line 10–15 mm from the tumor.
5. Perform a full-thickness wall excision.
6. After completing excision, irrigate with povidone-iodine solution to induce cytolysis.
7. After completing excision, mark and orient the specimen to ensure all margins are appropriately analyzed by pathology.
8. Close the rectal mucosal defect with technique to avoid stenosis of the lumen.

# Index




J. Kim and J. Garcia-Aguilar (eds.), *Surgery for Cancers of the Gastrointestinal Tract: A Step-by-Step Approach*, DOI 10.1007/978-1-4939-1893-5,

## M



## N

## O



## P

**R**

## U